PAIN
TRACKING

Additional Praise for *Paintracking*

"Deborah Barrett has generously shared the insights and methods she uses to manage her own chronic pain. The pearls throughout make it a must-read. I am recommending it to my patients."

—Jackie Gardner-Nix, MD, PhD
Author of *The Mindfulness Solution to Pain*

"Expertly covers every possible way to deal with pain. One needn't suffer from chronic pain, however, to benefit from this landmark work."

—Betsy Ress Jacobson
Fibromyalgia Resources Group

"This thoughtful and detailed self-management approach teaches readers to build on small achievements to have successful outcomes."

—Synne Wing Venuti, MSW
painACTION.com and PainEDU.org

"Masterfully bridges the mind/body dichotomy, captures the essence of chronic pain, and provides invaluable therapeutic information. Written in lucid language, it guides readers through the daunting journey for answers. Mandatory reading for patients and clinicians alike!"

—Denniz Zolnoun, MD, MPH
Director of the Pelvic Pain Research Unit at
the University of North Carolina at Chapel Hill

"This is *the* book I will recommend to everyone with chronic pain. I firmly believe it will serve as a rare tool to be used again and again."

—Margaret Robson
Regional coordinator, Fibromyalgia Association UK

PAIN
TRACKING

Your Personal Guide
to Living Well with
CHRONIC PAIN

DEBORAH BARRETT, PhD, MSW

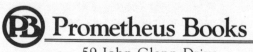
Prometheus Books

59 John Glenn Drive
Amherst, New York 14228–2119

Published 2012 by Prometheus Books

Cover image © 2012 Media Bakery
Cover design by Grace M. Conti-Zilsberger

Inquiries should be addressed to
Prometheus Books
59 John Glenn Drive
Amherst, New York 14228–2119
VOICE: 716–691–0133
FAX: 716–691–0137
WWW.PROMETHEUSBOOKS.COM

16 15 14 13   5 4 3

Library of Congress Cataloging-in-Publication Data

Barrett, Deborah, 1966–
    Paintracking : your personal guide to living well with chronic pain / by Deborah Barrett.
       p. cm.
    Includes bibliographical references and index.
    ISBN 978–1–61614–513–2 (pbk.)
    ISBN 978–1–61614–514–9 (ebook)
    1. Chronic pain—Popular works. 2. Pain—Treatment—Popular works. I. Title. II.
Title: Pain tracking.

RB127.B36165 2011
616'.0472—dc23

                                                                                          2011041550

Printed in the United States of America

Contents

Part 1. Paintracking

Part 2. Pain-Treating

Part 3. Pain-Living

Part 1

Paintracking

Chapter 1

My Story

This is the book I wish someone had handed me when I first encountered mysterious, overwhelming pain.

My pain began in June 1994, when I was twenty-eight and just weeks from completing a PhD in sociology at Stanford University. In a push to graduate, I spent long, intense hours at the computer keyboard, and, no surprise, my hands and forearms ached. I assumed this would pass with rest, and I daydreamed of the beach retreat I scheduled after graduation. But instead of easing, the pain worsened.

As a break from my graduate work, I had become active in capoeira, an Afro-Brazilian martial arts dance. During a fateful Tuesday evening class, despite sore arms from typing, I goat-walked the length of the gym on all fours, kicking up my legs behind me. As a fit, young woman with a naïve sense of invincibility, I regarded the mounting pain as a challenge to overcome rather than a signal to stop. The following day, I stubbornly persevered and lugged four bags of groceries the two and a half blocks to my apartment. By the time I reached the door, my pain was at the breaking point. I recall thinking it felt like the muscles in my forearms had been severed.

Over the days and weeks that followed, a burning sensation climbed up my shoulders and neck, across my back, and down the whole of my right leg. I had no idea what had hit me. My body seared with so much pain that I was unable to sleep and could barely take care of myself. My younger brother moved into my apartment and became my arms: he typed and cooked, and as the pain worsened, he even brushed my teeth. I summoned up the energy to visit multiple doctors, but each was baffled or dismissive. I was desperate for help.

Instead of starting the postdoctoral fellowship that awaited me at the University of North Carolina, I left San Francisco for my parents' home in Pennsylvania, virtually incapacitated. I was unable to hold a piece of paper or turn a doorknob. My parents became my caretakers, spoon-feeding me on my worst days. Over the next year, my mother, a family physician, assumed the role of medical detective, and my father became my stoic advocate. Together, we struggled to make sense of my mysterious, disabling symptoms. With my parents' support, I visited specialists who poked, prodded, and ran countless lab tests. Each visit raised my hopes, but none explained why I hurt so much.

My mother, distressed by the extent of my suffering, searched the medical literature until she found discussions of symptom patterns that mirrored my own. Her investigations led to the diagnoses of fibromyalgia and myofascial pain syndromes, which were confirmed by another round of doctor visits. While it was reassuring to name the demons, the diagnoses brought little relief. The prescribed medications produced more unpleasant side effects than comfort, and the hands-on therapies, although pleasant, failed to sustain any improvement. I ricocheted among pain-treatment programs, doctors, and physical therapy clinics, with little progress.

I read everything I could get my hands on about chronic pain and my specific diagnoses. Some of the advice helped some of the time, but just as often, my symptoms intensified. Take exercise, for example, which was described as essential to recovery. Often I felt good, even great, in the midst of a workout, but soon after, my pain would skyrocket, landing me in bed for days. Much of the advice seemed like empty words or unobtainable ideals. *How* was I supposed to accept my situation or improve my outlook—a common piece of advice—when I felt utterly miserable? I struggled so much, yet remained confused about what, if anything, helped. I had never been so frustrated.

Every now and then, I would experience a moment when my pain felt manageable. I rejoiced in these moments but had no idea what caused them. I was plagued with questions: Why would I experience a pain reprieve one moment and feel as if I'd been caught under a buffalo stampede the next? What made some mornings drastically better than others? Were there medications that would bring more substantial relief? What determined the length of my worst pain flare-ups? What sort of exercise would *really* help? And most important, how could I improve?

I came to see that the only way I could answer these questions was to don an investigator's hat and track my own experience. As a sociologist, I was accustomed to evaluating questions with systematic, empirical data. However, tracking my pain was easier said than done. I detested the worksheets I had been given by the pain clinic, which seemed to require me to detail my every waking hour. I hated to focus the little energy I had on my problems. Still, I made multiple attempts, and each time, I ended up tossing the worksheet aside in despair. I eventually realized the problem wasn't my lack of fortitude but the worksheets themselves. They demanded too much energy and neglected the pieces of the puzzle I considered most important. Fueled in equal parts by desperation and determination, I devised a simple tracking tool that I could fill out in a few minutes each day to capture my specific concerns. Finding an effective way to understand my experience has changed my life and is the basis of this book.

Chapter 2

Pain Positive?

Check all that apply to you:

- ❑ Living with my pain is exhausting.
- ❑ I hesitate to make plans because I don't know how I'll feel.
- ❑ I need more effective strategies to manage my pain.
- ❑ It often feels like pain controls my life.
- ❑ I feel isolated on account of my pain.
- ❑ My pain is often unpredictable.
- ❑ My pain can be overwhelming.
- ❑ Pain compromises my ability to work or to go to school.
- ❑ My pain makes it difficult to enjoy activities I would otherwise like.
- ❑ Pain interferes with my relationships.
- ❑ When it comes to my pain, I sometimes feel hopeless.

If you have checked any of the above, you test "pain positive," and this book is for you. You have likely become something of a reluctant expert on what it feels like to suffer, make sacrifices, and experience frustration and despair. You may feel misunderstood and at times misjudged by the people in your life.

Taking a Positive Approach to Chronic Pain

One reason chronic pain is so difficult to manage is the absence of positive messages on the topic. People who live with daily pain suffer not only from the pain itself but often from a lack of support and fear that they cannot lead a satisfying life. Hearing, "You just have to learn to live with it," for example, can be especially demoralizing. Moreover, our culture generally views pain as an aberration—something that is supposed to go away with time and proper attention. This is true for pains caused by transient problems like a broken arm, but not for pain that becomes chronic. Persistent pain is often regarded as a failure; its sufferer, as weak or inadequately committed to improvement.

Television commercials for medications regularly communicate this. They tend to open with someone in obvious discomfort, lamenting his or her inability to engage in a particular activity: a man wrings his hands, looking longingly at a tennis racket; a businesswoman holds her head in distress amid stacks of papers. Enter the helpful friend, coworker, or family member with the curative product. In the closing scene, the previously afflicted individual is engaging fully in the desired activity: the man smiles and serves the ball; the businesswoman presides over a meeting. Medicine has restored them, and life resumes as usual.

This quick-fix view of pain is deep rooted and pervasive, despite ample evidence to the contrary. At some point, the majority of adults will experience some form of chronic pain, whether from back trouble, disc disease, arthritis, a postsurgical syndrome, or one of the many other conditions that can involve debilitating pain. Still, pain is frequently portrayed as a temporary break in routine. Consider the rows of greeting cards that offer speedy recoveries and other get-well-quick messages. How often do you encounter cards wishing people strength in adapting to ongoing difficulties? People commonly take their health for granted until they, or people close to them, develop a chronic ailment.

In many cases, the difficulties of chronic pain are compounded by undertreatment and ineffective approaches. Prescription medications reduce but rarely eliminate painful symptoms and often come with negative side effects. Strategies recommended for particular conditions can be useful but may not address *your* specific needs. Healthcare professionals often experience frustration with the complexities involved in tackling chronic pain. It is not surprising that pain sufferers frequently spend considerable time, energy, and money searching for answers, including doctor shopping and experimenting with various treatments, and sometimes fall prey to scams.

This book offers a positive approach to life with chronic pain. What does this mean? Living positively with chronic pain emphasizes what you *can* do to improve your experience. In a nutshell, this involves identifying what helps most, then organizing your life accordingly. Self-knowledge brings power. The more you understand your pain, the less it interferes with your life. This comes through viewing each moment, even your very worst ones, as compelling data. When you treat your experience as an experiment, you not only tolerate difficulties more easily, but you learn from them. This requires that you take an active role in your own care. At times, this may involve rethinking strategies that you or your healthcare professionals had considered to be most promising or effective.

Why would you consider acting contrary to common sense or medical wisdom? To answer this, I first steer you to the compelling work of Dan Ariely, a behavioral economist who investigates how people make decisions.[1] In study after study, he has found that when people make decisions, they feel rational and in control, even when evidence shows they are not. People often base decisions on external factors and their current physical and emotional state, rather than a critical review of relevant data. While the results are sometimes trivial— such as the type of jam people buy or where they vacation—choices that affect pain level are not trivial.

Indeed, Dr. Ariely began his contemplations of human irrationality while enduring extremely painful treatments for severe burns that covered 70 percent of his body. During these treatments, bandages were removed quickly, based on the belief that faster removal would minimize his pain. He later conducted systematic experiments and found that this method actually made things worse because pain that is more prolonged but lower is tolerated better than pain that is shorter but intense. Since then, he has continued to study the many ways people make "wrong" decisions that feel perfectly rational.

This book invites you to figure out the "right" decisions for your specific situation through observation and experimentation rather than "common sense" or "medical wisdom." People with chronic pain face a confounding set of decisions, which are made even more difficult when pain fuels desperation and answers are not forthcoming. This book will help you assess data specific to your experience. Then, as you understand what does and does not actually work, you can improve how you manage your pain. To a certain degree, your experience will depend on whether you have received an appropriate diagnosis; the existing medical knowledge about your condition; and whether the condition's course is degenerative, stable, or time limited. But whatever is causing your pain, you will fare better by understanding the impact of your decisions on how you feel.

Who Can This Book Help?

People living with pain. If you are reading this because you live with chronic pain, you are far from alone. Unfortunately, millions suffer from chronic pains of one form or another. You may know others who, like yourself, look fine but feel awful. I hear from such people every day. Living with pain can be lonely and isolating. If you are frustrated, miserable, and unsure what to do, it is vital that you remain persistent and never give up. There is much reason for hope and optimism. That you are reading this book shows that you have already begun your journey. This book will provide a hands-on strategy for incremental improvement. Progress, however small, adds up. As you feel better in one area, you will become more able to experiment and tackle the next.

Look to part 1 to create a personalized PAINTRACKING tool for understanding how you are doing, conducting experiments to help you improve, and evaluating your progress. Part 2 describes pain-relieving strategies to consider in these experiments. Part 3 focuses on ways to apply what you have learned to your daily life.

People who care about someone living with pain. If you are reading this to help a loved one—thank you! Support goes a long way for people who suffer from frustrating and often invisible symptoms. Your interest itself may buoy the spirits of someone who has felt alone in his or her misery. By learning about their experience with chronic pain, you become a stronger advocate. Many of the recommendations about self-care apply equally to you as a support person. In order to help others without overtaxing yourself emotionally or physically, you need to care for yourself. Strive to keep your own life balanced, pleasurable, and fulfilling; develop a supportive network; and find a willing ear to listen when caregiving becomes stressful.

Providing support to someone with chronic pain holds many challenges. Despite a sincere desire to help, you may not know what to do or say. You may want to provide an empathetic ear, yet tire of hearing complaints. You might feel frustrated with the slow pace of improvement, yet fear that unsolicited advice will be perceived as criticism. You may want to be understanding, yet be confused by the dramatic fluctuations you observe in symptoms and abilities. You may want to respond nonjudgmentally, yet feel unsure when to coddle and how hard to push. Such guesswork can be exhausting. The best antidote is communication: ask the person you care about whether he or she is looking for suggestions, a sympathetic ear, encouragement, distraction, physical assistance, or comic relief. The person may not always be able to tell you what is needed. But take heart in knowing that this is a learning process for everyone.

Healthcare providers. If you are a healthcare professional working with people who suffer with chronic pain, please know that your role in the healing process is irreplaceable. Chronic pain syndromes can be very frustrating to treat. Improvements are often slow and incremental; setbacks are common; and treatments involve patience, experimentation, and attention. Don't let the slow pace or unevenness of progress derail your efforts. Remind yourself that the condition (not the individual) may be difficult to treat, and find satisfaction in your ability to persevere. Treating chronic pain often calls for an interdisciplinary approach. Make use of consultation with other healthcare professionals and referrals as needed to aid in your work.

That you selected a book on self-empowerment likely means you appreciate your clients taking an active role in their own care. Talk openly about what will help you work best as a team—such as how you prefer they share information with you during office visits or between appointments should problems arise. Your effectiveness will come through the therapeutic alliance you build together and your commitment to helping them improve. Your clients depend on your knowledge and expertise, and you depend on their accurate reports and adherence to prescribed treatments. Keep in mind that people who suffer from a confusing array of painful symptoms appreciate and crave support from a trusted professional. You contribute significantly through kind words, validation, respect, and encouragement.

Gaining Perspective

It can be useful to take a moment and put yourself in the other person's shoes. When pain feels overwhelming, it's easy to lose sight of how your experience might also be affecting others. If you live with pain, try imagining how you would feel if your partner, parent, sibling, child, friend, or colleague experienced your symptoms. Or, if you are caring for someone with pain, imagine trading places. This exercise can be especially helpful when your patience starts to wear thin. Empathy can help bridge the inevitable difficulties that come with relationship imbalances.

Final Note: It's Worth the Pain!

Living positively with chronic pain looks different for each person. Through your personal journey, you may discover gifts, such as deeper meaning, spirituality, or a refocusing on the people and things that matter most. Improvement involves a process. While it is not simple, it is worth the effort.

This book simplifies the process with tools and guidance. It presents information from medicine, social science, and psychotherapy in accessible language. Its goal is not pain-free living—an unrealistic pursuit even in the best of circumstances—but to allow you to predict the effect of your choices so that you can improve the ways in which you manage your pain. Developing this knowledge over time reduces the chance that you will test "pain positive" and instead allows you to assume a positive approach to your life.

As a wise doctor with fibromyalgia once shared with me, there's a significant difference between "being in pain" and "having pain." In other words, pain may be one of the many aspects of your experience without controlling or defining your life. This book offers a road map to create days you find satisfying. By being able to calculate the "pain cost," you can decide when it's worth it to spend pain on a particular pursuit and how to take full advantage of good moments and deliberately increase them. Part of this involves continually striving for improvement, while part involves accepting your current circumstances so you can advocate for yourself in an effective manner.

Chapter 3

Why PAINTRACKING?

The cornerstone of this book is PAINTRACKING, a self-study tool that will enable you to improve.

When you feel horrid, the idea of conducting research—even when it promises relief—may feel overwhelming. PAINTRACKING was created with this in mind. It is specifically for people who are exhausted by pain and don't have energy to waste deciphering complicated formulas. Let this book be your cheerleader and guide, walking you step by step through a process to create a personal research tool.

PAINTRACKING is necessarily customized. It would not make sense for me, or anyone else, to hand you a one-size-fits-all research instrument, however thorough or creative it might be. Many people have asked for a copy of the worksheet I used when my pain began—after all, it gave me back my life. However, its only magic was that it addressed *my* central concerns, and in a simple, personalized format.

Your PAINTRACKING tool can take any number of forms, depending on your individual strengths, style, and comfort. You may opt to use the online PAINTRACKING program that is a companion to this book. This program allows you to tailor your questions and responses, and your tracking can then be completed daily on your computer or other e-device. Or you may prefer to create your own system using a simple pen-and-paper approach, or craft a template you can fill out by hand, or track information in a computer spreadsheet. What matters is that you choose a system that you find easy and helpful.

The Payoff

It may be difficult to believe that studying your pain experience can transform your life, but this is the best method to learn what works. Consider how much of your suffering comes from uncertainty. I've heard from many people who are frustrated with the seemingly random nature of their symptoms; this unpredictability undermines their ability to make plans or feel in control, presents a confusing picture to others, and can lead to self-doubt.

In my case, PAINTRACKING helped me differentiate what helped from what didn't—revealing some surprising discoveries. By keeping and interpreting simple records, I could finally establish an exercise routine without painful setbacks. By sharing some of my findings with my doctor, we eventually discovered a trio of medications that reduced my pain and let me sleep through the night. As I felt better, smiley faces replaced the frowns on my tracking worksheet. There was a time when I could not have fathomed living well with chronic pain. But that is exactly what I am doing. Knowing precisely what causes my pain to soar (and how to prevent it), as well as ways to maximize my comfort and productivity, puts me in the driver's seat.

The specific adaptations that helped me, or anyone else, may not be relevant to you. However, the *process* that led me to my discoveries is relevant to anyone struggling with chronic pain. This is the basis of PAINTRACKING, which promises four things:

Promise 1: You will uncover the "larger picture." Seeing fluctuations in your experience over time provides a realistic view of your situation. You will be able to measure and interpret your progress (and take note of any backsliding). Making sense of your experience can be very reassuring. Understanding your patterns also frees you from the roller coaster ride of unpredictable pain. When you feel bad, you are at risk of pessimistic thinking, such as mistakenly believing your worst days are typical.

Promise 2: Painful flare-ups will no longer shock or overwhelm you. PAINTRACKING will help you discover the cause of flare-ups and turn them into predictable events, eliminating the misery of "out of the blue" pain. Knowing what incites pain provides you with valuable options. You can decide to avoid specific circumstances, adapt your behavior to reduce the pain, or march ahead with your eyes wide open. When you are able to consider a flare-up as an anticipated interruption, rather than a shocking turn of events, you can schedule recuperative downtime with your best coping strategies.

Promise 3: You will discover ways to feel better. Each of us has the capacity to feel better. Reflect on your ups and downs—what would it be like to learn how to elicit the "ups" intentionally? Assessing what helps (and what hurts) allows you to base your decisions on facts rather than guesswork. Then, as you identify effective therapies and behaviors, you can make them a part of your life. For example, knowing that a hot shower and a five-minute brisk walk alleviate morning aches is a terrific incentive to incorporate them into your daily routine. Through detective work, you will uncover your personal recipe for relief.

Promise 4: You will continue to improve. Your ability to improve is open ended. Even when you are doing fairly well, further progress is always possible. Through experimentation, you can continue to test new strategies. But change can be intimidating, even when you are not entirely satisfied with how you feel. You may worry about the effects of a new approach and your ability to judge its effectiveness. PAINTRACKING helps eliminate unnecessary discomfort or guesswork. Its daily tracking method encourages ongoing experimentation by offering decisive feedback on any changes or adaptations. If you experience a setback for any reason (and you will because life is unpredictable), you can feel assured in your capacity to learn from it and move forward.

Why PAINTRACKING Is Necessary

For years, we've been told, "Listen to your body," but with chronic pain, our bodies' messages can be deceptive. We face a disturbing paradox: intuition is often a poor judge of what we need. When people with chronic pain awake feeling as if they were pummeled in their sleep, or are too stiff to move, it may seem perfectly reasonable to stay in bed to recuperate. Or, when pain is low, it may seem practical to load up on activities. Unfortunately, these commonsense reactions often backfire. Morning pain and stiffness can worsen with rest, and overexertion, even when you feel fantastic, can incite debilitating pain. Without data to guide us, we are at the mercy of pain's cruel whims. This can be demoralizing! When you cannot trust your own instincts, the world becomes unpredictable and frightening.

Living well with chronic pain often involves acting *contrary* to your intuition. This paradox is useful when treating anxiety or depression. As a psychotherapist, I help people recognize when acting opposite to their impulses is actually beneficial. For example, you can decrease your anxiety by facing and not fleeing from the object of your fear, provided you do so safely. Similarly, people with depression often want to stay in bed with closed blinds; however, forcing themselves from bed and into engaging activity is more likely to lighten their mood. This principle is relevant to chronic pain as well. While intense pain may seem like a good reason to avoid feared activities or to stay in bed, it often improves with meaningful engagement.

Unfortunately, there is an additional wrinkle when it comes to pain. While going against your instincts sometimes brings just what you need, at other times, it can backfire, and your pain will soar in response. People with chronic pain tread the precarious line between too much activity and too much rest— and what constitutes "too much" is often revealed only in retrospect. How you feel in the moment is often a deceptive guide. You may feel great while engaging in exercise or activity, then later experience a dreadful flare-up in response. It can feel as if you are "damned if you do" and "damned if you don't." Without clear direction on what would be most effective, approaching these decisions is like trying to traverse a field of land mines.

Navigating this minefield requires data about your reactions—namely, the consequences of your decisions. While you may never be able to trust your gut instincts, you can develop a "new intuition," which is based on data you accumulate from deliberate experimentation. This will allow you to make decisions that are based on how your body tends to react. Over time, your acquired self-knowledge will allow you once again to listen to your body and interpret its cues—in this case, in light of relevant data.

Everything You Need to Know to Feel Better

How to live well with chronic pain is no secret. Across chronic pain conditions, the medical and self-help literatures promote the same strategies again and again. So, are you ready for the prescription for feeling better and for continuing to improve? (*Drumroll.*) Here it is:

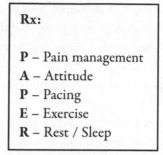

Rx:

P – Pain management
A – Attitude
P – Pacing
E – Exercise
R – Rest / Sleep

I use the acronym PAPER because "on paper" it sure looks simple. However, given the uncertainty and volatility of pain, each component poses a formidable challenge. The prescription's simplicity lies in stark contrast to the complexity of achieving any of its components. I can imagine what some of you are thinking:

> "You try to keep a positive attitude when you feel like you
>   were run over by a truck!"
> "What do you mean, exercise? My joints are killing me!"
> "How can I sleep with this much pain?"

No kidding! Chronic pain can make these goals seem unobtainable or at least really, really hard. If only we could fill this prescription at the corner drugstore—I'd gladly pay for a dose of fitness and a sunny disposition!

It's also challenging to figure out the right dose of each. How much and what type of exercise or medicine will diminish symptoms without adverse side effects? Unfortunately, the medical and self-help literature offers little guidance on dosage. Even the best clinical trials only demonstrate what works for some percentage of subjects, and anecdotes can be compelling but may not apply to you. Make this prescription work for you by PAINTRACKING. Let's consider each piece of the prescription:

P **for Pain management.** The marketplace for pain-relief treatments is growing by leaps and bounds. Without a tracking system, it would be virtually impossible to decipher the effects of multiple medications and other therapies that you are currently using or would like to try. PAINTRACKING provides simple techniques to track your responses to an otherwise overwhelming array of approaches and use this information with your doctor. If your pain is severe right now, skip ahead. Chapter 11 describes simple strategies to soothe your body, and chapter 17 describes medications commonly used for chronic pain. Before embarking on a journey toward long-term improvement, you need to be comfortable enough to relax, read, and think.

A **for Attitude.** Perspective affects well-being—a simple and intuitive idea that is also backed by extensive research. People who view their situation in a more positive light tend to be more resilient, flexible, and skillful when facing difficulties. But no matter how determined you may be, shifting your attitude can present a formidable task. The advice to "think cheery thoughts" is unhelpful, and for those with chronic pain, it can be downright insulting. A misplaced focus on attitude also risks implying that your pain is "all in your head" and would resolve itself if only you viewed life differently. At the same time, however, it would be imprudent to overlook substantial evidence that shifting one's attitude can in fact reduce suffering.

PAINTRACKING encourages you to use the data you collect to shape your attitude. The larger picture is often more optimistic than you may suspect, and this insight can be crucial when you most need it. In addition, you can test the effects of your efforts to lighten your mood. Chapters 10 through 12 describe empirically supported techniques to decrease your pain by calming your mind and body, controlling your focus, and shaping your self-talk. But don't trust me—use your PAINTRACKING tool to measure their effects.

P **for Pacing.** People in pain are typically advised to pace themselves judiciously. But figuring out *how* can seem virtually impossible. Perfect pacing requires perfect hindsight—only in retrospect can you evaluate the effects of your choices. PAINTRACKING allows you to extrapolate from past experiences and then deliberately test different pacing strategies. You can compare the results, for example, of approaching a busy day by including short recuperative breaks or a lengthy midday siesta. To pace effectively, you must first determine the rhythm that works best for you and then prompt yourself to slow down or push yourself as indicated. Chapter 13 describes strategies to use when you are need of a break or a boost.

E **for Exercise.** Research clearly supports the benefits of exercise on mood, thoughts, stamina, sleep quality, and pain level. Yet many people with chronic pain struggle to establish an exercise routine because it feels too difficult or triggers more pain. No matter how you feel, you *can* exercise successfully if you approach exercise as an ongoing experiment, rather than listening to personal trainers or other experts who may not be familiar with the capriciousness of chronic pain. Chapter 15 describes strategies to start slowly, then build up gradually while carefully monitoring the results. By tracking your exertions and their effects, you can build a successful workout routine.

R **for Rest.** Chronic pain and sleep problems are something of a chicken-and-egg dilemma: pain interferes with sleep, which intensifies pain and further disrupts sleep. Good-quality sleep reduces pain but with pain is more difficult to achieve. Medical literature on insomnia generally condemns napping because it can interfere with nighttime sleep—but what are you supposed to do when you face daytime exhaustion and nighttime sleeplessness? Plus, with certain pain conditions, morning pain and stiffness can be greater after a full night's sleep, confusing the idea of "good sleep." Chapter 14 describes strategies for you to try in your experiments to discover your optimal sleep routine.

Your Personalized Prescription

Your daily experience can make this prescription work for you, and not just on paper. Through experimentation and adaptation, you will discover how to personalize this prescription to your needs. Then, as you improve in one of the prescribed areas, you will likely improve in another. For example, as you manage your pain, your sleep will likely improve, which can enable you to exercise more, which may improve your attitude, further decreasing your pain, and so on. Tracking such progress is encouraging.

Chapter 4

Committing to the Process

Addressing the "yes, but…"

Because PAINTRACKING requires a commitment, make sure to address any resistance or ambivalence you may have. It is a very human response to have doubts about this approach, especially if you are wrung out by pain and overwhelmed by existing responsibilities. Use this chapter to cheerlead yourself through any doubts, and revisit it at any time you find your commitment wavering.

Take a moment and put any nagging thoughts into words, then look for your version of "yes, but" below. Then, read the rebuttal to help yourself re-engage with the approach and the promise it holds.

I don't want to pay so much attention to how lousy I feel! You may feel that you are already too preoccupied with your physical state and would rather forget about it than deliberately record it. These feelings are likely to increase on particularly good days, when you might feel too optimistic to be bothered to record data, or on particularly bad ones, when you feel too awful to bother.

- While you have to be aware of your experience to track it, recording meaningful data is distinct from dwelling on your problems. Dwelling—the rehashing of problems in your mind—is exhausting and emotionally draining because it often builds negative aspects to catastrophic proportions. In contrast, deliberate tracking is problem solving. Tracking today's experience will be rewarded by better tomorrows. Keep your improvement goals foremost in your mind.

I have so little energy—I don't want to spend it on record keeping! Pain and fatigue can hijack concentration and motivation. Anyone living with

27

chronic pain knows it can require monumental effort to engage in *any* meaningful activity. You will not be able to sustain record keeping if it feels too difficult, time consuming, overwhelming, or draining.

- PAINTRACKING's individualized system is specifically intended to keep energy and time expenditures to a minimum. What's more, as you uncover what helps, you gain energy. So, worries about low energy are more reason—not less—for tracking. If at any time your system feels undoable, revisit and simplify it.

I'm afraid to see how poorly I'm doing. The idea of logging your lived experience may feel depressing. You may be reluctant to confront how poorly you are doing or view details of your struggles, limitations, or travails. You may fear your worst suspicions will be confirmed.

- Facing reality can be scary, particularly when it's not ideal. However, in order to improve, you need to know exactly what you're facing and not live with an account based on hopes or fears. Objective data enable you to assess the areas needed for improvement and communicate more effectively with healthcare professionals.

I tried this before, and it didn't work! You may have had a bad experience with a similar exercise. Perhaps you tried to keep a journal, filled out an hourly logbook supplied by a pain clinic, or used another tracking tool. Journaling about your experience may have gotten things "off your chest" but not brought you any closer to answers. The intensity of a time-consuming practice may have been unsustainable. You may have started enthusiastically, only to quit shortly after.

- If previous attempts to chronicle your experience felt overwhelming, frustrating, pointless, or disappointing, more than likely the system you were using was inappropriate for you. Before assuming that you failed at the task, examine the approach you were using, which was either too labor intensive or failed to provide the results that would have made the effort worthwhile. PAINTRACKING is the right tool for the job because you design it specifically for yourself. Its system should fit the way *you* think, providing answers that make a difference in *your* life.

Now that I've missed a few days of recording, it feels hopeless to continue!
Record keeping can seem like yet another activity you can fail to accomplish.
Missed sheets may contribute to negative thoughts about yourself or your situation. Once you miss days, weeks, or even months of recording, you may feel
too defeated to resume the effort.

- The good news is that you can't be fired from this job! While systematic, daily records are ideal, all information helps. No matter how committed you are, missing some days is inevitable. As long as your tool feels
  appropriate, the question is less about preventing oversights than about
  what to do when they occur. Rather than flogging yourself, seize each
  day as an opportunity to learn. There are two mottoes to live by here:
  "Today is the first day of the rest of your life," and, more to the point,
  "Just do it!" There is no better time than the present to engage in an
  exercise to improve your experience.

I already know what affects me—there's nothing new to learn. If you've
already lived with pain for some time, you may be intimately familiar with your
experience. You may have already spent time as a detective, investigating what
helps. Or you may feel pessimistically that "nothing helps" and consider the
enterprise to be futile.

- Living with chronic pain involves a continual process of learning and
  adapting. You can gain insights by examining your current circumstances and experimenting with a new approach. Human memory is far
  from perfect; most of us struggle to recall the particulars of yesterday, let
  alone last week or last month. By collecting explicit data, you won't miss
  out on small changes and can also conduct experiments for additional
  insights.

I'm no scientist. How am I supposed to figure it all out? The idea of collecting and analyzing data may feel daunting, especially if you do not have
research experience. You may wonder if personal research will even be useful;
why not leave the research to researchers? After all, they are the ones conducting double-blind studies to figure out what works.

- Keep it simple. The research involved is only as complicated as you make it. You can focus on the one or two factors you most want to understand. While large-scale studies are essential in furthering medical understanding, what works for most people in any given study may or may not be effective for you. Your personal research is invaluable. Plus, nobody else can measure your experience as accurately or as thoroughly. Your daily measures capture expected and unexpected consequences as well as delayed responses.

An organization devoted to improving healthy behaviors through interactive technologies has among its goals helping people with pain conditions track their experience so they can communicate more effectively about it with their doctors.[1] They found, however, in survey research, that multiple barriers keep doctors and patients from discussing paintracking strategies or incorporating them into office visits. Top among these barriers was concern about its difficulty.[2] The takeaway points here are that tracking is valuable and must, must, must be simple to use. The survey research also found that people want tracking tools to be versatile and easy.

On board? Now, let's move on to the "how to."

Chapter 5

Envision Your Personalized PAINTRACKING System

Let's start with Roselyn. She's fifty-two and distressed about her pain. Following a car accident last year, she developed ongoing pains in her neck and back. She has a career, a solid marriage, and three teenagers. While she manages her active days for the most part, by the time she arrives home, all she wants to do is retreat to her bedroom. As someone who values her family, however, she struggles with guilt over this reaction. She feels that while she is managing well enough at work in her quiet office, her pain later interferes with her ability and motivation to engage with her husband and children. Each morning she tells herself that "today will be different," but she worries that nothing is changing. She has decided to track her experience to help her see the larger picture and find some solutions.

Roselyn wants a very simple tracking system and decides to use a blank appointment book, which she will keep next to her bed. When she awakes, she records the approximate hours slept because she suspects her sleep quality affects how she feels. In the evening, she records information on other factors that she thinks may be affecting how she feels: exercise ("H2O" for water aerobics class), weather conditions (represented with a doodle), medication (the number of prescribed "pain pills" she took that day), and any activities she did outside of work. Roselyn represents her daily well-being with a face doodle, augmented with exclamation marks. So far, her worst days look like this: ☹!! Her best have reached ☺! Take a look:

Roselyn's Calendar

Monday - September 3	Friday - September 7
11- 7 H2O 2P ☁ TV ☹	12- 6 H2O 3P ☀ TV ☹
Tuesday - September 4	**Saturday - September 8**
11–2; 4–6 3P ☁ TV ☹!!	11- 6 H2O 2P ☀ hot bath ☺! relaxed w/kids
Wednesday - September 5	**Sunday - September 9**
12- 6 H2O 2P ☁ read ☺	11- 7 H2O 3P ☁ hot bath ☺ chat w/Al
Thursday - September 6	**Notes:**
11–2; 3- 7 2P ☀ tea w/ ☺ neighbor	Hot bath helped! Feels good to get comfortable and chat.

Notice how Roselyn lines up her tracked items in each entry, which makes them easy to scan for patterns. So, what do her data say about her week? While she may feel like she comes home feeling awful *most* days, her data this week show otherwise: her smile and frown days were equal (three each), with one neutral day.

Next, take a look at her data to try to explain the fluctuations in her well-being. On the rainy Tuesday, Roselyn felt particularly poor—after having been up from two until four in the morning, not attending water aerobics, and taking three pain pills. In contrast, sunny Saturday was her best day—and she slept through the night, exercised, and took only two pills for pain. So, sleep, weather, exercise, and her need for pain medication, or a combination of these, may matter. But hold on. Let's explore further. Notice that her rainy Sunday was also a good day and that sunny Friday was not. This suggests that weather may not explain how she felt, and looking at her week, neither does whether she exercised that day nor the number of pills she took. However, one factor does appear related to how she felt: notice that Roselyn reported her worst days were the ones in which she spent her evenings watching television.

You may have a lot of questions: Did watching TV make Roselyn feel worse, or did she decide to watch TV precisely *because* she felt bad already? Or you could be wondering about the cumulative effects of exercise—while there's no evidence it mattered on a daily basis, what about over time? What sort of trends might we see in her well-being if she continued to exercise at this rate or increased its frequency or intensity? Or you may be curious about Roselyn's use of pain pills. Does her third pill indicate that her pain was higher, or might she be undertreating her pain on the other days?

Having questions at this point is just what you want. When you are trying to figure out something that can be affected by multiple factors, finding relationships between variables can provide a great *start*. Determining causality, however, often requires deliberate experimentation, and it is precisely these sorts of questions that encourage and inform the experiments that can produce answers.

Roselyn was similarly curious about the relationship between her behaviors and well-being. On Saturday, she noted on her tracking sheet that she had experienced relief from the hot bath and pleasure from chatting with others. The next day—a rainy Sunday in which she slept well, exercised, and took three pain pills—she decided to see if she could duplicate this result. She took a hot bath and then chose a comfortable place to chat with her husband, and once again, she rated her day more positively. But, you might have noticed, like Roselyn, that both days were on the weekend, so she may have felt better on account of the break from work. This question creates more reason to continue the experiment. Roselyn committed to a routine of a hot bath in the evening followed by some socializing (she had noticed the ☺ rating for Thursday, when she had enjoyed tea with a neighbor). She informed her family that she would be taking hot baths shortly after arriving home (and her older daughter even began running water for her when she heard her mother's car pull up), after which she would invite her family members to join her on their plush red couch.

In the following weeks, Roselyn noted a dramatic improvement in how she felt at home, which she clearly noted in the moment, then viewed as a pattern on her calendar. Once she was 100 percent confident that winding down in a hot bath was helpful, she decided to experiment with other, less wet alternatives to warm her muscles and calm her mind (described in chapters 11 and 12), and she found several to have good results. Roselyn still experiences pain and has times when her first thought after work is to hide out. However, the indisputable evidence that self-care and engagement will bring a better result (for everyone) helps Roselyn to choose what works even when she doesn't feel like it at first. She is now thinking ahead to similar experiments to determine the effects of the amounts she exercises and of her medication.

Notice the simplicity of Roselyn's tracking tool, with its numbers, doodles, and space for short notes. Unstructured calendars (or blank journals or notebooks, as long as you record the date) can be effective when you can keep the items you record fairly tidy. Their unstructured nature makes changes simple—Roselyn can add items to her system as she desires. But if she wants to collect more complex information, such as records on dosages of multiple medications, she might consider a template, spreadsheet, or online tool.

Now meet Terry. He's twenty-six, and until his lower back and pelvic pain began, he was a marathon runner and cyclist. Terry is single, and much of his life has revolved around his athletic pursuits with a similarly inclined group of friends. Now, however, when he tries to keep up with his friends, his pain soars and his spirits plummet. Given the importance of exercise in his life, Terry is determined to figure out ways to participate as much as possible. He commits to using a tracking system to evaluate the effectiveness of pre- and postexercise strategies that may help.

Terry decides to start his experiments with a three-mile run, opting to avoid biking for the moment because it hurts to sit. He understands that he is more likely to reduce (or even eliminate) postexercise pain if he starts even more slowly, but to a veteran twenty-six-mile runner, three miles seems nominal. He hopes to find a combination of strategies that can make this run sustainable so he can avoid having to cut back further. He decides to test the timing of his pain medication (before versus after running) and several pain-relief strategies that have been generally helpful for his back pain.

Terry wants a tracking system that he can fill out quickly by hand. He decides to create a template on the computer with categories that he can circle by hand or answer with short notes. He can fit one week of information per page, and he decides to print out two sheets, which he keeps on a clipboard on his desk. When he is ready to make changes to his template, he can print off the revised version.

Each morning, Terry records three pieces of information: the date (noting full information at the top of each week), his sleep-quality grade (which averaged a B this week), and a word on his mood. In the evening, he spends another minute entering data on what is most important to him—his run.

Terry's Template

```
Day/date Mon 10/1/12  sleep: A B C D F    morn pain: 1 2 3 4 5 6 7   mood: fine
Run: meds 3 miles  meds hot tub meditation / ice / massage / nap  post: 7
Activities: hung with James and Mun    else: the run felt great, then my back!!!

Day/date T 2        sleep: A B C D F    morn pain: 1 2 3 4 5 6 7   mood: down
Run: meds / 3 miles  meds / hot tub / meditation / ice / massage / nap  post: 6
Activities: watched a movie with Pat    else: good run, tired of pain

Day/date W 3        sleep: A B C D F    morn pain: 1 2 3 4 5 6 7   mood: ok
Run: meds / 3 miles  meds / hot tub / meditation / ice / massage / nap  post: 4
Activities: dinner with Andres    else: improvement

Day/date Th 4       sleep: A B C D F    morn pain: 1 2 3 4 5 6 7   mood: good
Run: meds 3 miles  meds hot tub meditation / ice / massage / nap  post: 3
Activities: hung with lil' Roy    else: feeling more optimistic

Day/date _____   sleep: A B C D F    morn pain: 1 2 3 4 5 6 7   mood: ____
Run: meds / ___ miles  meds / hot tub / meditation / ice / massage / nap  post: ___
Activities: _____    else: _____
```

Terry enjoyed his three-mile run on Monday but was blown away by the pain that followed, which was still at a seven even after a hot tub and a nap. On Tuesday, he prepared himself by scheduling a post-run massage, and he followed his run with pain medication and with meditation, a practice he began recently by sitting in his most comfortable chair and breathing slowly while relaxing his muscles and clearing his mind. This combination lowered his pain a notch, but not enough to keep up his spirits.

Note the improvement in Terry's experience in his next two runs. On both Wednesday and Thursday, he took pain medication before setting out rather than afterward. He also continued his meditation practice and on Thursday took a hot soak, which brought his pain to a three, a level that Terry finds fairly negligible. Seeing a four-point pain decrease in four days also buoyed his spirits. Terry plans to continue taking medication before his run, which he suspects may be a significant help, and testing post-run behaviors in different combinations. He also tracks activities outside of work and writes a note about anything that he wants to recall to provide a more comprehensive sense of each day. Terry hopes his approach will continue to show improvement, and if so, he plans to experiment with gradually increasing the length and pace of his runs.

Charlene is eager for change. After years of suffering from mysterious painful symptoms, at age twenty-two, she finally received an appropriate diagnosis. But, rather than experiencing relief that her symptoms have finally been named, she has fallen into despair over their chronic prognosis. Some days, she dwells on her troubles and sobs and sobs. While she recognizes that it can be therapeutic to let out her emotions and grieve, the long crying episodes leave her feeling depleted, congested, and exhausted.

Charlene decides to track the length of her blue periods and her response to them in an effort to decrease their frequency and intensity. This will allow her to experiment with different responses and evaluate their effectiveness. In addition, the act of recording this information will heighten her awareness about her experience and force her to contemplate alternate responses, even while in the throes of tears.

Charlene decides to use a printable spreadsheet in which she can list categories across the top and record information by hand in the cells. She likes the organization and flexibility of a chart format, and she plans to record data using a combination of numbers, letters, and brief notes.

Charlene's Chart

April 2012	time up	sleep	pain 1-10	mood grade	Cried?	responses	effect	activities	effect
Sn 1	6	lousy	8	D	2 hrs 10 min	-- hot bath	tired soothing	read	distracting
M 2	8	decent	6	C	30 min 20 min 5 min	hot bath, breaths self talk	relaxing calming good	brunch with Denniz	great!
T 3	7	ok	6	B-	30 min 20 min	music breaths	nice calming	h2O class	good
W 4	4 & 7	lousy	7	B	25 min 10 min	breaths self-talk	better ok	meeting, shopped, movie	tired (busy!)
H 5	7	ok	5	C+	20min 5min	breathing self-talk	calming better!	ate w/ neighbor	fun
Sa 6	6	ok	6	C	5min	breaths & self-talk	good!	went for walk	ok
Sn 7	6 & 9	good!	5	B+	X	☺!	☺!	called old friends	really nice!

On the first day of Charlene's tracking, she cried for two hours. During this tearful episode, she completely forgot about PAINTRACKING and her decision to test a deliberate response. Later that day, however, just as the tears began, she recalled the experiment and decided to try a hot bath. Before the tub filled up with hot water, her tears slowed considerably. She then climbed in for a soak, which she found to be soothing.

The next day, in the full throes of tears, she recalled the positive effect of the bath and turned on the hot water. She had two other crying episodes that day, during which she experimented with slow, deep breaths and speaking to herself in gentle, reassuring ways. Notice that the length of the episodes diminished over the course of the day as Charlene intervened more quickly and effectively. This pattern continued over the week with Charlene's experiments with various techniques to calm her mind and soothe her body. By Saturday, her tears lasted for five minutes, and Sunday was tear-free.

What can Charlene learn from her chart thus far? While it is not immediately apparent *which* of the interventions may be most effective, she sees evidence that the decision to intervene matters. Looking over the week, she is very pleased to observe shorter and less intense blue periods. In addition, the many other factors she is collecting—including the time she gets up; the quality of her sleep; her overall pain and mood rating; and her activities, which include social plans as well as exercise (and her perceived effect of these)—provide lots of data to mine when she is ready. At that time, she might explore the relationships among her pain, mood, and sleep and also focus more deliberately on the activities she chooses and their effects.

For Charlene, the very act of recording her depressive spells has helped her to feel more in control of them. She is starting to view her tears as data. Rather than seeing the flood of emotions as inevitable, she reacts to tearful thoughts by telling herself, "I feel a depressive episode coming on," and then considers her response. Noticing early signs of depressive feelings allows Charlene to think constructively about her ability to intervene, rather than getting caught up in the turbulence. She has been stockpiling a tool kit of strategies that help improve her outlook. She plans to start evaluating their effectiveness by sticking with one type for a period of time and then comparing it to others.

She is also interested in looking at her overall mood and seeing which factors seem most important. She suspects that aside from her quality of sleep, her moods are affected by the activities she chooses that day. She looks forward to planning and testing activities in a more deliberate way. In the meantime, she will continue to collect information that can help with future experiments as well as explain any unusual findings—she may observe, for example, that on days with poor sleep, high pain, and low mood, she is more vulnerable to tears, despite her best efforts.

Let's turn to consider Felipe. His worst problem is the unpredictability of the pain from his degenerative joint problems that have become pronounced in his thirties. Some days he feels reasonably well and able to be fairly active, yet on others, the pain interferes with his most basic needs. His worst days are those with the greatest variation—when, for example, he feels fine enough, and then, from out of the blue, severe pain stops him in his tracks. These days frustrate him most. It is getting to the point that Felipe is afraid to make plans because he fears he may suddenly feel incapacitated and vulnerable. At this time, Felipe is less interested in conducting experiments than having the opportunity to see trends over time and look for explanations of his pain flare-ups.

Because Felipe spends time every day at his desk computer (which he has set up for comfort), he has decided to use the online PAINTRACKING tool. To get started, he creates an account for himself at www.paintracking.com and reads the directions that walk him through how to create a personalized tracking system. Just like the handmade tracking tools described earlier, this online version offers significant flexibility and choice. Felipe decides to track his pain level, sleep quality, mood, exercise, activities, medication, and weather conditions. For each of these factors, he selects a range of possible responses from which he can later choose when recording his daily data. To record his pain, he chooses a ten-point pain scale and descriptive words that best describe his varying experience. He selects descriptions that resonate with him, like "unbearable," "burning," "crushing," and "exhausting," or he has the option of adding his own when he has one that better depicts what he feels. To make sure he fills out his sheet at approximately the same time each day, he requests a daily e-mail reminder.

After collecting a week or so of data, Felipe decides to search for trends. He requests graphs to illustrate the relationships among the different variables. From viewing these, hypotheses arise. He sees that he may be less vulnerable to pain flare-ups on the day *after* he has exercised. He also sees preliminary evidence that the weather and his sleep quality matter. The possibility of identifying patterns underlying his "unpredictable days" fills Felipe with hope. As he identifies the conditions associated with the variation in his experience, he will conduct experiments to enhance his understanding. He also looks forward to testing strategies to pace himself on the days when he expects to be most vulnerable.

Now It Is Your Turn.

Start by deciding on the format that would fit best with your lifestyle. Would you be most comfortable using a simple paper-and-pencil option? Are you adept with charts or computer templates? Or would you rather experiment with the interactive online tool offered as a companion to this book?

It can also help to envision the location and time of day that would be easiest for you to record data. Would you be more inclined to record data while at the computer or while relaxing in your recliner in the evening? Pick something you can stick to on a consistent basis. Keep in mind that tracking itself is an experiment. At any point, you can decide to change the format. Whatever format you choose, an effective system is:

Easy to use. No system is helpful if you don't feel up to using it. An effective system must fit well into your usual routine and be intuitive, easy to use (even at your worst), and require less than five minutes a day to fill out, with minimal contemplation, energy, or emotion. If recording feels like a chore, adapt the instrument. For tracking to work, nothing should stand in your way.

Adaptable. The best tools are flexible and interactive. Much of their therapeutic power comes from allowing you to conduct experiments and adjust them. When questions arise, you want to be able to alter your instrument without fuss. At certain points, your daily log may become as simple as a check mark on your calendar to affirm that you're still on track.

Consistent. Strive to make tracking data a part of your daily routine, such as brushing your teeth. While it is not always practical to record at the exact same hour each day, settling on a general time of day improves the accuracy of your entries. If you are generally optimistic in the morning and grumpy in the evening, for example, then recording sometimes in the morning and other times in the evening could produce dramatically different pictures of similar days.

Sometimes it can help to record certain information at different times of the day, as in some of the earlier examples. As needed, you might want to jot notes during the day, such as how you felt immediately after exercise; however, avoid turning tracking into an all-day activity. As you become more familiar with the process of tracking, you will develop the practice of making purposeful observations for later recording. You might say to yourself, "Man, this afternoon hurt," or, "That was a fantastic massage," to help the information stick. If you travel frequently or otherwise have a fairly inconsistent schedule, consider a system that is portable, or devise a plan B that mirrors your plan A as much as possible.

Relevant to you. It does not matter if others can decipher your system, as long as it stays relevant and understandable to you. To make sure you will be able to look back and understand exactly what you meant, even years later, create a "key" for especially quirky shorthand. Once you have decided the general format of your tracking tool, consider what you want to include in it. Your tracking tool should reflect your specific questions and way of thinking. Otherwise, it is unlikely that you will commit to daily recording, despite its benefits. Use measures that are meaningful to you and can quickly become second nature. Chapters 6 and 7 describe in detail variables you might include in your tracking sheet and ways to capture them.

The goal of creating your own tracking tool is to make one that is uniquely suited to you. However, it may feel intimidating to start from scratch. In my case, I created my first effective tracking worksheet after struggling with one that wasn't right for me and tweaking it until it was. For this reason, and because people often request a starter tracking sheet, I am including two example templates at the end of this chapter. You can fill in the spaces however you decide—with doodles, numbers, or descriptive words and abbreviations. Template 1 provides some categories for you to rate. Template 2 emphasizes your daily experiment—there's a place to note how you feel at different parts of the day; the test you are trying (such as a change in treatment or behavior) and your response; as well as any other factors that may be affecting your day. If either approach works for you, great! If neither does, also great! Channel your frustration into creating one that does. Or log on to the companion website to this book and let it walk you through the process, which will also follow in lockstep with the next chapters.

Example Template 1

Day/Date _____   Meds _____
Sleep _____   Pain 1 2 3 4 5 6 7 8 9 10   Fatigue 1 2 3 4 5 6 7 8 9 10
Nap _____ Weather _____ Mood _____   Exercise _____
Else _____

Day/Date _____   Meds _____
Sleep _____   Pain 1 2 3 4 5 6 7 8 9 10   Fatigue 1 2 3 4 5 6 7 8 9 10
Nap _____ Weather _____ Mood _____   Exercise _____
Else _____

Day/Date _____   Meds _____
Sleep _____   Pain 1 2 3 4 5 6 7 8 9 10   Fatigue 1 2 3 4 5 6 7 8 9 10
Nap _____ Weather _____ Mood _____   Exercise _____
Else _____

Day/Date _____   Meds _____
Sleep _____   Pain 1 2 3 4 5 6 7 8 9 10   Fatigue 1 2 3 4 5 6 7 8 9 10
Nap _____ Weather _____ Mood _____   Exercise _____
Else _____

Day/Date _____   Meds _____
Sleep _____   Pain 1 2 3 4 5 6 7 8 9 10   Fatigue 1 2 3 4 5 6 7 8 9 10
Nap _____ Weather _____ Mood _____   Exercise _____
Else _____

Day/Date _____   Meds _____
Sleep _____   Pain 1 2 3 4 5 6 7 8 9 10   Fatigue 1 2 3 4 5 6 7 8 9 10
Nap _____ Weather _____ Mood _____   Exercise _____
Else _____

Day/Date _____   Meds _____
Sleep _____   Pain 1 2 3 4 5 6 7 8 9 10   Fatigue 1 2 3 4 5 6 7 8 9 10
Nap _____ Weather _____ Mood _____   Exercise _____
Else _____

Example Template 2

Day/Date _____ Rate AM _____ Midday _____ PM _____
Test _____ Response _____
Other factors _____
_____

Day/Date _____ Rate AM _____ Midday _____ PM _____
Test _____ Response _____
Other factors _____
_____

Day/Date _____ Rate AM _____ Midday _____ PM _____
Test _____ Response _____
Other factors _____
_____

Day/Date _____ Rate AM _____ Midday _____ PM _____
Test _____ Response _____
Other factors _____
_____

Day/Date _____ Rate AM _____ Midday _____ PM _____
Test _____ Response _____
Other factors _____
_____

Day/Date _____ Rate AM _____ Midday _____ PM _____
Test _____ Response _____
Other factors _____
_____

Day/Date _____ Rate AM _____ Midday _____ PM _____
Test _____ Response _____
Other factors _____
_____

Chapter 6

Tracking Your Well-Being

The first and most crucial piece of data to track is your well-being. Although you may have a sense of when you feel better or worse, what is it exactly?

When people inquire, "So, are you any better?" how do you know? Think about it. If you have not clearly defined what it means to improve, you may miss signs of improvement. Generally, the decrease or even disappearance of a particular pain is much less dramatic than its presence. Consider, for example, how quickly you can forget an irritating buzzing sound once it stops (until it reappears). Similarly, you are more likely to notice new pains than the absence of old ones. It's also common to judge how you feel against how you think you *should* be feeling, rather than how you felt last week or last month. To conceptualize your well-being, ask yourself:

1. What is my worst problem (the thing you cannot stand or find most debilitating)?
2. What do I most want to change?
3. What best indicates how I am doing?
4. What lets me know whether I'm feeling better, worse, or the same?

Your answer to any of these questions helps provide a way to evaluate how you are doing. This will serve as a gauge of your well-being and the central target of your experiments to improve. In scientific terms, this piece of information is called a *dependent variable* (because it *depends* on a host of other *variables* or factors, such as your environment, behavior, and therapeutic strategies). For Roselyn, it was the extent to which she could enjoy her family; for Terry, it was his ability to run; for Charlene, it was reducing crying spells; and for Felipe, it was predicting (and later controlling) pain flare-ups. Once you decide how to define your well-being, the next step is to consider how to measure it. As both research subject and investigator, you can create a personalized measure that captures your daily reality.

OK, sounds good, but how do I go about measuring my well-being? I need help! Coming up with a rating system for quality of life may feel like a foreign concept. But don't worry. You don't have to start from scratch. This chapter provides many examples of well-being and simple ways to measure them. Scan the headings (and subheadings) below for categories that resonate with you. I cannot overstate the value of creating measures that feel personal and intuitive.

Bear in mind that your concept of well-being will likely change over time, as you accumulate self-knowledge and improve, or as new situations and questions arise. Focus on the here and now and select what you *most* want to understand and change at this point.

No matter how you conceptualize well-being, select a measure that

1. captures the aspect of well-being most salient to your experience;
2. you can evaluate quickly and without excessive deliberation; and
3. you can rate in a reliable and consistent way.

Pain

Your experience with pain is likely to be connected to your sense of well-being. People with chronic pain inevitably develop an intimate relationship with their pain. You are the only one who can evaluate at any moment whether your pain resides in the background or foreground or whether it feels manageable, difficult, or overwhelming. Pain varies in severity, location, sensation, duration, character, and the degree to which it affects your abilities or fills your day. When *you* think about your pain, what comes to mind?

Numeric Pain Scales

Among the most common ways to depict pain severity is with a ten-point scale in which one is negligible discomfort and ten represents the worst imaginable. One benefit of adopting this ten-point scale is its universality. In the United States, medical professionals are encouraged (and in some cases required) to inquire about pain using this scale, a data point sometimes referred to as the fifth vital sign (after temperature, blood pressure, pulse, and respiration rate).[1] You have likely seen ten-point scales with accompanying facial expressions posted on the wall at your doctor's office or other medical clinic.

As Eula Biss describes in her essay "The Pain Scale," it is much less taxing for doctors to hear someone describe their pain as a "ten" than as a "hot poker driven through their eyeball into their brain."[2] Quantitative pain scales are clear and simple; they sanitize all the horrid details of our experience. Using numeric scales also allows you to analyze trends over time; numbers allow the options of graphing trends, calculating average pain ratings for a given period of time, and seeing the percentage you have improved (described in chapter 8).

Use the standard ten-point pain scale if and only if you can select a number that captures your experience without having to deliberate. Ideally, you want all measures in your tracking tool to be quick and easy to rate. Because pain is subjective and personal, the scale is not meant to be interpreted as a thermometer; your five might be someone else's seven. The value of the numbers is that they allow you to compare your own experience at different moments. It should be meaningful if you move from a six to a three or a four. Because pain levels tend to range significantly over the course of the day, you may decide to depict the day with a range, such as a "2–5 day," rather than assigning it a single number.

If you are committed to numbers, but not the standard ten-point scale, devise your own. It can help to assign meaning to each number and use fewer categories:

1 = minimal / 2 = uncomfortable / 3 = intense / 4 = excruciating
0 = no problem / 1 = annoying / 2 = tough / 3 = need to lie down / 4 = destroyed
1 = light / 2 = medium / 3 = bad / 4 = severe / 5 = unbearable
0 = OK / 1 = hurts / 2 = hurts a lot! / 3 = HURTS*#@!!!!
1 = tolerable / 2 = challenging / 3 = intolerable

Pain scales typically depict severity, but you can scale any aspect of pain that is meaningful to you, such as:

the degree to which pain is affecting you:
   1 = negligible / 2 = a little / 3 = moderately / 4 = a lot / 5 = extremely

how manageable your pain feels:
1 = manageable / 2 = some difficulty / 3 = very difficult / 4 = unmanageable

the extent to which pain interferes with your day:
            1 = hardly at all / 2 = challenging / 3 = total interference

Pain Descriptors

Another way to capture pain is by describing it. You may observe that your pain has distinct qualities that are fundamental to your well-being. Noting that you "hurt a lot" or have a pain rating of six may capture your experience less well than selecting the appropriate words, such as:

aching	mild	tender	intense	crushing
shooting	blinding	irritating	stabbing	pinching
burning	metal-claws	constant	crampy	nagging
deep	throbbing	dull	periodic	excruciating
piercing	tight	gnawing	radiating	tingling
hellfire	hammered	shocking	tortuous	superficial
vise-grip	smashed			

You might choose descriptive words if you experience pain by its characteristics. Your day may be significantly different when your pain feels "gnawing" versus "radiating," or "achy" as opposed to "burning." Reflect on your pain. Do you have two or three meaningful words that come to mind when you assess the variation in your pain? If so, consider how you might include these in an open- or closed-ended item in your tracking system. Or, if you tend to be a visual person, you may decide to capture your pain with simple informative doodles (e.g., smiles, frowns, bright suns, dark clouds, lightning rods, etc.).

Pain Location

Many of us have multiple pain sites. Your experience may depend most on where you hurt on a given day. You may have been asked by a pain specialist to shade areas on a line drawing of a body from front and back views to indicate your pain. While these pictures convey much information, they are impractical daily measures because of the time and effort required. (Plus, all that coloring can bring on a flare-up for some!) If location seems most salient to you, consider simpler, less labor-intensive ways to capture it. Perhaps you alternately experience localized and generalized pain, or feel baffled by the appearance and disappearance of leg pain, or evaluate your day by the extent of pain in specific areas, such as your jaw, pelvis, head, arms, or back.

You could indicate, for example, whether your pain feels local or all over, or estimate the percentage of your body affected. On your best days, pain may include 25 percent of your body, while your worst may be 75 or 100 percent. Or you could note the places that hurt most, such as your neck, legs, or lower back. Sometimes your worst days may be when a particular part of your body gives you trouble—such as those terrible "burning back" moments.

Overall Pain Experience

Your overall experience with pain may feel distinct from any particular aspect of it. You may experience days in which your pain feels all consuming and other days when it feels manageable, regardless of its intensity or features. Or you may lack a clear sense of what makes your pain more (or less) of a pain. If this describes you, consider how you might represent the "whole" of your experience with global categories, such as:

$$T = \text{tolerable vs. } I = \text{intolerable}$$
$$\text{OK/Not}$$
$$L \text{ (livable) vs. } NL \text{ (not livable)}$$

Come up with your own pair of terms that captures your experience and with a shorthand method to incorporate this information into your tracking tool.

Fatigue

Many pain conditions involve fatigue, and this symptom may define much of your well-being. You may experience fatigue as cognitive, as physical, as emotional, or, most likely, as some combination. It can be helpful to reflect on what you say to yourself or how it may manifest as behavior, such as enticing you onto the nearest couch, too exhausted to move. If fatigue defines much of your experience, consider its most salient aspect:

How able are you to think, focus, concentrate, or understand?
How well can you sustain activity?
What is your current energy level?
Is it difficult to stay awake?
Do you feel that you can drive safely (or engage in other activities)?

When you ferret out what matters most, consider how you would like to represent it.

Numeric Fatigue Scales

Numeric scales to rate fatigue are less common than for pain; however, the same logic applies.

1 = minimal / 2 = fairly tired / 3 = very tired / 4 = exhausted / 5 = smashed

0 = decent / 1 = somewhat run-down / 2 = run-down / 3= totally run-down!

1 = light / 2 = medium / 3 = intense / 4 = nearly asleep

1 = fairly clear / 2 = cloudy / 3 = foggy / 4 = brain-dead

0 = OK / 1 = tired / 2 = tired! / 3 = Tired!! / 4 = TIRED!!!!

1 = tolerable / 2 = challenging / 3 = intolerable

If you decide to include scales for pain and fatigue, consider using the same metric. In other words, if you are using a five-point pain scale, create a similar one for fatigue. This can make your scales more intuitive (the less thought, the better), and quicker to interpret later. For example:

0 = negligible pain	0 = negligible fatigue
1 = some pain	1 = some fatigue
2 = irritating pain	2 = irritating fatigue
3 = aggravating pain	3 = aggravating fatigue
4 = intolerable pain	4 = intolerable fatigue

The word "fatigue" may seem like a poor representation of what you experience, which may feel more like "complete exhaustion" or "obliteration." Use categories that capture your daily experience.

Some descriptive words for cognitive fatigue:

foggy	cloudy	vacant	brain-dead	mushy
cotton-headed	slow	out of it	zonked	blender-head
confused	dizzy	zombielike	fuzzy	muffled
absent	confused			

Some descriptions of physical fatigue:

tired	sleepy	floored	exhausted	destroyed
heavy	weak	drained	smashed	run-down
spent	weary	near collapse	pummeled	flulike
head bobbing	eyes closed	droopy		

Energy Level (Timing and Duration)

Energy levels vary over the course of the day. For people contending with chronic pain and fatigue, these variations can be dramatic. If you desire greater insight and control over your energy, collect details on the ebb and flow of these cycles. For example, you can record the times of day your energy is at its highest and lowest, or the duration and frequency. Some questions to consider:

- When do you experience your worst fatigue?
- How long do these periods last?
- How difficult is it to arise from sleep in the morning?
- How often do you flop down on the couch (or bed or office floor)?
- When does your energy seem to peak?

Think about the most salient aspects of your fatigue and the question, description, or scale to capture it.

Mood

Some days, your emotional response may feel more significant than your pain or fatigue. While it is understandable to think that pain determines mood—the more pain, the unhappier you feel—they are not perfectly correlated. We've all had days when we felt upbeat despite pain or struggled despite minimal symptoms. If your emotional states or responses feel central in determining your well-being, track them. Documenting depressive symptoms can also help establish the need for professional help (see chapter 18). It is equally important to identify the conditions under which you experience joy, peace, optimism, and other positive emotions in order to increase these.

Consider feeling words that capture your experience:

satisfied	content	appreciative	hopeful	happy	delighted
ruminating	fretful	anxious	irritable	blue	fatigued
sad	blah	in the dumps	unhappy	ticked-off	tearful
weepy	crying	unmotivated	hopeless	ambivalent	apathetic
angry	stuck	depressed	dejected	paralyzed	fed up
cut off	numb	weepy	blunted	scared	explosive

You could record the frequency and duration of times when you feel particularly hopeful or hopeless. Just as with the indicators of well-being, you can measure your mood with a scale or descriptive words. A few examples:

1 = joyful / 2 = content / 3 = neutral / 4 = sad / 5 = depressed
1 = hopeful / 2 = okay / 3 = hopeless
1 = excellent / 2 = fine / 3= struggling / 4 = down

Another option is to record your mood with a simple doodle—as they say, a picture is worth a thousand words. In this case, no artistic skill is required. The simpler and faster, the better. Rudimentary facial features can depict tremendous variations in mood. The difference between ☺ and ☹ speaks volumes, and you can add exclamation marks for intensity. You can also augment a simple face by varying the size of its smile or frown or by opening the mouth for emphasis. Additional changes in the size and shape of the face and its features offer limitless options.

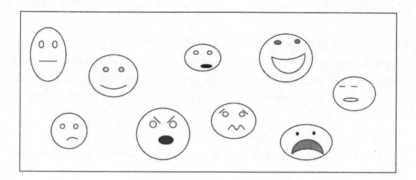

Overall Well-Being

You may decide to include a more positive concept that measures your overall well-being instead of, or in addition to, measures of pain, fatigue, or mood. No matter how you feel, no symptom or set of symptoms wholly defines your experience. It may be more honest and realistic to note your general sense of the day. Plus, you may not know *why* a day was good (or bad), just that it was. Selecting a positive measure of well-being, such as happiness, contentment, satisfaction, or your level of fulfillment, also encourages you to look for and reinforce the aspects of your day that you appreciate and want to continue and increase. The approach you take in order to create days that feel more fulfilled, for example, may differ in some ways from an approach to reduce physical symptoms. Moreover, research shows that engaging in positive experiences can reduce your perceptions of pain and enrich your overall experience. You might decide to record the extent to which your day felt satisfying or fulfilling:

S = (satisfying) / U = (unsatisfying)
F = (fulfilling) / U = (unfulfilling)

Add nuance with simple symbols, such as plus and minus signs. An S++ day might be "extremely satisfying," while a U– might be "very unsatisfying" or "very unfulfilling." Or you could grade your days, such that:

A = outstanding / B = good / C = fair / D = really hard / F = terrible

Use plus and minus signs for emphasis. A+++ days would be something to celebrate (and experiment to reproduce), while F– days deserve serious scrutiny.

Another way to consider the big picture when rating your days would be to create a question to capture your experience, such as:

- If all days were like today, how would it feel?
- If today were my average day, how would my life be?
- If all days were like today, could I live with it?

Your response to such questions can be coded with a scale or simple categories.

1= unacceptable / 2 = OK / 3 = fine / 4 = good / 5 = great
1 = unlivable / 2 = tolerable / 3 = livable
OK (O) / not OK (N)
1= yes / 2 = sort of / 3 = no

Come up with your own abbreviations or a numeric system to limit recording time if you need to write or type in a response.

Other and More Positive Measures of Well-Being

Don't be surprised if you develop ideas about what matters most to you when contemplating your day that were not covered here. You may have something you say to yourself as the day draws to a close. Or a particular behavior, thought, or ability may stand out as a personal measure of your well-being. You might be less concerned with symptoms than with how well you coped or what you were able to accomplish. For some, the ability to work or engage in another activity may stand in for more general satisfaction. In that case, consider questions such as:

- What was I able to accomplish this day?
  (1= nothing / 2 = some / 3 = a lot)
- How satisfied am I with how I coped?
  (1 = little / 2 = some / 3 = very)
- To what extend did I engage in meaningful activity?
  (0 = none / 1 = some / 2 = enough / 3 = lots!)

Or you may consider your relationships most meaningful, given the extent that pain and fatigue can make relationships vulnerable (see chapters 23–25). There is evidence that improving one's relationships reduces suffering of all kinds.[3] You might decide to record such things as:

- your level of intimacy and satisfaction with your partner;
- your ability to enjoy, listen to, empathize with, or focus on your partner, children, parents, friends, or coworkers;
- whether or not you felt you treated others well; or
- the extent to which you engaged with others socially.

You can measure any of these with open- or closed-ended questions, using abbreviations, doodles, categories to circle, or other quick and intuitive ratings.

When you are desperate to understand and reduce painful symptoms, it makes sense to measure them as a central part of your well-being. However, there is also good reason to consider more positive measures of well-being—what you would *like* to experience rather than what do would like *not* to—particularly as you begin to improve. Focusing on your ability to enjoy yourself or feel closer with people in your life, or focusing on your accomplishments, helps shift your attention to these heartening occurrences. Unlike symptoms, which during your best moments would be measured by their absence or as "zero," positive experiences offer open-ended upper scores. You can then focus on experiments to see if you can continue to raise your "feelings of intimacy" or other positive aspirations. Goals to reduce painful symptoms and enjoy a rich life are interrelated. Decreases in pain may help you engage more fully (and easily) in life, and achieving satisfaction and positive engagement in areas that matter most to you may reduce your perception of pain. Experiment and see.

IN REVIEW

Select a measure of well-being that

1. represents how you are doing;
2. reflects what you most want to understand and influence; and
3. can be measured easily and consistently.

Chapter 7

What Matters

Measuring Explanatory Factors

S o far, your tracking system includes a measure (or measures) of well-being. Quite often, exercises to understand chronic pain end there. While charting your well-being over time provides essential information, it does not explain *why* you feel as you do. However long you have lived with pain, you no doubt have questions:

1. Why was last week so much better than this one?
2. Would I respond better to a different medication or dose?
3. What would ideal pacing look like for me? How much can I do without doing "too much"?
4. What type and amount of exercise would help most?
5. What can I do right now to feel better?

Answers come from collecting data on the factors that may be affecting how you feel and seeing how they relate to your well-being. These are the pieces of the puzzle that you interpret and, whenever possible, tweak until you experience sustained improvement. Or, in scientific language, they are *independent variables*, which can explain the variation in your well-being (the *dependent variable*).

Why You Feel the Way You Feel

To identify factors that matter, brainstorm about what appears significant, confusing, or otherwise connected to how you feel. We all have stories or hunches about our experience. These hunches are your hypotheses. Some examples:

- It seems that my pain is more manageable when I engage in a moderate level of activity.
- My pain seems to intensify when I drink red wine.
- When I plan something enjoyable, I think I actually feel better.
- I may have greater stamina when I schedule in rest breaks.

Collecting data on your hypotheses then allows you to test what you may suspect and to respond accordingly. This chapter describes explanatory factors that you can explore in your tracking-system tool. As you consider what to include, resist the urge to solve everything at once. A tracking tool that is too laborious for daily use is not helpful. Instead, consider a small handful of categories that you think matter most. As you discover their impact on how you feel, you can add or change your variables and increase your understanding.

Begin with Environmental Factors

Certain environmental factors can make you feel particularly vulnerable to pain. It is important to understand these, even if they lie outside of your control or you already understand (or strongly suspect) their effect. Why? Because tracking their impact ensures that you see the full picture.

Let's say that as part of your strategy to improve, you embark on an exercise program and see in your tracking data that your first week at the gym was miserable. That week also happened to be chilly and rainy, and you generally fare better on warm, dry days than on cold, damp ones. Without collecting data on the weather, you may not be able to tell the extent to which your pain increased on account of exercise, weather conditions, or some combination of both. Thus, to pinpoint the effects of the exercise (or other behavior), you want to be able to examine the effects of exercise on days that are cold and wet as well as warm and dry. Having data on the weather can keep you from drawing false conclusions about other causal relationships. In scientific terms, the weather functions here as a *control variable*—that is, you want to *control* the effects of the weather to identify the true impact of exercise. Make sense?

Another reason to track conditions you think are important is that our beliefs are not always based in fact. If you find that weather has no effect on your well-being, there's no need to track it (and you can start rethinking your approach to weather conditions). If you do find that weather is significant, you might desire greater detail, such as whether your pain increases with the arrival of a cold front, a drop in barometric pressure, or increased humidity, as well as the specific weather conditions that bring relief. This information can help you mitigate the effects of foul weather, take advantage of fairer skies, plan your ideal vacation, or help you assess arguments for moving to a different climate.

When including environmental factors of interest in your tracking system, keep it simple. You might record the precise temperature if you have a thermometer hanging in plain sight or built into your tracking application; but don't turn on the Weather Channel or search a website in search of data. Instead, record your impression of the weather, such as with simple doodles or descriptive notes:

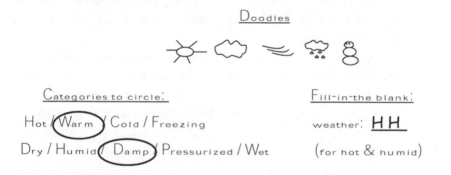

Or combine doodles with a note for a quick and comprehensive record, such as for cold and sunny, warm and rainy, hot and cloudy, and snowy and windy.

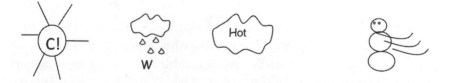

Similarly, you can devise a scale to summarize any other environmental factors—such as from peaceful to chaotic, or a scale of environmental friendliness. When the effects of environmental factors are significant, change those you can. And continue to track significant factors, even when they are beyond your control, if they will help you evaluate the effects of other variables, such as a new medication, therapy, or behavior. It would be a shame to discontinue a beneficial therapy because you neglected to note something in your environment that significantly affects how you feel.

Consider the Choices You Make That Impact Your Well-Being

Let's move ahead to the strategies you are using, or could use, to influence your well-being. This is where you include and personalize the prescription for improvement summarized in chapter 3 with the acronym PAPER (pain management, attitude, pacing, exercise, and rest). By testing these factors in your tracking tool, you can adjust them for optimal benefit. This self-knowledge is key to sustained improvement.

OK—sounds great—but how do I go about understanding all these factors? I need help! First, remember to start with only those factors you want to understand most. As you find answers, you can exchange them for others. As with the previous chapter, skim through the headings to select the variables you want to include. Select ideas that feel most relevant, and skip those that don't. Let the examples stimulate your thinking.

P Is for Pain Management

Medicines and Supplements

When testing a new medication or considering current ones, the big question is "How is this working for me?" Most people with chronic pain try many medications, often in combination. Systematic records are far superior to memory or best guesses in evaluating your reactions. They also allow you to collaborate with healthcare professionals to determine what works, eliminate anything ineffective, and adjust doses to provide the greatest relief and least side effects.

Sometimes it's a challenge to remember whether I took my medication, let alone record every single time I take a pill! Recording full information every time you ingest a pill is neither realistic nor helpful. Collect only what you need for the insights you seek. This may be the dose, frequency, time of day taken, or your responses or side effects. Dosage may be relevant if you are evaluating a new medication or the best way to take "as needed" prescriptions. Timing likely matters if you are determining the best time of day to take a medication—whether, for example, you benefit more from taking pain medication in the morning versus evening; before versus after strenuous activities; or on a regular basis versus only during significant pain episodes. You may decide to collect data on side effects to evaluate a new medication, dosage, or schedule.

> **Note:** The following examples are illustrative only. They are **not** intended to represent advice on any specific medication or dosage. For a more comprehensive discussion on the use of medication, see chapter 17.

If you are creating a template or using the online PAINTRACKING tool, you can include full information on each medication. If you are noting them by hand, use abbreviations—but make sure you keep a full record of the name and current dose of all medications and supplements you take. While you may believe you will always remember C equals thirty milligrams of Cymbalta®, nobody has a perfect memory. More than likely, your medications will change along with your needs and discoveries and as new ones enter the market. It is invaluable to be able to reflect on what you were taking years earlier. Create a key that corresponds with your tracking tool. Prescription medications have a brand name and a generic one; brand names tend to be capitalized (as in Klonopin®), while generics are written in lowercase (as in clonazepam). You can choose whether to record the name as it appears on your prescription label or by the one most familiar to you.

> Keep a key that includes full information.
> Track the medications that change or vary.
> Use simple shorthand to record their names and doses.

Syd's medication. Syd has been taking three prescribed medications: Serzone®, Ultram®, and Sonata®. While his doses remain consistent, their frequency varies. Each morning, Syd takes Serzone and Ultram to alleviate morning pain. On days when his pain persists, Syd sometimes takes additional Ultram; other times he decides to "tough it out." Because Syd is interested in the effects of this decision, he records his daily doses of Ultram so he can evaluate its impact on his well-being. He sometimes takes Sonata on the nights he has trouble falling asleep; he similarly records the variation in his use of Sonata so he can evaluate its effects on how he feels the following day.

Syd's record of medication taken each day

Day, Date	Template 1	Template 2	Key:
M 11/6:	Sz, U	Sz U (1) ~~So~~	Sz = Serzone 100mg (morning)
T 11/7:	Sz, U	Sz U (1) ~~So~~	
W 11/8	Sz, Ux2, So	Sz U (2) ~~So~~	U = Ultram 100mg (morning, and as needed)
Th 11/9	Sz, Ux3, So	Sz U (3) So	
F 11/10	Sz, U	Sz U (1) ~~So~~	So = Sonata 5mg (bed, as needed)

As you can see, Syd created a key with full information on his medications, and he uses the abbreviations in his tracking system. In his first template, Syd used open-ended notation and wrote in abbreviations to represent the medications he took and their frequency, such as "U×2" to indicate two doses of Ultram. He later changed his template to include the abbreviations on the template itself. So, instead of writing in abbreviations for the medication, Syd records the number of Ultram in the parentheses and crosses out Sonata when he doesn't take it. Syd likes to see all his medication, including Serzone, in his template; however, if his list of medications were substantially longer, he might include only those that varied.

Syd's sheet reveals that on Wednesday and Thursday he took additional Ultram, the same days he took Sonata. By examining his data over time, Syd discovered that he feels significantly better when he responds promptly to pain with additional medication, rather than "toughing it out," and that this positive effect continues into the next day. He brought this information to his doctor for feedback.

Side Effects

Every medication carries a list of potential side effects. Some you may never experience, others may be a minor nuisance, and still others can be prohibitive. Unpleasant side effects influence people's decisions about the desirability of particular medications. When you start a new medicine or change doses, the equation is whether the benefits outweigh the difficulties. By tracking the positive and negative effects over time, you work with your doctor to assess a drug's efficacy (see chapters 16 and 17). Consider open-ended spaces to specify effects for new medications, or closed-ended ones for medications you have used before or for which you otherwise have a sense of their potential side effects.

Open-ended	Closed-ended
7/1 Cy, Px2, G _dizzy, nausea_	7/1 Cy, P, (2), G (diz) (naus) tired diarh
7/2 Cy, P, G ____runs____ ☹	7/2 Cy, P, (1), G diz naus tired (diarh)

One Change at a Time, Whenever Possible

Ideally, it's best not to change more than one thing at a time when evaluating medication because simultaneous changes make it more difficult to pinpoint your response. In practice, however, this may not be feasible or even recommended—your doctor may advise you to taper off one medication as you increase another. When multiple factors fluctuate, you can still disentangle their specific effects by examining daily records over time (as described in chapter 8).

Pamela's experience. For the past seven years, Pamela has been taking three medications: one for pain (Percocet®) and two for sleep (clonazepam and Ambien®). Her medication routine has been stable, so much so that she simply enters "PCA" in her tracking worksheet. While Pamela believes she is managing "adequately," she and her doctor (aided by her records) have decided to try Lyrica® to see if she improves further. If Pamela responds well, they hope to reduce and possibly discontinue her other medications, starting with clonazepam, then Percocet and Ambien. Pamela feels anxious about changing medication, especially about how her body might react without her nightly dose of clonazepam. Keeping careful records feels reassuring to Pamela. She has a plan with her doctor to check in should she note any difficulties during the transition period.

As you see below, Pamela started recording Lyrica in its own column with the plan to group it with her other medications if the trial goes successfully. (For space reasons, these records are displayed in *weeks* rather than as the *daily* data she collected.) The first week Pamela took Lyrica, she recorded its full name and dose. Subsequently, she shortened it to "L," noting its dose only when it changed. Because Pamela tolerated her initial doses of Lyrica, she increased it as advised while decreasing clonazepam. For each change, Pamela diligently noted the new dose, highlighting it with an asterisk. Because Pamela did not experience any setbacks as she increased her dose of Lyrica and decreased her clonazepam, on week 12, she discontinued clonazepam altogether—note that "C" no longer appears in subsequent entries, and "L" joins the grouping of her now usual medication regimen.

Tracking Pamela's changes in medication

	Medication	
Week 1	PCA	Lyrica (25mg x3)*
Week 2	PCA	L
Week 3	P C(.5) * A	L (50mg x3)*
Week 4	PCA	L
Week 5	PCA	L
Week 6	PCA	L
Week 7	PCA	L
Week 8	PCA	L
Week 9	PCA	L
Week 10	PC (.25)*A	L (100mg x 3)*
Week 11	PCA	L
Week 12	PA*	L
Week 13	PLA	
Week 14	PLA	

Key:
P= Percocet ½ Tablet 4/day
C= clonazepam 1 mg (bed)
A= Ambien 5 mg (bed)

Because of the long half-life and physical dependency that can develop with clonazepam, Pamela will continue to evaluate how she feels in the upcoming weeks. If she sustains her improvement for an agreed-upon time period with her doctor, she will start tapering off Percocet, then Ambien. If at any time Pamela finds she fared better on a previous dose, she and her doctor can return to her earlier combination or search for an alternative. Whatever medication Pamela ends up taking will be based on actual empirical results rather than an emotional reaction.

Pamela's chart illustrates one way to record changes in medication. Feel free to come up with your own, as long as you include what you find most important. Your medication regimen could be more complicated than in Pamela's example: You may be starting a new medication while taking several others as needed for pain, sleep difficulty, anxiety, or other fluctuating symptoms. Plus, you may want to evaluate how each can provide the best outcome. The more discretion you have in how you take your medication, the more important it is to test what works best: Are you reaching too often or too infrequently for your pill box? What is the ratio of unpleasant side effects to benefits? How do your symptoms respond to different medications, schedules, and combinations?

Representing Daily Variation in Medication and Dose

Detailed questions require more detailed data. The first step is to prioritize—don't tackle all your questions at once. But even if you decide to assess a complicated puzzle with fairly elaborate data, the fuss can be minimal.

Example of minichart for multiple medication and data points

Date: _____	AM	Day	Eve	Nite
Savella®	—	—	—	—
gabapentin	—	—	—	—
Sonata	—	—	—	—

Minicharts allow you to collect several layers of information by varying the number of columns and rows and what they represent. The above example includes categories to track information at four time points: morning, midday, evening, and night. Tracking general times of the day is substantially easier than trying to record the exact hour. Putting an X in the appropriate boxes, for example, would be all you need if your interest is the time of day you took each medication. For greater detail, you could fill the boxes with dose information or the effects you experience at that time. Or, rather than noting time of day, you might list other categories of interest, such as before, during, or after relevant activities. If your questions require multiple observations, consider how you might adapt this simple but versatile system to fit your specific needs and style.

Other Pain-Management Strategies

Chronic pain creates consumers eager for relief. The list of nonpharmacological therapies and products is long and diverse, with alternatives continually introduced. Professionals offer physical therapy, massage therapy, therapeutic hypnosis, biofeedback, yoga, and acupuncture, among many other services. Products range from elixirs to electronic gadgets to self-help instructions for stretching, meditations, and guided imagery, among other approaches. Each requires an investment of time; money; and, often, emotion, as our hopes may be raised and sometimes dashed. Consult with trusted professionals when deciding to try something new, and then carefully track its effects. This helps you approach what may seem like an overwhelming market of possibilities as a manageable set of experiments.

Tracking nonpharmaceutical strategies is similar to tracking pharmaceutical strategies, but with much simpler records of "dose" or "frequency"—as appealing as it sounds, few people enjoy more than one massage or soak in a hot tub per day. Tracking pain-relief strategies can be as simple as noting what you used that day.

Example template:

Day: _____ PT / massage / heat / meditation / stretching
Day: _____ PT / massage / heat / meditation / stretching
Day: _____ PT / massage / heat / meditation / stretching
Day: _____ PT / massage / heat / meditation / stretching

Including a list, as above, to circle or check is not only easy to fill out, but it also provides a daily reminder of potentially helpful strategies. To evaluate the effects of strategies you have tried, create a rating system. Pick something easy, such as thumbs up / thumbs down, alphabetic grades, a numeric scale, or face doodles, as in the examples below. If some of the benefit is the pleasure or relief it may provide in the moment, include a place to note this.

Examples of notes with feedback

Day 1 <u>mass 30m Allen ☺ !!</u>	PT / Med/ HT / Ms/ Str	👍 (ok) 👎
Day 2 <u>hot tub 10m ☺ great!</u>	PT / Med/HT/ Ms / Str	A B C D F
Day 3 <u>mass 60m Dana (sore!)</u>	PT / Med/ HT /Ms/ Str	++ +[–] – –
Day 4 <u>stretch (ok)</u>	PT / Med/ HT / Ms /Str	☺ - 😐 - ☹
Day 5 <u>physical therapy</u>	PT/ Med/ HT / Ms / Str	0 1 2 3 (4)5

Consider how you want to capture your experience of strategies intended to relieve pain. Including pertinent details such as the length of time or specifics about a therapist or technique helps make sense of inconsistent results, such as why a massage may have been helpful one day but not another. In addition, comments such as "loved that!" or "I feel great!" are valuable notes to read when you slip into pessimistic thinking.

Knowledge about what worked can change your behavior and your experience. Discovering, for example, that five minutes of slow, deep breaths, or ten minutes in the hot tub, or a half-hour massage with a particular therapist consistently alleviates your pain is encouraging. This information helps you to act decisively and increase your comfort rather than feel dejected about a pain flare-up. Tracking therapies over time also provides data on any longer-lasting effects.

A Is for Attitude

Research shows the significance of attitude on our experience (see chapter 12). Negativity transforms pain into suffering, while optimistic self-talk turns lemons into lemonade. Hearing that your outlook matters, however, is much less powerful than seeing this effect for yourself. This is precisely why tracking is vital. Tracking your mood may not guarantee a sunny disposition, but looking at trends over time pinpoints the positive (and keeps the negative from drowning it out) and provides a way to test the effect of strategies that may shift your thinking. This information helps you view your situation in a realistic light, avoid mistakenly concluding your worst is your usual, and take action to lift your spirits. Instead of wallowing in the awfulness of how you may feel, you can choose a strategy that *you* have found to be effective. Consider ways to depict your outlook. Some examples:

Numeric scales:	0–10 (from hopeless to fantastic) /
	1–2–3 (positive / OK / negative)
Doodle scales:	☺! / ☺ / ☺ / ☹ / ☹!
Descriptive words:	despair / sad / OK / positive / cheery
	acceptance / nonacceptance

Recording a daily measure of attitude also raises your level of awareness about what you say to yourself. We all know the same glass can be half empty or half full. As described in chapter 12, the ability to change your attitude depends on your awareness of self-talk. Our thoughts often occur at lightning speed, and we may remain unaware of them or their impact. In an instant, you may tell yourself, "I can't stand this pain," which intensifies your struggles. On the other hand, a reassuring thought, such as "I have experienced pain in the past, and will get through again," can keep a setback in perspective. Your tracking system can help you modify distressful, negative thinking.

In addition to noting your attitude, record your responses to any negative thoughts or mood, as in Charlene's example in chapter 5. If you suffer from bouts of sadness, you could include your reaction to such bouts and the effectiveness of the reaction. This system holds you accountable by demanding that you record steps taken and evaluate them, which can lead you to discover what works.

Or, on a more positive note, you may choose to note your successes with affirming thoughts and their effects. Positivity begets positivity—and more so when you have data documenting its benefit.

P Is for Pacing

Although chronic pain can make people feel like sitting out or hiding in bed, active engagement is generally more beneficial. Unfortunately, however, not all activity is helpful, and too much of it causes setbacks. By tracking activities and their effects, you can calculate the "pain cost" of given activities and distinguish those that incite pain from those that are more rejuvenating. Tracking your response to activity and rest can also help you discover your optimal rhythm. You can deliberately choose activities that promise to be more fulfilling than depleting.

Steve's dilemma. Steve was invited for dinner by friends he adores. Unfortunately, Steve feels exhausted, aches all over, and fears that a social engagement will make matters worse. At the same time, he appreciates these friends and worries that if he turns them down—yet again—they may stop inviting him. He doesn't know whether he should bite the bullet and visit his friends, or risk offending them. He's also puzzled by the fact that social visits sometimes lift his spirits and other times deplete him. Will he feel worse and regret going? Will the warmth of his friends feel more compelling than his symptoms? Or will the positivity of the evening actually diminish his pain and fatigue? His uncertainty about the effects of his decision makes it especially challenging and confusing. Steve realizes he needs data to guide his decision, and he adds social activity to his tracking sheet. He decides to treat the invitation as his first data point for this category, knowing that whatever he learns will inform future decisions. In his tracking tool, Steve includes a measure of social activity (yes / no), specific factors that may be relevant, whether he leaves "early" or "late," and a measure of whether or not he regrets his decision.

Fri: activity: [yes]/ no specifics: ☺ <u>games</u> early /[late] regrets: **none!**

Sat: activity[yes]/ no specifics: **<u>cold, bad chairs</u>** [early]/ late regrets: **40%**

Steve planned an early-exit strategy for Friday but was enjoying himself so much with friends that he stayed fairly late. As his log reveals, his experience on Friday was so positive (no regrets!) that he decided to venture out the following night. On Saturday, he met friends at a club, which felt overly air-conditioned, with hard metal folding chairs. This time Steve decided to bow out early, which tempered his regrets. In the future, he'll call ahead about the venue so he can come prepared, such as by bringing a warm sweater or a padded seat cushion.

Steve is eager to continue this experiment, with its promise of uncovering ways to build a more active (and comfortable) social life.

Like Steve, as you understand the effects of specific activities and conditions, socializing becomes more energizing and positive. Knowledge allows you to predict when participation will feel worth it. Consider what you might want to include in your tracking system to help you evaluate the effect of social situations—such as the activity itself, the people involved, environmental factors, and strategies to bolster your coping and comfort.

It may also be helpful to include a place to record your prediction of how you expect to fare. This lets you test your predictions against your experience and learn whether you tend to err on the side of optimism or pessimism. You might include separate measures of your mood and comfort level because at times, people feel lousy but enjoy themselves. Like Steve, you might want an outcome variable, like "regrets" or a more positive framing such as "enjoyment" or "success."

Annie's evenings. Annie wants to expand her social life. On account of pain and exhaustion, she has become something of a recluse, staying in most evenings to watch TV in her comfy chair, warmed by a heating pad on her back. While she finds this soothing, she craves company. At the same time, she is afraid of taking on too much and feeling trapped or exhausted in the company of others. Like Steve, she decides to use her tracking tool to figure out how to create a social life.

Annie decides to record whether she goes out or stays in, specifics about the activities and participants, her expectation for the event ("exp") and how it turned out ("was"), along with a space to note additional factors that seem relevant.

Fri:	out (in) Jeff&Barb	exp: hard	was: fun!	what: reclined,laughed
Sat:	(out)/ in movie, cafe w/ Ben	exp: ☺	was: ☺	what: A++ movie, cushion
Sun:	(out) in TV	exp: fine	was: fine	what: relaxed

Before developing rheumatoid arthritis, Annie loved to entertain and throw elaborate dinner parties. She decided to start small and invite two friends for dinner Friday night. As Friday approached, she worried she might not have sufficient energy at the end of her work week for this undertaking. She predicted it would be "hard" but kept to her plan. To her surprise and delight, she had a wonderful time. After dinner, Annie reclined in her favorite chair, and she and her friends shared stories and laughter. She realized she benefited from making herself comfortable after dinner (ignoring the dirty dishes). She is eager to extend another invitation to test whether the pattern holds with a different set of friends. Had the evening been too taxing, Annie might have amended her approach, such as serving on paper plates, ordering in, or preparing something in advance that she could heat up.

On Saturday, Annie joined her friend Ben for a movie that had received rave reviews, and she came equipped with a seat cushion. She did not expect it to match the comfort of home—thus predicting an OK (☺) but not great (☺) time. The movie was extremely engrossing, a perfect distraction from her pain. She felt so upbeat afterward that she joined Ben for tea at the café next door. Annie had intentionally left Sunday unscheduled to engage in her usual TV watching, which was "fine," as expected, but much less isolating than usual, following two social successes.

As you consider ways to make changes in your social calendar—whether to increase or decrease events' quantity or change their qualities—it helps to know:

- the extent to which you find different situations "worth it,"
- which people you find energizing versus enervating,
- the places (or types of places) that provide the most comfortable environment,
- factors that increase your (dis)comfort, and
- any obstacles that may interfere with your comfort (such as your own feelings about asking for what you may need).

Engaging in activities that "should" be pleasurable but instead emphasize your pain can feel demoralizing. You can increase the odds that you will really enjoy yourself by knowing the sorts of activities that provide comfort, selecting people you enjoy, and negotiating the conditions of the event in a polite and skillful manner. Chapters 10 through 18 describe strategies to increase comfort; chapters 23 through 25 offer suggestions on negotiating relationships, including how to express your needs.

Other Activities

You can approach the other activities in a similar fashion. If your current goal is to engage in more activities, you might simply indicate activities you undertook. The level of specificity of your categories depends on your objectives and abilities. You might select from a list included in your tracking tool, such as:

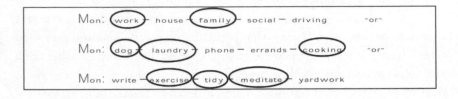

You can also include more detail about the extent or effect of an activity. Among the most difficult aspects of chronic pain is figuring out how to pace yourself. Note the example below with its places to record activity intensity, consecutive activities, and rest breaks. This can help you figure out if you fare better when you schedule a rest break between morning and evening activities, for example, or limit the number of consecutive activities.

Example measures of activity level:

Level:	high / moderate / low
Estimated time:	_____
Parts of day:	am / noon / pm / mid-N
Consecutive activities:	_____
Rest breaks:	_____

You can also experiment with the kind of rest breaks that are most restorative. You can compare whether you feel better when you spend a certain amount of time meditating in your car, lying down and listening to classical music, practicing biofeedback or self-hypnosis, propping up your feet in front of the TV, or taking slow, deep breaths. You may also find, counterintuitively, that the more often you schedule breaks, the *more* you can do. Discover your most comfortable, productive rhythm by tracking patterns of activity and rest:

Recording Pacing

Activity __gym__	Rest __medit (15m)__	Activity __errands__	Rest __car 10 min.__
Activity _____	Rest _____	Activity _____	Rest _____

You can include whatever characteristic you find most important.

> For activity—how much, what type, any special accommodations or circumstances?
>
> For rest—how long did you rest, where, or under what circumstances?

Experimenting with activity and rest breaks leads to a more sustainable pattern and ideally to a second wind, or maybe a third, fourth, and fifth!

E Is for Exercise

Regular exercise and fitness offer many benefits. Yet people with fibromyalgia and other pain syndromes live in constant fear of overdoing it, as even modest workouts threaten to intensify pain. Unfortunately, we often discover we did too much only after the fact. It is common to feel great while exercising but later suffer in agony. The way out of this distressing cycle is to develop an acute awareness of your responses to exertion.

Exercise machines can gauge intensity and duration: StairMasters®, treadmills, and other aerobic equipment often include timers, estimates of calories burned, distance walked or climbed, and sometimes heart rate. For lower-tech exertions, such as walking or jogging in your neighborhood, record your exertion by distance (e.g., number of times around the block), time spent (in minutes or number of songs listened to), a sense of effort (high, moderate, low), or other estimations. Strength training can be measured by weights and repetitions. If you are taking a class or exercising to a video, you could note how hard you pushed, such as whether you felt you were "keeping up" or "holding back."

Equally important is tracking your response. For people with pain, monitoring how it feels following exercise is essential in creating a sustainable level.

Jim's story. Jim suffers from chronic pain and fatigue due to an untreated case of Lyme disease. While exercising in the water, he feels fabulous. He enjoys relief from pain and the ability to stretch and move in ways he only dreams about on land. Immediately afterward, he feels energized and ready to take on the world. Within the space of two hours, however, Jim starts to feel drained and beaten, as if it would take monumental effort just to cross the room. He can scarcely believe how good he felt earlier that day. "What did I do to myself?" he wonders. Because his postexercise pain and exhaustion are so overwhelming, Jim resolves to stop exercising altogether.

Unfortunately, this story is not uncommon. Negative repercussions of exercise can overshadow the promises of benefit, and many people give up rather than endure what feel like inevitable flare-ups. However, because Jim knows exercise *could* help and because he loves how he feels while in the water, he decides to take one last stab at it. This time, he cuts way back, with the plan to build up slowly and deliberately over time.

Jim's water aerobics log:

Mon:	exercise: **W5** ☺	2 hrs. after: ☺	evening: ☺
Tues:	exercise: **W5** ☺	2 hrs. after: ☺	evening: ☺
Wed:	exercise: **W7** ☺	2 hrs. after: ☺	evening: ☺
Thurs:	exercise: **W9** ☺	2 hrs. after: ☺	evening: ☺

Jim tracked how he felt at three time points: (1) while exercising, (2) two hours afterward (when his postexertion pain is typically in full force), and (3) in the evening. On Monday, he engaged in water exercises for only five minutes, which required tremendous restraint. Because he tolerated the exercise with no setback, Jim repeated it the next day. He increased by two minutes on Wednesday, and again on Thursday, without negative repercussions. Never before had Jim successfully participated in water aerobics on subsequent days, as he typically required several days to recover from overexertion. With the aid of his tracking system, Jim committed to increasing gradually (and scaling back as needed) until he could participate in a full hour-long class. For the first time, Jim feels realistically optimistic about achieving his exercise goals.

Winnie's workout. After developing lupus, Winnie experienced fatigue and sore joints, which prevented her from her favorite exercise—kickboxing. Realizing that she wanted to be able to exercise again, Winnie developed a less strenuous exercise routine, which she can do indoors (in the event that the weather is sunny and hot, which flares her lupus), and which provides a mix of strengthening and flexibility. She built up to going to the gym every other day, where she walks for fifteen minutes or takes either a yoga class or a water aerobics class. This has worked well for her for more than a year; however, she would like to increase her activity level further.

By experimenting and noting how she felt, she found a schedule that provides the best result. Winnie's notation is simple: "W" for her walks, "Y" for yoga, and "A" for aqua aerobics.

Winnie's cross-training exercise program:

Mon: **W**

Tues: **W A**

Wed: **W Y**

Thurs: **W**

Fri: **W A**

Sat: **W Y**

Sun: **W**

Winnie discovered that she benefits from the fifteen-minute walk each day, even when combined with yoga or aerobics classes, and appreciates yoga the day after aqua aerobics. She also discovered, however, that back-to-back days of aqua aerobics or trying aerobics and yoga on the same day caused a flare-up in her symptoms. After maintaining this new schedule for a period of time, Winnie plans to increase her walks *slowly* to test what her body tolerates.

No matter what your experience, you, too, can exercise effectively (really!). Be open about what it means to exercise. It may not mean scaling mountains, although it can feel that intense. By tracking your exertions and responses, you can discover exercise that is achievable and satisfying. With chronic pain and fatigue, this involves creative experimentation and a willingness to start as slowly as needed. Bear in mind that two minutes a day is much more than nothing. (Chapter 15 provides specific points on how to approach exercise with chronic pain.)

R Is for Rest

Rest is essential in reducing pains. Achieving sufficient rest, however, can be challenging—it may be that you experience difficulty falling asleep, frequent or periodic awakenings, fitful sleep, early awakenings, or trouble returning to sleep once awakened (whatever the hour). Or you may toss and turn due to pain; awake exhausted after a full night's sleep; or suffer from continual fatigue, regardless of how much you have slept. Tracking your sleep reveals patterns and their impact on your well-being. Consider which of these matter to you most:

- the number of hours you sleep at night
- the time you spend in bed
- daytime fatigue / alertness
- nighttime awakenings
- the longest stretch of sleep you achieve each night
- nighttime sleep quality
- daytime napping (or urge to nap)
- how refreshed you feel in the morning

Make sure to track your sleep in a way that won't interfere with it. At night, your attention belongs on sleep-enhancing behaviors. If you awake during the night, recording this fact may be more important than specifics such as the exact length of time you were up. It is counterproductive to check the clock every time you awake or contemplate sleep difficulties while you are in bed, eager for sleep. If you want to record the hours you slept, you could note the time you go to bed and the time you arise in the morning. To measure sleep quality, use impressionistic measures that would be easy to consider in the morning.

> Make sure your measure and method do not interfere with sleep!
> **Your impression of how you sleep is more valuable than the exact number of hours you sleep, particularly if charting such a number would interfere with sleep.**

Some additional nondisruptive questions you can consider in the morning:

- How refreshed do you feel upon waking?
- What is your sense of the quality of your sleep?
- How satisfied do you feel with how you slept?

Consider questions that can provide a reliable reflection of your experience, as well as a simple way to rate your response—whether symbols, letter grades, numbers, or descriptors. On a technical note, when recording sleep, be clear about the twenty-four-hour period to which you are referring. For example, Monday's tracking sheet can include how you slept on Sunday night and how you feel Monday morning. This is important when it comes to interpreting your data.

Cathy's sleep record. Cathy knows that sleep affects how she feels but not which aspect of her sleep matters most. To keep things simple, she decides to record the time she goes to bed, the time she awakes, and a one-word description of how she feels upon awakening:

Bed <u>11:00</u> Up <u>7:00</u> AM <u>decent</u>

From her sleep data, Cathy learns she feels her best (less pain, more energy) when she spends 7.5 hours in bed—significantly less sleep, and she suffers the rest of the day, and significantly more intensifies morning pain. This information makes it easier for her to commit to an eleven thirty bedtime, given that she has to get up at seven for work. While this is helpful, Cathy notes exceptions—sometimes, despite 7.5 hours in bed, she awakes feeling awful. She decides to investigate what may differ on these nights. She depicts unsettling dreams with a skull and crossbones and frequent awakenings with an up arrow. Each morning, Cathy takes a moment to reflect on her night:

Bed <u>11:30</u>☠↑ Up <u>7:00</u> AM: <u>awful !!</u>
Bed <u>11:30</u>↑ Up <u>7:00</u> AM: <u>tired</u>
Bed <u>11:30</u>☠ Up <u>7:00</u> AM: <u>tolerable</u>
Bed <u>11:00</u> Up <u>7:00</u> AM: <u>decent</u>

Her records reveal that she felt her worst (awful with two exclamation marks) after a fitful night of bad dreams and awakenings. She was tired when she awoke frequently but had peaceful or neutral dreams. Her best (and only "decent") morning followed a nightmare-free night in which she slept solidly. These discoveries shift Cathy's focus to the next puzzle—how to improve her sleep quality and, specifically, how to reduce nightmares and awakenings.

Sleep is affected by many factors—diet, exercise, medications, comfort, emotions—all of which can be tracked for answers. By including sleep in your tracking system, you can test the effect of sleep on your well-being as well as strategies to enhance your sleep (see chapter 14 for more on this). Sleep and pain are inextricably linked. You may be surprised by the extent to which your sleep affects your pain level and other aspects of your well-being.

Other Factors

Aside from those included in PAPER, you may have additional questions. You can modify your tracking system to include any factors that seem relevant to you. Some examples:

Diet

If you wonder, "Am I what I eat?" you may want to test the effects of your current diet or specific foods or drinks on how you feel. Recording everything you consume would require too much effort and provide superfluous data. Strive to narrow your question to something that feels most relevant and testable, such as the effects of when you eat your biggest meal or of specific substances such as alcohol, caffeine, or nicotine.

You can represent narrow questions with simple, single measures. For example, if you experiment with a particular diet, include a daily indicator of whether or not you followed the diet (whether it's Weight Watchers®, low fat, low carb, or "no eating after seven p.m."). The same applies for the effects of particular foods, drinks, or substances—indicate the extent to which you drank alcohol, smoked, or consumed caffeine (found in coffee, tea, soft drinks, and chocolate) or products purported to improve your well-being.

Buddy's diet. After steadily figuring out ways to improve, Buddy decided to turn his attention to his consumption patterns. At the moment, Buddy is on a low-carb diet he adheres to sporadically. He also enjoys coffee, beer, and an occasional cigarette. His notation is simple: he notes the relevant categories each day.

LC diet _____   coffee __✓__   beer _____   cig. __✓__

Because Buddy strayed from his low-carb diet, "LC diet" remains blank. He checked "coffee" and "cig." because he smoked with his morning coffee, but he had no beer. As Buddy searches for relationships between his consumption and his well-being, he may decide to include greater detail, such as a count of beers, coffees, or cigarettes consumed each day, or a description such as "many" or "few."

Patty's diet. Patty has become interested in the possible effect of food and drink on her sleep. She suspects her evening behaviors are most significant and wonders about the effects of when she eats her largest meal and the effects of alcohol, caffeine, and sugar. Patty suspects her morning coffee is beneficial but wonders whether caffeine in the later part of the day may affect her sleep. She decides to track her consumption of alcohol, caffeine, and sugar; the time each day of her drinks; her last source of caffeine (including chocolate); and her largest meal.

Alc: __2 @ 8pm__   Caffeine: __0 > 3pm__   Sugar: __1__   Large meal: __5pm__

Patty's log shows that she had two alcoholic drinks at eight p.m., no caffeine after three p.m., and one candy bar, and that her largest meal was an early dinner at five p.m. Over time, Patty explicitly tested the effects of each by deliberately varying them one by one.

A personal account. Early in my experience with pain, I decided to track my alcohol consumption to explore any effect on my pain level. I had long enjoyed red wine with dinner, and once my pain began, the wine also offered pain relief, which I particularly valued when eating with friends. I was floored to discover in my tracking system that *any* amount of alcohol consistently increased my pain for *two days*, regardless of any other factors. This news dramatically changed my taste for alcohol.

Knowing the full effect of the food, drink, and other substances you consume allows you to make informed decisions. Like me, you may be surprised by what you find. This does not have to mean giving up things you otherwise enjoy; it instead allows you to plan according to the cost and benefits.

Stress

We commonly hear about the effects of stress on well-being. You may suspect your pain varies by your stress level, but you want to be sure—you want specifics. If this is the case, track it. Begin by figuring out what you mean by "stress." It may be something that pervades certain days or may be more situation specific. You may experience stress when your schedule feels demanding, or around certain people, environments, or emotionally charged issues. To depict your stress, however you conceive of it, you can use a rating scale, descriptive words, or symbols. For example:

75%   UGH!   High   + +   ☹

Or you might simply include the word *stress* and embellish it accordingly—by crossing it out, underlining it, circling it, or emphasizing it with exclamation marks: Alternatively, you may want to indicate something about the type of stress you are experiencing, such as the extent you experience stress at home or at work.

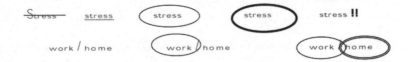

As you gain a better understanding of how stress affects your well-being, you can include behaviors to reduce its effects. Keep in mind, too, that even positive life events, such as having a baby or moving to a new house, increase stress levels. While it is unrealistic to eliminate stress, you can influence your response to it.

Take a Breath . . .

This chapter covered many examples to consider in your quest to track what affects your days. If this feels overwhelming, take a few slow, deep breaths. **Sift through and select the few pieces that feel right for you.** You may have a lot of information in front of you that you would like to include in your tracking tool. When you are exhausted with pain, this can seem overwhelming. Do not fret that you may not be up for this task or that you may be missing something! Remember that you have your whole life to learn and improve; indeed, that's the intention of this method—to continue to learn and improve, then to learn and improve some more. Avoid judgments about what tracking "should" look like. What's important is that you open yourself up to experimenting to see what may help you feel better. You might benefit most from starting with just *one* piece of information, such as focusing exclusively on your sleep. This would be plenty. You might jot down a daily measure of your sleep quality and note how this relates to your well-being. This exercise may lead you to discover an important pattern, which could inspire a small change to enhance your sleep, which could improve how you feel more generally. Take it in small steps. As you become more comfortable and confident about the tracking process, you can always revisit the many examples described for further ideas. Okay?

Next, we turn to making sense of whatever data you collect.

Chapter 8

Learning from Your Own Experience

This chapter describes how to use the data you collect to improve how you feel. Specifically, you will learn how to:

1. discover and make sense of the patterns in your experience;
2. test hypotheses and figure out what helps (and hurts); and
3. conduct experiments to determine how best to improve your pain management.

While larger amounts of data provide greater grist for the mill, you can begin to interpret your experience as soon as you record your first pieces of information.

1. Making Sense of Patterns

Identifying patterns in your experience is important for seeing the bigger picture and finding an accurate answer to the question "How am I doing?" You can measure the extent to which your symptoms have improved, maintained, or worsened; the number of days you felt your best (or worst); the degree to which good (or bad) days occur in batches; or other patterns of interest.

Patterns provide you with the first "aha" insights. Seeing how your days vary—whether measured by your pain rating, mood, or satisfaction level—helps you acknowledge the reality of your situation. Without such observations, tunnel vision can set in, skewing your perspective through the lens of your most recent experience. In other words, when you feel lousy, you are more inclined to think you always feel lousy, even when you recently enjoyed several good days, weeks, or months. Records of your ups and downs supply a reality check to prevent selective amnesia. You gain an accurate sense of experience, including times when you soared and plummeted; the length of flare-ups and reprieves; and the frequency of "crash and burn" cycles. These observations allow you to work simultaneously to accept your situation without exaggerating or minimizing it and to set targets for change. This also allows you to zero in on information worthy of further investigation as well as changes that may be subtle but significant. As you discover ways to improve, revisiting earlier data shows how far you have come.

Exploring patterns is as simple as you make it. The key is to focus on the variation in your well-being (described in chapter 6) using one of three simple techniques:

Eyeball your data. You can learn a tremendous amount by simply looking at your data without any numbers, statistics, or graphs. Remember, the goal is to find answers while keeping the process simple and doable. You can start your search as soon as you record a few days' worth of data. Look for fluctuations and patterns. Do your days look as you had suspected? If not, what seems different? Do you notice better days tend to cluster together or occur at certain times of the week? Information gained by eyeballing trends increases your self-knowledge and informs the next steps in improvement.

Count and compare. If you desire greater detail about overall trends, you can analyze more deeply by counting and comparing your observations. This simple method answers specific questions, such as:

- How long do my worst bad spells last? What about my best periods?
- Do I experience any weekly patterns?
- Did I have more bad days or good days this week? This month?
- How do my weekdays compare to my weekends?

This analysis does not require a degree in statistics. Simply start with a question and then turn to the data for answers. For example, if you want to know if this week showed improvement over previous ones, tally up the number of good days and compare with the number during previous weeks. What constitutes a good day depends on how you measure well-being; you may count good days by how often you select "good" on a "good / OK / lousy" scale, or judge your pain as less than five, or record a ☺ rather than a ☹. This allows you to find, for example, that you have had four good days this week, compared to only one to three during previous weeks. Or you may discover that your good days have not increased, but the intensity of your worst ones has.

By counting and comparing the quality of your days over time, you gain a clear sense of patterns and changes in your experience. This not only elucidates what you have been going through, it also pinpoints areas you need to analyze further and target for experimentation.

Calculate averages or percentages. If your questions about trends are more sophisticated—say, you want to know your average number of "unacceptable" days—your data can deliver on this, too. Keep in mind that you can make effective use of your data without ever calculating a percentage or an average. The power of collected data is that you can revisit them at a later time should you desire more specificity. For example, you may want to present your experiences accurately and succinctly to your doctor, to strengthen your claim for disability compensation, or to reassure yourself of improvement. Knowing your "average pain rating," or the percent of the time your pain felt "intolerable," and how this has changed over time allows you to communicate the severity of your symptoms in objective terms. Or, if you are having a particularly bad day, it can help to know, for example, that bad days occur only 20 percent of the time (and not 90 percent, as it can seem when you are down).

Do just what is needed to answer your current questions. The following chart describes examples of using each method on two different measurements of well-being—a quantitative (1–10) pain scale and a descriptive mood rating (noted with a facial expression) to illustrate general trends.

Examples of exploring trends in two different types of well-being measures

Method	Pain level measured with scale (1–10)	Mood depicted with doodle ☺ ☺ ☹
Eyeball trends	Explore the ups and downs in your number ratings. Look for notable patterns, such as consecutive days with roughly the same pain rating or short periods with dramatic fluctuation, or parts of the week or month with significantly higher or lower pain ratings. If you are using the online program or a computer spreadsheet, you can generate graphs to scan for patterns. Otherwise, keep it simple and eyeball the numbers for trends.	Explore your doodles for remarkable sequences. Search for clusters of ☺s or ☹s or ☺s, or other patterns, such as whether ☹s seem more likely to follow other ☹s or another mood record. If you have also assigned numeric ratings to your doodles, such as ☺ = 3, ☺ = 2, and ☹ = 1, you have the choice of using graphing functions to display trends.
Count and compare	Use this method when you desire greater information about specific patterns in your pain rating. Let's say you want to know the frequency of your worst days (7 and above) or your best (4 and below). Start with the most recent record and move backward, tallying up relevant days. This reveals the number of your best or worst days in a particular week or month. Or you might want to count the largest string of good or bad days. You might discover your best month was March, which had five sequences with at least four good days in a row, compared to your worst month, December, when four good days in a row occurred only once.	Consider counting and comparing the trends you noticed while eyeballing your data, such as the specific extent to which your mood appears to lift over the course of the week. To do this, you could count the number of ☺s early in the week and compare them to your reported mood at the end of the week or as the week progresses. This can reveal, for example, that as the month progresses, you have noted

		three ☺s on Thursdays, Fridays, and Saturdays, but not one on a Monday. Or you may find just the opposite: your longest string of ☺ days occurs at the start of the week.
Calculate averages or percentages	You can calculate your pain "average" by adding up your daily ratings and dividing by the number of days in question. You might find, for example, that your pain averages 4 on weekends, compared to 6 on weekdays, or that your average pain rating has been decreasing over time, with 7 in February, 6 in March, and 5 in April. The online program, as well as spreadsheets, will generate these statistics for you. Reserve this method for times when you want more specific information on your pain rating, such as to communicate precisely to your doctor or for a disability assessment. Otherwise, keep it simple.	You can calculate the frequency of descriptive categories, even when you have not assigned them any numeric category. If you want a monthly average, you can simply count up the occurrence of each rating that month and divide by the number of days in the month. For instance, if you count six ☺s in a thirty-day month, this means that ☺ days occurred 6/30 times or about 20 percent of the time. You might find that you felt ☹ 30 percent of the time, and more neutral, or ☺, the remaining 50 percent. You can then compare percentages in previous and future months to pinpoint change.

Knowledge about the patterns in your experience—whatever the level of specificity—demonstrates how you are faring over time. Stopping with patterns, however, does not provide reasons for the variation. You wouldn't understand, for example, whether a decrease in your average pain rating was due to a seasonal change or a specific intervention. Let's move to testing causal hypotheses to understand the reasons behind your fluctuations—*why* lousy days seem to follow wonderful ones, or weekends are harder than weekdays, or December was 20 percent worse than other months.

2. Test Causal Hypotheses to Learn What Affects How You Feel

Most of us have stories, or theories, about what causes flare-ups, such as specific weather conditions, overdoing it, poor sleep, inconsistent exercise, stress, or an interruption in our usual routine. These speculations, or hypotheses, are directly testable by examining potential explanatory factors (described at length in chapter 7). When you decided what to track, you were guided by causal questions, such as:

- What level of activity results in my best days?
- What would an optimal exercise routine look like for me?
- To what extent does my sleep quality affect how I feel?
- How much is my pain medication helping my symptoms?

These questions focus on the relationship between your well-being and other significant factors, such as your sleep quality, medication, or pacing. To understand causal patterns, you must look at the variations in your well-being in relation to the other relevant factors. Testable hypotheses are likely to emerge as you find patterns in your data. For example:

- What causes my best days to cluster together?
- Why are my best days followed soon after by flare-ups?
- What accounts for my longest stretches of ups (and downs)?
- What occurred during my worst days or just before them?
- What has changed over the past few months, resulting in more flare-ups?

To explore the relationship between your well-being and other factors, use two simple techniques:

1. study one piece of information over time in relation to your measure of well-being; and
2. study everything in selected short periods in relation to your well-being measure.

By alternating between these two methods, you can develop an increasingly sophisticated understanding of *why* you feel the way you do.

Study one thing over time. Focusing on the relationship between how you feel and *one* other piece of data, such as sleep, exercise, medicine, weather, or pacing, over a long stretch of time provides multiple data points to compare. If you are testing the effects of exercise, for example, you can see how you felt on the day that you exercised and the days that followed, week after week, month after month. The lengthy time span allows you to evaluate the effect of unusual events—such as increased fatigue associated with a particularly rainy March—and increases your certainty about your findings. By studying the effects over a long period, you are able to uncover a pattern that endures despite fluctuation in other factors, such as the weather.

Start with the hypothesis you most want to explore. Let's say you want to understand how your activity level affects your pain. First, identify days with high (and low) pain ratings, and then examine what you did on those days and the ones directly preceding them. Check whether you engaged in any unusual type or amount of activity or paced your day in a particular way. You can also choose days with unusual levels of activity and then examine your pain level on and around those days. The goal is to understand the relationship between pain and activity and figure out, for example, whether your pain corresponds with more activity or less, or with a particular pattern or type of activity.

You may find, for example, that your worst pain consistently occurs directly after high-activity days, while on longer stretches of good days, your activity level remains more moderate. This finding would support an "overdoing it" hypothesis—your pain appears to climb when you have been especially active and lessen when you slow your pace. This observation helps you gauge and moderate your activity level. It can also encourage you to conduct experiments to test this theory and find your optimal amount of activity (more on this coming up).

Example of relationship patterns between activity and pain level

	"Overdoing it" Pattern (Activity → Pain)	Contrary Pattern (Activity → Pain)	Inconsistent pattern (Activity → Pain)
Day 1	High → High	High → Low	High → High
Day 2	Med. → Med.	Low → High	High → Low
Day 3	Low → Low	High → Low	Med. → High

Or you may find, contrary to expectations, that your activity level is inversely related to pain. In other words, you reported low pain during high-activity periods and high pain when you'd done the least. This could reflect a tendency to push when you feel your best and lie low during pain flares. However, it could also mean that your fuller days operate as effective distractions from pain, while on slower days, your pain roars more loudly with less to drown it out. This distinction is crucial in guiding your responses. You could then conduct experiments to see when pushing through pain is helpful or destructive.

Finally, you may find an inconsistent relationship. Activity level may explain some of how you feel, but not all. Your worst days may sometimes stem from overexertion, yet you may also find you feel your best on jam-packed days. Such inconsistent findings may mean that your activity level and pain are unrelated or, more likely, that additional factors are at work. This is excellent fodder for experiments to figure out the conditions under which busy days deplete or nourish you.

When data seem confusing or run counter to your expectations, see these quirks as gifts. Counterintuitive findings can focus your attention on factors you may have otherwise overlooked. Noting the instances in which explanatory factors did a particularly poor job of explaining your well-being can raise questions and discoveries: "Why did I feel so good after such a lousy night of sleep?" "What else happened on that perfectly sunny day to make me stay in bed?" Let counterintuitive findings motivate you to delve deeper: "What else is going on?" To answer this, examine more than one factor at a time—which brings us to our next method of data analysis.

Study everything in select short periods. Select a key moment that you want to understand. Then zero in and consider *everything* you've recorded during this intriguing snapshot of time. This may include environmental factors, sleep, stress level, exercise, changes in your medication or other therapies, and any unusual activity or circumstances. While it is virtually impossible to evaluate every factor over a long stretch of time, it is fairly easy to do this for short periods. To select key moments, you may want to:

a) Compare your highest and lowest periods.

Explore your best day (or cluster of days) and then compare with your worst day (or cluster of days). First, see what, if anything, your good and bad periods have in common. Then set the commonalities aside for a moment and delve into their differences. Do bad periods tend to have more activity or less, more sleep or less, and so on? In addition to examining the specific days in question, search for differences that occurred *just before* your recorded upturn or downturn. Don your investigator's hat as you observe the multiple data points around your best and worst days.

By focusing closely on a short period, you can examine multiple factors with a fine-tooth comb. You may discover the constellation of events that tend to occur with your best days, such as a good night's sleep; moderate exercise; and combining engaging, meaningful activities with planned downtime. By exploring the data in different key moments, you can see whether the patterns you noticed hold up at other times.

b) Explore moments of dramatic change.

When a great day is followed by a rotten one, this raises the question "What happened?" To answer this, see if anything else has changed. You may find evidence that on your great day, you took on a much more ambitious array of activities than usual, which may have led to the next-day crash. Or you may have stayed up later than usual or slept especially poorly, either of which could contribute to feeling run-down the following day. Or you may find evidence that the increased optimism from your great day led to less tolerance for the return of pain. Often, dramatic shifts stem from a combination of factors. They may have nothing to do with your behavior and everything to do with the arrival of damp weather, stressful houseguests, or a nasty cold. Once you identify a potential explanation, whatever it may be, look to other dramatic moments of change to test whether the pattern applies there as well. The longer the series of data you have collected, the more opportunities you have to test your theories on other, similar periods.

c) *Study days that are unexpected, counterintuitive, or surprising.*

You can use your hypotheses to discover moments when they fail, such as days that were terrific despite cold, damp weather; a stressful schedule; or lousy sleep. If you find that *every* time you stay out late, you feel worse, then you have your answer. If not, you have discovered evidence of "the dog that didn't bark," to use Sherlock Holmes's famous phrase. In other words, you have stumbled onto more counterintuitive findings: late nights and poor sleep may *not* be a surefire formula for increased pain. These "explanation failures" open up new avenues to explore.

You may find that your greater-than-expected resilience occurs when you make use of self-care activities, such as a massage or meditation, or pleasurable activities like connecting with a good friend. As you formulate new hypotheses about the forces behind your unexpected resilience, check the data in other periods to see whether self-care or fun activities similarly headed off setbacks. You may find that when you engage in rejuvenating activities, you fare better, even after a particularly busy or sleepless night. You can continue to return to counterintuitive periods to probe deeper and retest your sharpened theory. And, as you develop new hypotheses about self-care activities, you can return to the method of comparing one thing over a longer period of time to examine the relationship between self-care and well-being.

Alternating between studying one thing over time and delving more deeply into key moments can provide a more complete picture. It doesn't matter which you do first. Each generates questions that can be explored by the other. You can alternate between these approaches as your investigation takes shape. For example, if while examining clusters of data a particular factor appears significant, you can then explore how it relates to well-being over a longer stretch of time. Or, if counterintuitive or confusing findings arise as you study single factors, you can select significant moments and assess all potentially relevant data.

These methods allow you to identify the factors associated with your being at the top of your game or in the throes of a painful crash. Yet looking back over past records suffers from the old chicken-and-egg dilemma. What you have been viewing as a cause may in fact be an outcome of what you're trying to explain. Suppose, for example, that your records reveal a day in which you felt lousy and stayed in bed all day. Did you stay in bed because you felt lousy? Or did you feel lousy, in part, because you stayed in bed? To solve this puzzle requires deliberate experimentation, which brings us to the most exciting part of PAINTRACKING—experimentation. You can craft specific experiments to verify what actually helps (and hurts) and how much, then adjust for greater and greater improvement.

3. Actively Experiment with Each Factor and Deliberately Improve How You Feel

Your PAINTRACKING tool is a dynamic, living system. You can test the insights you gain from examining your data by deliberately testing and tinkering with them. You can build such experiments directly into your tracking tool and adjust interventions until you discover what works best.

Experiments offer a kind of feedback loop: with each new discovery, you can improve your situation and then test again for greater specificity. If you find that a hot shower or a brisk stroll helps you feel better when you wake up feeling crummy, you can incorporate these activities into your daily routine and your tracking system. This allows you to feel realistically confident about the effects of these behaviors; also, when they do not bring the anticipated result, you have fodder for a more nuanced experiment or analysis. Finding out what helps and seeing it in your data encourages you to do what works.

Experimentation can also be a state of mind. Let's say you are unsure whether you will feel better if you exercise for thirty minutes today. Whatever you do provides data. If you exercise, record this and reflect on your findings. If you decide not to exercise, record this and reflect on your findings. Each decision generates data. Viewing your behavior (and life) as a continual experiment makes it easier to proceed when you cannot predict the outcome of your choice. When you approach your life as a series of experiments, whatever the outcome, you learn something valuable. One of the ways we locate our limits is through testing them. No day, regardless of how rotten it may feel, occurs in vain if it supplies you with valuable findings.

Phase 1: Test it out! Let's say you want to determine your optimal exercise regimen. But when you examine data on your prior attempts to exercise, you find a fairly complex pattern. You consistently reported that exercise feels great in the moment (as did Jim) but within a few hours, you felt drained and pained. However, you also notice that on the subsequent day, you tend to report a boost in energy, stamina, and mood—strong evidence of the benefit of exercise. But you want more; in particular, you would like to figure out a strategy for approaching exercise that does not involve ruining your day with debilitating pain and fatigue in order to improve the following day. So you plan experiments:

1. to test the effects of the time and intensity of exercise; and
2. to test the effects of a planned restorative break following exercise.

In the first experiment, you approach exercise, as described in chapter 15, by starting slowly—perhaps a five-minute walk. You build the experiment into your tracking system by including measures of your exertion and response. If you do not feel "pained and drained," you have the green light to continue at that level the following day. After several green-light days, you may increase slightly and test the effects. By monitoring your experiment over time, you can test how hard you can push before inciting unpleasant side effects.

In the second experiment, rather than adjusting your exertion, you decide to test the effect of various recuperation activities. You build into your tracking tool a measure of exertion, recuperative activities, and subsequent pain level. You may find that lying down after exercise and engaging in slow, deep breathing for thirty minutes not only feels good but also restores you. You can vary this practice and test the amount and timing of this calming activity to see what is most rejuvenating.

Experiments teach you in real time about your body's responses. You can deliberately test the effects of your exertions and your responses to these exertions and make prompt changes. In addition, framing your behaviors as experimental data makes daily fluctuations easier to bear and allows you to retrain your own reactions.

You continually face opportunities to test (and retest) the effects of a change, whether in your therapeutic regime, your schedule, or your self-talk. Before you begin an active experiment, consider your baseline data. This does not mean you have to *wait* to start the experiment until you see how you have been feeling. Just take a look at your measures of well-being before you begin.

The natural variation in your life can also present something of a natural experiment. By looking over time, you can discover associations between variations when change was not intentional. The strength of each experiment lies in your ability to observe the effects of your behaviors. Then, as you derive new and more developed ideas about what works, record these experiments and compare the outcome with earlier periods.

Experiments are most accurate, according to the scientific method, when you change one factor at a time. If you change medications, for example, data evaluation is easier if you do not make additional changes at the same time. This constancy provides greater assurance that variation in your well-being is due to medication and not something else. Of course, life is messy, and it is not always possible or even desirable to attempt to keep your days identical. You may be desperate to feel better, wanting to make multiple changes at once. Plus, many fluctuations are beyond your control—such as the weather or the demands you face. That's OK. You can tease out the effects of a medication (or other factor) by using the techniques that evaluate the relationship between variables. By looking over time at your main test variable (in relation to your well-being), you can pick out significant patterns, and by studying key moments, you can evaluate the effects of multiple variables.

Phase 2: Keep it up! Over time, the results of your experiments will reveal the best ways to approach your life, including decisions around work, social and family activities, exercise, medication, sleep, activity and rest, and self-care. As you discover what helps, the next step is clear: do more of what helps and less of what does not. Slowly and deliberately, you can restructure your days to incorporate the most helpful behaviors. While this may seem obvious, multiple obstacles (some of our own making) can interfere. You may have days when you *don't feel like* engaging in the behaviors you know would increase your comfort. Or you may have times when competing priorities make adherence challenging.

As you see your pain ratings diminish, your mood improve, your abilities climb, or your life satisfaction increase, day after day, then week after week, your new regimen will become more intuitive. Plus, by sticking with what works, you will be able to continue to measure and witness the benefits. This knowledge provides vital fodder for realistic self-talk that can help you incorporate beneficial approaches into your everyday life (see chapter 12). It also provides motivation to override even strong urges to push harder than would be effective or lie low when you would benefit more from participating.

A strength of PAINTRACKING is that you learn to predict specific outcomes of your choices, whatever they are. When you decide *not* to stick to your least-pain or best-mood regimen, this, too, is a choice. In fact, knowledge about the outcome of such choices makes it easier to contend with the times when you select a path you know will result in additional pain. You are not forging into the unknown but, instead, deciding to accept a certain amount of discomfort in exchange for a specific effect or freedom. Deliberately choosing pain-inducing activities also operates as an experiment. You can record these deviations in your tracking system and measure their outcomes, as well as pair such experiments with a test of recuperation strategies.

Experimentation is ongoing for many reasons. Even when you have discovered a very effective routine, at some point, your circumstances or wishes are likely to shift:

- You may encounter a therapeutic strategy you would like to try, or you may want to revisit something you've tried in the past.
- You may be undergoing a dramatic change in your lifestyle or schedule—perhaps due to a new baby, a job change, a relationship shift, retirement, or a return to school—and want to test different strategies.
- A new pain medication may have been introduced that interests you (and your doctor).
- You may have experienced a setback due to an accident or an illness and need to readjust your routine to meet your current abilities.
- You may decide to try to seek further improvement in an area that had felt "as good as it gets."

How long should your experiments run? If they are working, they can run forever. Don't groan! Your first attempt to find answers will look very different from later ones. Once you figure out how to feel your best, subsequent tests and adjustments are much less complex and require less notation and effort. When you are doing well for a stretch of time and feel confident about what you are doing, you may decide simply to track your well-being. Ideally, you will reach a point where you have a very thorough understanding of what helps you feel your best (and worst) and feel satisfied with this information. Tracking this, then, can be as simple as including a notation in your daily calendar (or online tracking tool) to indicate that you are on track.

If you notice a decline, or want to make minor adjustments for any reason, you can always reintroduce measures of relevant factors that determine how you fare. You may wonder how you would feel going to bed fifteen minutes earlier or later. Or you may have a satisfactory exercise routine but want to test what would happen if you increased the number of days you exercise. Or you may find that age-related changes have altered your experience, meriting a trip back to more thorough tracking.

When an experiment does not seem to be working, what then? If the experiment involves medication, this is something to discuss with your doctor; some medications should work within a couple days, and some take longer (see chapter 17). For other experiments, you have to rely on your own judgment: how you feel, your confidence in your hypothesis and conclusions, and the extent to which other factors may be influencing the experiment. But for people in chronic pain, the phrase "no pain, no gain" is often ill-advised. If you find your experiment unhelpful or worse, it's time to stop and rethink your strategy.

However, even when your inclination may be to discontinue an experiment altogether, don't be hasty. It may be that your hypothesis was on target but you need to rethink the magnitude of the intervention. For example, if you hurt terribly after increasing your exercise program, consider cutting back to a more modest starting point and increasing as your tolerance increases. This is the beauty of a living, breathing experiment. You can adapt as you go and measure the results. Analyze what you find and retest as needed until you feel confident of the answer. Then, continue to tweak your experiment until you find the combination of interventions that works best for you.

Some Ideas for Experimentation

This experiment is about your life. You are both the guinea pig and the scientist in charge. Be inventive! Sometimes you may not feel like doing what may work best, and this can influence your choices for experimentation. You may have to challenge yourself to act opposite to what your body is telling you, then test the result. Remember, chronic pain can undermine your instincts. You will benefit from trusting your data and the outcomes of your experiments more than your initial or more automatic assumptions based on how you feel.

Tracking your experience can then supply a new intuition. Consider some examples that run counter to common sense that can be tested and retested:

1. Stop while it feels good. Trust your data and not your adrenaline to determine your optimal exercise routine. The same goes for taking on a very busy schedule. For some chronic pain conditions, exercise and other activities that feel terrific can result in significant flare-ups. Use your tracking system to discover your body's limits. The opposite can also be said:

2. When you feel lousy, get up and get going. Turn to your data when deciding when and whether to arise from bed. It may well be that you awake feeling smashed, pummeled, or exhausted but will fare better if you arise and make meaningful plans for the day. You can experiment to find the extent to which staying in bed quells the pain, as well as the effects of your efforts to create a day that feels meaningful. Use your tracking system to figure out your best response when you feel miserable and the activities that most invigorate you.

3. Less can be more. Scheduling rest breaks on your most demanding days can allow you to accomplish more. Use your tracking system to test the conditions under which you benefit more from pushing yourself or from taking frequent breaks. You can also experiment with the rhythm of activity and rest that provides you with the most stamina.

4. Keep comfort a priority. Don't forget that your pain level fluctuates. Relinquish any all-or-nothing thinking about your options, and seek new ways to engage in activities you value. Use your tracking tool to experiment with changes to see what helps most; these can be simple, such as treating a soft cushion as your constant companion, keeping a lawn chair handy, or committing to a midday stretch or meditation break. Let your data emphasize that there is no "one way" to do things, and find the ways that increase your comfort as you move through your day.

5. Sooner rather than later? For those who take pain medications as needed, it may be worthwhile to compare the effect of using medication proactively rather than waiting until your pain kicks into high gear. Be sure to discuss your specific medications with your doctor. Then, using your tracking system, test the differences in how you take your medication. You may find you require lower doses when you take them

prophylactically (in anticipation of the pain) rather than waiting until your pain mounts and is harder to control.

In Sum

The value of your PAINTRACKING data comes in the analysis and application to your life. This section described methods to evaluate trends so that you can have a realistic picture of your experience and of the relationship between your well-being and behavioral and environmental factors, as well as strategies to experiment to improve your comfort and abilities. Through understanding, you can take control of your life. The very idea that you can make informed choices is empowering. Living with chronic pain can feel like you are a raggedy doll, tossed about by conditions beyond your control. By facing and experimenting with your experience, you learn not only to understand your situation but also to manipulate it to your advantage.

We turn next to strategies and approaches that you may want to test out in your PAINTRACKING system.

Part 2

Pain-Treating

Chapter 9

Products, Practices, and Professionals

Where to Begin?

What can you do when you feel particularly lousy? It is easy to feel powerless in the face of chronic pain. Knowing where to turn makes a tremendous difference. Part 2 describes strategies to test out for your PAINTRACKING tool kit. Chapters 10 through 15 describe self-care techniques that can soothe aches; relax your body and mind; and improve your sleep, outlook, and physical stamina. Chapter 16 gives advice on building a therapeutic alliance with your doctor and sharing what you have learned through your tracking efforts. Chapter 17 describes medications commonly used for chronic pain and how to understand and assess their effects. Finally, chapter 18 describes the important role of mental healthcare when contending with chronic pain and how to make use of and evaluate its offerings.

General Tips

When thinking about trying any products, practices, or professionals:

Be safe. Not every intervention is medically appropriate or even safe for every person. Behavioral strategies to improve one's outlook or sleep quality are generally risk-free. Yet other seemingly benign interventions, such as massage or applying heat or cold, may be unsafe for individuals with particular health conditions that can make them vulnerable, such as diabetes or a heart or skin condition. Before embarking on something new, consult with your physician.

Mix and match. Effective pain-relief strategies most often include a combination of medication with behavioral and/or cognitive approaches. Be open to experimenting with multiple strategies.

Act proactively. Incorporate strategies into your daily routine to keep your pain manageable. Interventions are generally more effective once pain has escalated. Try to break the pain cycle early, before it intensifies.

Be prepared. As you discover what works for you, keep your favorite remedies at hand. Before venturing out, make sure you will have easy access to whatever helps.

Have a contingency plan. No matter how well you plan or predict your circumstances, unexpected flare-ups occur. When people feel their worst, they are less skillful at creative problem solving, yet this is when they need it most. By having a contingency plan, you can take action to improve the situation without having to deliberate.

Calculate costs. When people feel desperate, they are more prone to try anything and may act rashly. During calm moments, consider your ability to afford new products and practitioner visits. Keep in mind that costs vary considerably—and higher fees do not necessarily bring better outcomes. Research any practitioners (online or by asking current clients) before scheduling appointments with them, and, whenever possible, try to test products before investing in them. Always check return policies and keep receipts (also for tax purposes).

Take heart. No matter how lousy you feel or how unfriendly your current circumstances, there is *always* something you can do for yourself.

Paintrack! Look to your personal tracking data to evaluate anything you decide to try. Each of us can react dramatically differently to the same medication or approach. What you find through your own careful tracking efforts matters more than the evidence of an approach's general success rate. After a fair trial, stick with those that bring fairly consistent improvement and rethink those that do not.

Caveat Emptor!

Unfortunately, people seeking to alleviate or manage chronic pain can be vulnerable to deception and quackery. The desperation that can accompany suffering, coupled with the lack of quick fixes, creates a pool of consumers who are eager for promising news. Amid the helpful advice and useful products is unscientific information as well as unscrupulous treatments and practitioners. Reliable approaches tend to call for patience and compromise, which increases the appeal of easier methods, however questionable they may be.

The weight-loss industry provides an analogy. Everyone knows what it takes to lose weight—you need to consume fewer calories and increase exercise, which burns calories and increases metabolism. Aside from drastic surgeries, there's no magic involved. Experts agree that effective, sustainable weight loss requires a commitment to mindful eating and exercise. Nonetheless, a multimillion-dollar weight-loss industry continues to profit from people seeking alternative methods. We've all seen products advertised that promise to shed pounds without diet or exercise. These are often promoted by individuals who claim to be medical experts, alongside testimonials and dramatic "before" and "after" photos. These advertisements hold great allure for people who are desperate to slim down. Yet the bottom line remains: healthful and sustainable weight loss comes from lifestyle changes rather than from a pill, a gadget, or a cream.

The same can be said for chronic pain. At present, no miracle cures exist. If your pain is the result of a structural problem (such as a ruptured spinal disk), you may gain tremendous relief from specific surgery. But for the vast number of people whose pain is inoperable (and may even have been caused by surgery), solutions are multifaceted. Medications can reduce chronic pain but do not cure it. Significant and sustainable improvement comes from successful experimentation, patience, and significant behavioral change. Just as dieters benefit from knowledge about nutrition and exercise and from having a supportive community, people with chronic pain benefit from reliable information about their condition and treatments and from social support. In both cases, deceptive gimmicks only rob people of precious money and time while giving false hope.

Unfortunately, distinguishing legitimate approaches from illegitimate ones is not always straightforward. Peddlers of modern snake-oil gimmicks can be quite sophisticated—they may be supported by medical degrees, have a list of publications, or belong to a clinic. Advertisements for unproven or nefarious products can appear in respectable mainstream media outlets. Moreover, chronic pain can affect people's concentration and judgment and make them more vulnerable to the most remote possibility of promising results.

Falling prey to scams can happen to anyone—something I know from personal experience. On a particularly lousy day, I purchased a product that turned out to be a pernicious credit card scam. With the benefit of hindsight, I see that my judgment was clouded by my intense longing for a way to boost my energy, which allowed me to overlook the red flags that later appeared fairly obvious.

To safeguard yourself from fraudulent products, practices, and professionals in your search for relief, familiarize yourself with the following red flags. These flags signal approaches that promise more than is reasonable. Often these flags occur together, revealing an even greater likelihood of deception.

Red Flags

(1) Products and practitioners touting cures

Beware of any advertisements or practitioners that promise a cure. The discovery of a cure for chronic pain or your particular pain condition would be breaking news. You would not encounter it in an obscure source, a "personal" e-mail from a stranger, or an advertisement. With the millions of people suffering with chronic pain, news of a cure could not remain a secret known only to the company or clinic marketing it. Many very competent professionals stay abreast of research and treatment options. News of this magnitude would be well publicized to physicians and the public. Word would spread as quickly as news of a saucy political scandal or a breakthrough treatment for impotence. Be extremely suspicious of ads that announce such miracles with CAPITAL LETTERS and exclamation marks!!!!

(2) Product vendors

Be skeptical when the promoter of a product directly benefits from its sale. A common justification offered by vendors of multilevel marketing is that they believe in their product. Such pyramid schemes can provide principal (but unprincipled) sellers with significant profits. Although not all vendors of questionable products are crooked, they are at best biased advisers. This group includes infomercials (paid advertisements that appear to be informative programs) and practitioners who profit from the sale of products they recommend, as well as those who are paid a fee to promote a product. In a perfect world, financial decisions would not sway a practitioner's choice of treatment for a patient. Be wary of practitioners who sell products, particularly if they are reluctant or unable to offer a source other than their own front desk for purchasing the remedy.

(3) Personal testimony as evidence

Personal stories, especially those most similar to your own, can be very convincing. Testimonials about treatments for chronic pain follow a predictable pattern. They begin by portraying how compromised an individual had been before finding the advertised treatment, then describe a dramatic improvement or complete recovery. Because of my Internet presence, I receive a steady stream of "personal" e-mails from individuals describing how they found "the answer" to chronic pain, as well as clinic ads filled with glowing testimonials. Hearing that someone with similar difficulties is now "pain-free" can be quite compelling. But testimonials are the worst type of evidence to determine whether something is effective.

Personal stories are anecdotal, meaning they are based on one person's experience, which may or may not pertain to you. Your situation may actually be quite distinct—despite apparent similarities—and the story may be embellished or completely fabricated. But even when a story appears credible, what worked for one person may not work for another. Moreover, the individual may be mistaken about what helped. Chronic pain conditions are multifaceted, and symptoms wax and wane. Evaluating your own experience is challenging; evaluating someone else's is infinitely more complex, especially without any systematic data. Plus, a "spontaneous remission" may occur for any number of reasons and may have little or nothing to do with the product or practitioner described. Reliable data come from systematic trials that can take into account the multiple factors involved.

Our society may have become inured to testimonials because we encounter them throughout the Internet as increasing numbers of domains open up to personal comments and reviews, many anonymous. However, the repercussion of valuing someone's experience with a movie or recipe is relatively harmless. The stakes increase dramatically when it comes to your health and well-being. Think critically when you encounter heartstring-tugging stories that promote products or practitioners, including correspondence disguised as personal e-mail messages. Testimonials tend to raise additional red flags, as they tend to include claims about a secret cure (flag #1) and profit those marketing them (flag #2).

(4) The lone scientist

Beware of reports of a lone scientist, persecuted by mainstream medicine, who tinkers in his or her lab for years until developing what nobody else could—the miracle cure. Again, if this genius (however marginal) had really discovered the proverbial fountain of youth, we'd all be lined up for a sip. Do not be deceived by any statistics presented. Lone scientists may be quite successful in *selling* their product, regardless of whether it works. Hope sells. Some "lone scientists" may have a vocal group of followers who offer personal testimonials. Lone scientists may themselves be fictitious, fabricated by self-interested companies attuned to what it takes to market their schemes. Lone scientists tend to be associated with additional red flags: their claims tend to be grandiose (flag #1), profits go to the lone scientist or the company that invented him or her for marketability (flag #2), and, more than likely, personal testimonies are presented as evidence (flag #3).

(5) The panacea

Remember the traveling snake-oil salesmen of yore who peddled an elixir to "fix what ails you"? It's no wonder they had to keep traveling. Many of us may be willing to try a "panacea" once—fewer of us, twice. While some things are generally healthful—a balanced diet, restorative sleep, moderate exercise—no product treats everything. The more problems a product allegedly treats, the wider its potential market and the less creditable its claims. Let your skepticism grow with the length of the list of conditions a product allegedly cures. One advertisement I received via e-mail that touted a cure for fibromyalgia also claimed to remedy asthma, nail biting, constipation, and a long list of other, dissimilar problems. Treatments that are allegedly "good for everything" also offer cures for never-before-cured ailments (flag #1), rely on personal testimonials (flag #3), and hail from a secret place or practitioner (flag #4).

(6) Offers for a free trial

The popular adage "There's no such thing as a free lunch" is generally worth heeding. Most of us would enjoy getting something for nothing or next to nothing—and sometimes we do, such as product samples that arrive in our newspaper, are served in our grocery store, or are provided to our doctor by pharmaceutical companies. Companies offer such samples in hope that you will like the product and become a future customer. Activate your skeptic's antennae when free samples are offered for products that promise to improve your health, stamina, or well-being. Be especially wary if they require any investment on your part, such as paying for shipping and handling, or request your credit card information.

"Free" should mean free: no strings! Giving your credit card or bank information for supposedly free items can expose you to fraud and identity theft. At the least, you may be billed for subsequent orders if you don't cancel by a certain date; worse, you may be charged for items you did not order. A common form of online credit card fraud involves disreputable companies, often located overseas, that seek to gain access to your credit card information through advertisements for "free trials" of a product. Some go to great lengths to look legitimate, even including warnings about scams and differentiating themselves from "fraudulent offers." Most often, these "free trials" include other red flags: they promise miraculous health benefits (flag #1); use personal testimonies, often in the form of "before" and "after" pictures and even under the guise of investigative journalism (flag #3); often include "medical testimony," sometimes accompanied by a photo of a "scientific expert" (flag #4); and very often describe their products as helpful for everyone (flag #5).

Think Scientifically

The chapters in part 2 describe strategies for improving life with chronic pain that have evidence supporting their usefulness, such as using heat or cold, meditating, pacing your activities, taking prescription medications, exercising judiciously, and cultivating a positive attitude. The strategies included in this section are by no means exhaustive. There may be strategies not covered here that you want to try—including the latest fad or alternative treatment. But whatever you consider, beware of red flags and check their safety with your doctor before initiating them. Even "herbal" remedies can have dangerous, even lethal, interactions and consequences. Spending your time, money, and precious hope on promises of a quick fix may result only in additional suffering. Whenever you decide to try a product or practice, test its effects. Keep in mind that chronic pain symptoms tend to wax and wane, so be careful not to jump to conclusions about particular strategies or therapies without a reasonable trial (or unless unreasonable side effects develop).

Chapter 10

Strategies to Focus and Calm Your Mind

Fostering deliberate awareness can shape your focus, including on how pleasant (or unpleasant) you find something, and emphasize the choices you can make in a given situation.

When I'm in pain, I'm in pain! How would trying to change my focus matter? Think about what happens when you are stuck in standstill traffic. The surest way to maximize your suffering is to ruminate over the unpleasantness and inconvenience of the situation. Focusing on worries or second-guessing the routes you *should* have taken will increase your distress but do nothing to speed up your trip. You will arrive at precisely the same time if you think about something pleasant and calming or if you focus on your pain and regrets, which will make the trip seem longer. From this vantage point, it's easy to see the uselessness of fretting. You might as well try to find a better way to use your waiting time.

In difficult situations, it's common to focus on our distress, making bad things worse. Being in pain is like sitting in traffic—both experiences are unpleasant, but it is your choice how you spend each moment and the extent to which you make the situation better or worse.

Consider childbirth classes, which have proliferated in the past decades to give women greater control over their experience of labor. These classes teach women to direct their focus as a way to control their pain. The specific strategies vary by childbirth philosophy. Some focus on breathing techniques; others, on the pain itself—but all teach ways to cultivate a deliberate or mindful focus rather than being controlled by the vicissitudes of labor. In your own experience, how has your focus influenced how you felt? Have you ever noticed that:

109

- your pain increases when you feel scattered from chaotic or demanding circumstances?
- your pain plummets when you are able to slow down and focus?
- your pain intensifies when you are worrying about it?
- your pain decreases when you are engaged in an activity you enjoy?

If so, experiment with the following strategies to calm your mind and reduce your pain.

Deliberate Awareness of the Present Moment

Mindfulness is the decision to pay attention and embrace the present moment with intention and without judgment. Think of mindfulness as providing a flashlight, and you can decide where to shine the light. At every moment, you experience multiple inputs, including pain, that compete for your attention. By being mindful, you can decide to focus your attention on a particular experience, whatever it may be. When you approach a delicious dessert, for example, it's your choice whether to savor each bite; to undermine your pleasure by worrying about its calories as you eat it; or to gulp it down, oblivious of its flavor. How you approach the dessert affects the quality of your experience. In practicing mindfulness, consciously and calmly direct your attention to a subject of your choice. Strive to maintain your attention on the chosen subject, gently returning it whenever it wanders.

So, how can I use this to change my experience of pain? Research on mindfulness-based approaches demonstrates its effects on reducing people's suffering, increasing their sense of control, and enhancing general well-being.

Decreased pain. When you are tuned in to your bodily sensations, you are more inclined to observe signs that it's time to slow down, take a break, or change activities. In contrast, mindlessly pushing through pain may result in your ignoring mounting pain until it is severe. When people are experiencing pain but are too busy to register this fact, they are more likely to lose their patience, misunderstand or snap at others, or react in ways that do not represent their best self, only to realize later that their distress stemmed more from neglecting their pain than anything else. For me, an ungentle response to my husband usually indicates that I am taking on too much and need to slow down and focus.

Increased pleasure. Being mindful also increases the likelihood that you'll be in a position to take advantage of life's sweet moments and small pleasures (and with pain as a companion, pleasure is precious). Parents with grown children often impart advice to parents of young children: "Enjoy them now; they grow up so fast." The frequency of this comment may reflect that the chaotic pace of life with small children can rob parents of the feeling that they were fully present. The more preoccupied people feel, the harder it may be to experience the beauty and fullness of the present moment. Pain can feel all encompassing. By focusing on the challenges of pain, such as worries about the future, regrets, or losses, you may miss opportunities for sweet indulgence. Don't let negativity interfere with your chance to share laughs with friends, notice newly opened flowers, enjoy the song of birds, engage in valued tasks, or savor a bite of chocolate. No matter how lousy you may feel, being mindful can help you direct your attention to places besides your pain. Experiment with transforming everyday activities, such as listening to music, putting on hand cream, flossing your teeth, walking outside, or washing the dishes. As you focus on ways to increase your engagement, see if your pain takes a backseat.

Fewer judgments. Being mindful reduces the likelihood of negative snap judgments that can intensify your suffering, such as thinking, "This pain will ruin my whole day!" When you monitor your thoughts, even for a short period, you may be surprised by the extent to which your mental space is taken up by such snap judgments. Recall the futility of negative rumination in traffic. When people operate without awareness, they can confuse automatic thoughts with the actual experience of pain. Mindful awareness allows you to identify your thoughts for what they are—mere thoughts—or replace them with more helpful ones. (More on this in chapter 12.) As you become aware of evaluative responses with potentially negative effects, practice letting them go and replacing them with more neutral, descriptive observations. This allows for greater acceptance and choice in your response. When an activity is not what you expected, you can spend your time and attention focused on what is *missing* or *not* as you anticipated, or you can experience it *just as it is*. Focusing on people and situations in a nonjudgmental manner allows you to be more present.

Thoughts as thoughts. Suffering often emerges with the thoughts and emotions that arise around pain. Worrying about the pain of an anticipated dental appointment, for example, will increase distress long before the appointment even begins. During a breakthrough therapy session, one of my clients discovered that it was his *fear* of leg pain, more than the pain itself, that kept him from engaging in activities. His pain flare-ups, when they occurred, had become fairly manageable; however, his apprehension about future pain was continuing to cause distress. As he learned to focus on the present moment—and not worry about the next one—his experience became significantly more tolerable.

Remember: "Just because you think it does not mean that it is true." This discovery can be liberating. Practice identifying negative thoughts as "just thoughts" and not facts, thereby decreasing their effect on you. Mindfulness allows you to respond to thought patterns as you come to recognize them. Through practice, you can refrain from journeying along with the thoughts that can drag you down. When you observe a particularly pessimistic thought, for example, gently refocus your attention, rather than feeding or indulging in the thought. You can assign thoughts descriptive labels such as "my depressive thought," making it easier to see it for what it is and let it go.

Separating sensation from suffering. Mindfulness also offers tools to separate the actual sensation of pain from the thoughts and emotions that give it more substance. You can observe your pain as it takes place without judgment. For example, rather than labeling a variety of sensations collectively as "pain," practice describing your physical sensations in more nuanced ways. Gently notice what you feel in your body using neutral, descriptive terms: a circle of pressure on your back, a feeling of warmth pulsing down your arms, some stiffness in your neck, or heaviness in your legs. Try to acknowledge your pain without bias or interpretation, as in, "I feel tightness in my right calf and a burning across the shoulder blades," instead of judging, as in, "This pain is horrible. I can't stand it." Just as in the traffic-jam example, you contribute to defining your experience. Once you isolate your pain (in objective terms) from the thoughts and emotions that exacerbate it, pain becomes just pain, not a narrative of suffering. Viewing pain as one aspect of your experience, composed of physical sensations, reduces the likelihood that it will feel all encompassing.

Awareness of body. Sometimes focusing on your pain itself—its location, its intensity, its quality—helps diminish it. Experiment with ways to reduce painful sensations through deliberate awareness. Begin in a comfortable position, and breathe slowly and deeply until you experience inner calmness. Then, take note of the physical sensations that you experience and your ability to change their quality and intensity. You can incorporate meditative techniques such as mentally breathing into the locations of your pain or imagining healing colors or temperatures that reduce feelings of pain, or you can use relaxation strategies to release perceived tightness in your muscles.

Engaging your senses. Research has revealed the significant effect of our senses on our experience, ranging from the therapeutic effects of touch and pleasant music to the power an image can have on mood and perception of pain.[1] Experiment with ways you can alter your experience by engaging your senses. Here are some suggestions:

- *Touch.* Slowly and gently rub lotion on your hands or other parts of your body; give or receive a massage; wrap yourself in a soft, warm blanket; engage in sexual pleasure.
- *Scent.* Surround yourself with aromas you find pleasing (soaps and lotions, candles, herbs) or objects with positive scent associations.
- *Sight.* Feast your eyes on the beauty in your midst; gaze at pictures with positive associations, such as loved ones (including baby pictures and pets), happy occasions in your life, or particular locations or artwork that inspire or calm you. Allow yourself to bask in the positive feelings that emerge.
- *Sound.* Listen to sounds of nature—enjoy the birds outside your window or a recording of beach or other sounds that transport you. Select music that evokes good feelings—belt out the lyrics to a favorite oldie, enjoy the calming effect of a soft melody, or listen to songs with strong positive associations.
- *Taste.* Indulge in food and drink that bring you pleasure. The trick here is quality, not quantity. Rather than turning to food or drink as an escape, be mindful of each bite or sip of things you find delicious. Close your eyes, relax, eat slowly, sigh, and savor the small pleasure. This approach can turn eating into a sensual indulgence.

Experiment with activities that engage your senses to find ones that help shift your mood and thereby decrease pain. The effectiveness of these activities depends to some extent on how deliberate you are in your focus.

Psychological grounding. Mindfulness has become an increasingly common focus within psychotherapy. It is central to some approaches, such as dialectical behavior therapy, mindfulness-based cognitive behavioral therapy, and acceptance and commitment therapy, and it has been entering other approaches as well. All mindfulness-based psychotherapies share the idea that mindfulness helps individuals feel more grounded, more accepting, and less judgmental, which allows them to improve their relationships, emotional well-being, and tolerance for distress.

Controlling Your Pain by Calming Your Mind

Mindfulness practice can also counter what often feels like an otherwise mindless or automatic response to stress, which tends to increase pain. When your distress alarm is activated, your muscles tense, your breathing speeds up and shallows, and you become on edge, at full readiness. Although this sort of hypervigilance can be valuable in a crisis, as a response to daily stresses, it unduly taxes your system. With many chronic pain syndromes, distress also triggers increased pain, which can persist long after the source of stress recedes. Sources of distress can be emotional—such as from anxiety, interpersonal conflict, or overstimulation—or physical, such as from having to stand in line while pain mounts or from seemingly benign stimuli such as loud noises, cold air, or bright fluorescent lighting.

The following mindfulness practices are focused on relaxing your mind, which in turn can improve your experience and perceptions of pain. Additional advantages may include reductions in insomnia and anxiety, which are both highly correlated with chronic pain. Research shows that relaxation has positive effects on mood and outlook as well as people's sense of control and acceptance of their pain experience.[2]

Calm your mind. Pain can interfere with your thought processes. When you notice yourself feeling frayed or frazzled, use mindfulness to slow down and calm your body and mind. You can augment mindfulness with meditation, focusing on breath and body awareness. Excuse yourself as necessary so you can sit in a quiet, comfortable place. Take slow, deep, calming breaths. Focus on the rhythm of your breath. Do not be in a hurry. As your mind clears, you will become better able to find more constructive ways to respond. (Contrast this with reacting "mindlessly" to whatever may be bothering you.) When you calm your body and mind, you also heighten your awareness of the present moment. As you go through your day, notice when you feel calm and focused and when you feel most scattered. You can train yourself to be mindful in response to the first signs of distress, or at designated times or in response to environmental cues, such as whenever you stop at a red light or enter a room.

Slow, deep breaths. Focusing on your breath offers a mindful way to feel grounded and present. And consider this: Your breath is always accessible, no matter where you may be. And breathing has no negative side effects. You can attend to your breath whatever you are doing and without inconveniencing anyone. As described in chapter 11, slow, deep breathing can reduce muscle tension. Consider the following variants in your experiments to find a breathing practice that helps when you notice you are starting to feel scattered, or throughout the day to enhance your focus:

- *Count while you breathe.* It can be calming to count as a way to keep your breaths slow and your mind focused on your breath. The speed of your counting should feel calming—you may decide to inhale and exhale to a certain number of beats or assign a number to each breath.
- *Exhale with sound.* You might foster relaxation by emitting a gentle, relieving sound as you exhale, such as a sigh, moan, or whatever comes.
- *Observe a pattern to your breath.* It can be helpful to imagine your breath as a shape, such as an oval or a square, and imagine moving along the shape with each breath. Experiment with different patterns, such as breathing in as you travel up the edge of a rectangle, holding your breath across the top, exhaling down the right side, then holding across the bottom.
- *Aim to increase the length of your out breath.* Relaxation may intensify as you slow the speed of your exhale. Gently and gradually experiment with slowing down your exhale to exceed the length of your inhale.
- *Use an internal mantra.* It may help to say something calming to yourself as you breathe, such as, "Breath in, I relax," and, "Breath out, I'm calm." Experiment with words that enhance your relaxation and help you feel safe and grounded.
- *Visualize your breath.* Use your imagination to picture your breath, such as inhaling swirling, cool blueness and exhaling with fiery reds and oranges.
- *Relax on the exhale.* Just as with stretching, allow your body to relax upon exhalation. Scan your body for tension and exhale as you relax.

There are many other ways to practice mindfulness to breath, such as simply noticing your breath without trying to change or control it. See what might work for you.

Meditation. Meditation is simply a way to clear your head and quiet your thoughts. People with chronic pain are especially vulnerable to feeling overloaded from undertaking too much. Meditation is a form of mindfulness that offers a way to rest your mind and free yourself from racing thoughts and internal commotion.

Most religious traditions include a form of meditation. In recent years, the Western medical community has been incorporating meditation for relaxation and pain control, among other health benefits. At the forefront of the movement that has brought mediation into mainstream medicine is Jon Kabat-Zinn, a scientist, meditation teacher, and prolific writer whose work has led to the creation of programs that use meditation for stress reduction. Kabat-Zinn began teaching mindfulness-based stress reduction classes in 1979 at the University of Massachusetts Medical School. This approach teaches people to separate the physical sensations of pain from the way they think or feel about them. Among his books, *Full Catastrophe Living* in particular chronicles the use of meditation in the treatment of chronic pain. Increased research attention examines the effect of meditation on chronic pain. One such study found meditation to be as effective on pain intensity, distress, mood, and overall life quality as a multidisciplinary pain strategy.[3] The following provide basic instructions on meditation to get you started:

(1) *Find a quiet, comfortable place.* As much as possible, choose a time and place that feels safe, private, and free from distraction. Consider hanging a "do not disturb" sign on your door for the duration of your session. Turn off your phone or any other devices.

(2) *Make yourself comfortable.* Meditation does not require you to twist yourself into a lotus or any other challenging posture. Assume a position that feels comfortable, such as reclining in a supportive chair or lying down amid pillows. Minimize possible sources of discomfort—avoid trying to meditate on an empty stomach or in a room that is too hot or too cold. Your eyes can be open, gently closed, or at half-mast—whatever feels most relaxing, but not so much that you fall asleep!

(3) *Select a focal point or anchor.* The goal of meditation is to quiet your mind by focusing your attention on something specific, such as:

- *Your breath.* Breathe slowly and naturally and pay attention to the sensations as you inhale and exhale. You can use diaphragmatic breath to relax more deeply, or any of the suggestions listed earlier, such as counting your breaths.
- *A sound, a mantra, or music.* Quiet is often desirable, but you may prefer to meditate by focusing your attention on sound, such as the trickling of water, the hum of your exhaled breath, a calming word or short phrase that you chant, or a relaxation tape.
- *A bodily sensation.* Concentrate on a feeling of warmth, an experience of colored light, or any other pleasant sensation you can conjure up. Imagine moving the sensation slowly throughout your body and notice how this feels. Send your sensation of warmth or color to soothe areas with pain or discomfort.
- *Touch.* Focus your attention on the sensation of touch, such as your hand on a smooth surface. Close your eyes and slowly run your fingertips over an object, such as a rock, or a part of your body (such as your ear). Move very slowly and experience the sensation in your fingers and palm as you breathe slowly and deeply.
- *A visual aid.* Focus your gaze on something in your environment that engages you, such as a picture, an item in the room, or a lit candle. Stay focused on the item as a way to anchor your thoughts.
- *A visualized image.* As you breathe, conjure up an image of a place you find comfortable and safe. Engage your senses to flesh out the scene— the more detailed, the more effective. If you select the beach, for example, listen for the crash of waves and cries of seagulls, smell the salty sea air, feel warm sand conforming to your back, and taste a spray of salt water.
- *A taste.* Jon Kabat-Zinn offers the example of devoting several minutes to eating *one* raisin.[4] His patients are instructed to notice its packaging, aroma, appearance, texture, flavor, and how it feels in their mouth. This simple example reinforces how much can be discovered through mindful attention.

The idea is to ground yourself in some deliberate way that can allow distractions in your environment or thoughts to recede.

(4) *Quiet your mind.* This is the most challenging part of meditation.

Because our minds are naturally busy, it is inevitable that disruptive thoughts will creep in, such as your to-do list, worries, judgments, or other mental noise. Observe what comes into your mind without engaging in it (refrain, for example, from running down your to-do list). Imagine watching your thoughts and emotions come and go. When you notice yourself engaging in your thoughts or emotions, gently guide your attention back to your breath or other focus of your meditation. Distractions are inevitable; do not berate yourself for them. For the more persistent intrusions, experiment with visualization exercises to let them go—such as wrapping each thought in a bubble that glides away, envisioning your thoughts floating down a river or over a waterfall, or catching each thought with a butterfly net and releasing it downwind. As needed, tell yourself, "I do not need to think about that right now," with the awareness that you can decide to revisit your thoughts at a later time.

(5) *Be mindful of judgments.* There is no right or wrong way to mediate. Try to remain impartial about your experience. Evaluating how your meditation is going can increase anxiety. Instead, try to let things just happen, and accept however you may feel. Gaining comfort with meditation takes time. Try to accept your experience just as it is. Strive to let your mind be.

(6) *Pace yourself.* Keep your first meditation session short. Even a few minutes can be effective in creating a calm feeling. When you finish a session, take a slow, deep breath as you become aware of your larger surroundings. Be gentle with yourself; don't stand up too quickly. You may want to stretch. As you gain comfort, you can increase the time or frequency of the sessions as seems helpful. As you become accustomed to meditating, you can also try these head-clearing techniques while walking or while otherwise engaged.

Guided imagery. This technique helps generate a mental image or series of images that fosters a feeling of safety, comfort, and relaxation. Research has shown that imagining pictures or thoughts linked to positive feelings has pain-relieving effects. In guided imagery, the guide—whether an instructor as part of a group or class, a therapist, a video or audio recording, or a script—helps you enter a relaxed, focused state by creating in your mind's eye a scene that embodies tranquility, warmth, the absence of outside pressures, and a deep feeling of safety and comfort. The more you engage your senses, the increasingly real it will feel. It may be a place where you have been and felt particularly relaxed, such as soaking in a hot bath, lying under the sun's rays at the beach, or engaging in a tender intimate moment. It may be a journey to an idyllic place where you feel cushioned and pampered. As with other techniques, you can adapt it to your unique preferences. Most guided imagery sessions will describe a place where you feel comfortable, safe, and peaceful. But don't feel hemmed in by a prescribed setting; if the thought of lying on the beach reminds you of chafing sand rather than relaxing warmth, select another.

Once you develop imagery that you successfully associate with relaxation, you can go solo and guide yourself there whenever desired. At first, you may need to practice this exercise in your most comfortable environment. But, with practice, you may be able to conjure up this imagery as needed, even while in less peaceful surroundings.

Hypnosis. Hypnosis may sound mysterious, even magical, yet achieving a hypnotic state is actually a fairly mundane event. You know that feeling when you are driving and you suddenly realize you've not been paying attention but have arrived at your destination? This is a hypnotic or "alpha" state. Individuals in hypnotic states are fully awake and focused but with a decrease in peripheral awareness. In other words, while in a hypnotic "trance," you have a heightened attention in one area and significantly less in the others. By deliberately inducing a trance, you can transcend your body when you require a break from unpleasant sensations. As you focus on relaxing and letting go of distractions, the conscious part of the brain temporarily tunes out. When a person is effectively hypnotized, alpha brain waves increase and physiological changes take place, such as decreases in pulse and respiration.

Mental health professionals with specialized training in hypnotherapy (as opposed to hypnosis for entertainment) can help you achieve this altered state. Contrary to popular belief, nobody can be hypnotized without his or her consent or awareness. Instead, trained professionals can assist you in entering a hypnotic state and teach you self-hypnosis. The process is similar to other relaxation techniques. You begin in a position that is comfortable but not so relaxing that you fall asleep, and you take slow, deep breaths. The hypnotherapist assists you in focusing your attention on specific thoughts, tasks, or sensations, often using a guided visualization exercise to achieve a heightened state of awareness, which temporarily blocks out peripheral input. You can become more open to specific suggestions and goals, such as modulating pain, improving your outlook, or otherwise enhancing your life. Research has shown sustained pain relief through hypnosis that is at least as effective, or more effective, than other relaxation exercises.

With self-hypnosis, you can create for yourself a relaxing environment you can enter. Breathe in a slow, relaxed manner. Make sure you don't hold your breath. Self-hypnosis feels like you are in a daydream and deep in concentration, relaxed, and removed from your immediate circumstances. For example, I often use a hypnotic technique when my pain is high and I want to be able to concentrate on my writing. For me, this involves staring straight ahead and breathing slowly while very gently rocking my head back and forth. I imagine myself transcending my body while I continue to concentrate on what I am writing. As I write these words, I am engaged in this practice.

Mindfully Accept the Pain

There may be times in which your efforts to reduce the pain fall short. The pain may seem too intense and overwhelming to mollify, or you may not feel able to focus mindfully on anything else. Sometimes, pain can ransack your attention and crowd out other thoughts, feelings, and sensations. When this happens, use mindfulness to embrace the whole of your experience and accept it for what it is right now. Paradoxically, you may find that by fully accepting the pain, you reduce its intensity. You may also find that, like some of my clients, your more creative expressions emerge during such intense moments.

Embrace pain as part of life. Pain is an inevitable part of life. Fighting this fact intensifies suffering, while expected pain is easier to bear. Acknowledging pain can also lead to deeper philosophical and spiritual connections. It can help you accept the eventualities of existence: people grow old, develop illnesses, and die. While these facts are obvious, they can get lost in our cultural fixation on youth and health. Rather than tormenting yourself over difficulties, imagine ways to make room for them, along with your other varied experiences. Happiness and joy come from fully experiencing the present moment, not the absence of negative experiences or feelings. In other words, you can enjoy beauty or joy while simultaneously feeling pain or sadness or anxiety. Being fully alive involves embracing the richness of life. As the Buddhist monk Thich Nhat Hanh suggests, you can relieve pain by mindfully embracing it—even imagining it as a baby in need of your care.[5]

Chapter 11

Strategies to Soothe Your Body

This chapter focuses on ways to improve your physical comfort. Look for new ideas to test and reminders to revisit any old favorites.

Heat

Heat is a natural analgesic, and its relief can be instant. For many of us, heat soothes. It can provide comfort to sufferers of irritable bowel syndrome, migraines, fibromyalgia, and lower back pain, among many other pains. For neuromuscular problems, heat promotes relaxed, supple muscles, which are easier to stretch. It can have longer-lasting effects by increasing blood flow, which promotes healing and reduces muscle spasms. Comfort from heat can also enable you to engage in other beneficial behaviors.

So, how do I find heat when I need it? Many sources of therapeutic heat are common knowledge, such as heating pads and hot baths. Yet we can forget to take full advantage of these. Another significant obstacle comes from not treating your comfort as a priority. Beware of any judgmental thoughts that arise around making time for yourself. If your experiments reveal benefits, commit to using heat on a regular basis.

Experience your shower as a pampering spa. The flood of hot water from the shower can help you stretch areas that irk you most, such as tight neck muscles that can cause tension headaches. (Consult with a physical therapist for the most appropriate and productive stretches for you.) The promise of such kind treatment can serve as a powerful incentive to drag an aching body from a cozy bed. Similarly, the anticipation of a leisurely hot shower at the end of the day can make difficult moments more bearable. By warming the bathroom with a space heater or heat vent, you can extend the time in which your muscles are warm and thus engage in a longer stretching routine.

Prolong the heat in your tub. A relaxing hot bath can reduce muscle tension and encourage sleep. Enhance your comfort with peaceful music, pampering bath products, an inflatable pillow to cradle your head and neck, or soft foam for underneath. (Check out the bath products at your local drugstore or in specialty shops and catalogs.) An additional tip: Unless you have a gracious water heater, fill the tub partway with warm water, then increase the heat as you go. This way, you won't squander precious hot water or risk running out before the tub fills. Yelling for someone to boil a kettle to heat up your tub is not conducive to relaxation. As you soak, add hot water as needed to maintain your desired temperature.

Consider upgrading your bathtub. Modern bathrooms often have large tubs, some with built-in massage jets along the side. If you are so lucky, put it to good use. Or, if you find hot water especially helpful, investigate such upgrades. The range of what is available is wide—from built-in whirlpool tubs, sometimes referred to by the brand name Jacuzzi®, to whirlpool kits available at home improvement stores. Many have integrated heaters that keep the water hot. Before investigating a bathroom remodel, make sure to test their effect. Perhaps a friend or local hotel has one you can try? If trying out a whirlpool kit, check the return policy.

Bigger can be better. Hot tubs (also referred to as spa tubs) are multi-person units that can be housed inside or outdoors and remain filled with hot water. You may be able to test their effects at a local gym or health spa (most provide at least one free visit) or even at a hotel, either locally or while on vacation. If you find that a soak in the hot tub significantly reduces your pain, consider this among your reasons for joining a particular gym or health club. Personal-use hot tubs may be worth the investment if you can accommodate one. Their large size also enables you to stretch tired, sore muscles. During certain phases, I practically lived in my hot tub—climbing in at both ends of the day and taking an occasional dip under the moon. While my need has dramatically decreased, I still appreciate its effects.

Hot tubs vary considerably in price and features. Many dealers have showrooms with demonstration models for potential buyers to test, so pack your suit. If you don't want to take the plunge in a showroom, at least climb into an empty tub and test the ease of entry and exit, the comfort of its seats, and the placement of its jet nozzles. Or you may find a good deal on a pre-owned hot tub. Beyond the initial investment, costs include energy bills (approximately equivalent to a refrigerator), chemicals, and water bills. Check out your home's wiring to make sure it can handle the electrical demand of the tub you have in mind. Maintenance involves changing the water every few months and maintaining chemical balance to keep it clean and clear.

The maximum temperature of a standard hot tub is 104°F. Consult with your doctor about the safety of high temperatures, particularly if you have a heart condition, may be pregnant, or have any other medical concerns. If you are someone who benefits from very hot water, and your doctor approves, it may be worthwhile to talk with the manufacturer about increasing the capabilities by a couple degrees.

Try out a hot room. Another way to heat your entire body is with a sauna. Saunas are heated rooms—either dry heat enclosed in wood, or the humid, steamy, tiled variety. Both are commonly found at gyms and health spas and provide a therapeutic place to relax and stretch. Home versions, which come as a one-piece unit, are also available through home improvement stores. Larger, built-in home saunas may make sense if you are building a house or planning a major home remodel. As with the hot tub, check with your doctor before investing in or using a sauna.

Treating yourself to a total body warming—whether in a tub, shower, or sauna—can be wonderful. If your experiments reveal significant pain relief, respond accordingly. For times when access is limited, consider the following heat sources, which can warm you virtually anywhere while fully clothed.

Microwaveable heat sacks. Heat sacks offer heat anywhere you have access to a microwave. These cloth bags, which I affectionately dub my "happy sacks," have the consistency of beanbags and can come in any size or shape. Many versions are available commercially or can be homemade. To craft a rudimentary sack, scoop a few cups of dry rice (or dried beans or grains such as buckwheat or feed corn) into a tube sock or cotton pillowcase and knot it closed. Heat it in the microwave, and you have a malleable heating pad that conforms to the contours of your neck, lower back, or any other nagging area. Wrap it in a towel, and it will remain hot for at least thirty minutes and feel warm for hours.

Experiment to discover the right temperature. The length of microwave time depends on the size of the sack, the strength of the microwave, and your preferences. Because they are not electric, they are safe to use in bed or when napping in a chair. (Do not put the hot sack directly against your skin.) If you find aromas soothing, consider adding sprigs of spices or dried herbs (such as lavender or lemon thyme) or a few drops of aromatic oil. If you have access to a sewing machine or to a friend who sews, you can customize your sack—long thin shapes for your neck and shoulders, lightweight squares for your face and jaw, large rectangles for lower back or stomach pain, and so on. Select fabrics to suit your decor and lift your spirits. Thick cottons work best, and cotton velvet can add a luxurious touch. Avoid synthetics because they may be unsafe for microwave use. Consider designing one for your office chair, another for your bed, and another for travel. I stash "happy sacks" wherever I am a frequent visitor.

Microwave heat sacks can be used virtually anywhere there is microwave access, including during travel. Heat one (or two) just before embarking on a car trip; along the way, convenience stores at gas stations often have microwaves (wrap your sack with paper towels to keep it food-free). Think creatively. Most airports also have microwaves, and I have found airport bartenders to be quite obliging with an odd request (politely asked) to heat a sack. You should be able to use the same sack for months. Just make sure the rice stays dry (or you'll end up with cooked rice), and keep it separate from food to avoid odors. If it does start to smell bad, pour out the old rice, launder the cover, and refill it with fresh grain.

Revisit the hot water bottle. For those too young to recall, water bottles are actually rubber bags—traditionally red—that hold hot water. Many drugstores continue to carry them. They are simple to use: just unscrew the plastic cork, fill with water that is hot (but not boiling), and refasten the cork. Release excess air before closing to let the bag conform to your body. The less water you use, the more malleable its form. Water bottles remain hot for up to an hour. For comfort and safety, wrap a towel around the bag rather than placing it directly on your skin. Like heat sacks, hot water bottles cool during use, making them safe to take to bed as long as the cork is securely closed. (Cautionary note: never use water bottles with electric heating pads, heating blankets, or any other electrical devices because contact between water and electricity can result in shock and even death.)

Newer versions of the hot water bottle use alternative materials, sizes, and shapes, and may come with covers. Among the most remarkable is a clear, thin plastic bottle that is the size of a standard pillowcase and fits conveniently inside one). When empty, these are very lightweight, like plastic bags, and fold up for easy portability. Lying down on one can be sheer bliss—as close as you can get to immersion in hot water while completely dry—because they can cover a large portion of your body. I found these to be particularly wonderful when I was pregnant (not too hot!) and for use during postpartum massage, when lying facedown was otherwise uncomfortable.

Plug it in. Most people are familiar with electric heating pads: typically inexpensive plug-in gadgets, available in most drugstores, department stores, and discount outlets. They provide a constant source of heat, are lightweight, and can be used wherever there's an electrical outlet. Consider strapping a large pad to the back of your chair at work (I have one against my back as I write this), while relaxing, or during a meditative break. Some heating pads offer moist heat with a thin layer of spongelike fabric that you dampen and insert into the pad sleeve. Most new versions have automatic shutoff features, and most have adjustable temperature settings. Still, be mindful to unplug the pad when you are finished. Heating pads are not recommended for use when you may doze off because of the risk of skin irritation, burns, and fire.

Heat your seat. In addition to the standard heating pad, a growing array of products can provide a warm seat in different settings. Heated seat cushions for cars plug into car lighters (or power ports). Deluxe versions offer features such as zoned heat and massaging vibrations. You can also plug standard heating pads into your car with the help of an adapter, available in auto stores. There are also many car models that come with heated and even cooled seats as well as lumbar support features. You can also find a variety of heated seating, such as heated folding chairs (to ensure you a warm seat in any situation) and heated hammocks (to provide tropical-style relaxation). Specialized products address multiple purposes such as heated massage lumbar cushions, designed to provide low back support and warmth while they massage your lower back muscles, or heated massage machines for other areas, such as your neck and shoulders. Consider what would enable you to be most comfortable and warm—chances are, a product exists!

Single-use heat packs. There is an array of single-use products that can provide heat for several hours. These include therapeutic bandage–like wraps that adhere to parts of the body, stick-on pads that can fit surreptitiously under your clothing, or small packs that you can slide into a pocket or hold in your hand. They come in different shapes, sizes, and forms and can retain heat for up to several hours. Their unique advantage is that they are not dependent on electricity or hot water. Consider packing one for outdoor excursions. Topical creams, particularly those with pepper (capsicum) oil, can provide a similar feeling of heat by increasing blood circulation where applied. (Be careful to keep the spicy oil away from your eyes and other sensitive areas.)

Hot water massage with your clothes on. Hydromassage units, located at some health clubs and shopping malls, offer an innovative combination of massage and heat therapy. They use heated water and jets (similar to a hot tub) but are completely enclosed in plastic, able to provide a full-body heated water massage while you remain completely dry. The unit resembles a tanning bed— you lie down inside, fully clothed, and the clamshell top is lowered. You can control the pressure, pulse rate, and travel speed of the jets along your back and sides. Home-use machines are now available; as these are relatively new and expensive devices, test and research these well before considering purchasing one.

Cold

Ice is the treatment of choice for newly injured muscles to prevent or reduce inflammation. For chronic pain, cold can function as a local anesthetic, numbing sore tissue and slowing nerve impulses in the area. Beyond treating initial injuries, there is no hard-and-fast rule about when to try cold versus heat. Chronic pains that involve inflammation, such as rheumatoid arthritis, may respond better to heat than to cold. But this is highly individualized. As long as your doctor sees no danger in treating yourself with cold, test your response. To avoid damaging your skin (think frostbite), make sure there's a barrier between you and anything frozen and limit exposure to fifteen or twenty minutes a session. If you respond well to cold, consider the following delivery systems.

Keep it simple. Applying cold can be as simple as rummaging through your freezer. A bag of frozen vegetables works in a pinch, as does a bag of ice (add water if desired). Commercial cold packs stay cold longer and can be refrozen after each use. Some hot water bottles are also freezer safe (check the label). To apply an ice bag or ice pack, wrap it in a small towel and position it on the affected area. Frozen hand towels offer additional malleability. Simply fold a damp towel and place it in the freezer in a plastic bag; after fifteen minutes, remove the towel from the bag and drape or wrap it around the affected area.

Gel packs offer versatility. Commercial gel packs come in many forms, from the supermarket variety to specialized therapeutic versions. Gel packs conform to your body better than ice and stay colder longer. Therapeutic versions come in many forms and styles, including specialized wraps that fasten around specific joints (popular among athletes) or circular packs that conform to breasts. Gel packs often come with washable covers and pads for additional comfort and safety and to retain their temperature. Many varieties are available that deliver heat as well as cold; you can alternate your desired temperature by using your pack from the freezer and later heating it in the microwave or in hot water.

Ice massage can offer frozen bliss. With ice massage (unlike cold packs), the ice should come in direct contact with your skin. The aim is to numb the area completely. Ice massage can be done with an ice cube or a bag of ice. Keep the ice in constant motion over the affected area to safeguard your skin from burn. A simple and effective method involves freezing water in a disposable cup, then peeling back the cup top an inch or two to expose the ice surface. (Disposable foam cups, while unkind to the environment, works well for this purpose because it keeps your hand warm and dry and is easy to peel.) If you have someone who can provide you with an ice massage, great! Most often, however, ice massage is something you can do for yourself, provided the area is within reach, such as your lower back or neck. Either way, assume a comfortable position, avoid rubbing the ice over the bony areas of your spine, and limit the massage to five minutes to avoid frostbite. For times you may want a cold massage but are far from a freezer, single-use cold packs produce twenty to thirty minutes of cooling relief.

Cold and hot water. If your body feels swollen with pain, a jaunt in a cold tub or shower can be restorative. Some people benefit from alternating between hot and cold, a common practice in European spas.

Muscle Relaxation Techniques

The following techniques are intended to relax your muscles and reduce your pain. See which, if any, work for you, and incorporate the winners into your routine.

Slow, deep breaths. One of the most powerful techniques to calm the body involves your breath. It may sound silly, but how you breathe matters. "Take a few deep breaths"—isn't that what we say to encourage others to calm down? Other common expressions speak to the relation between breathing and anxiety: "Don't hold your breath," or waiting with "bated breath." Emotional distress affects the way we breathe, which, in turn, affects our tension level. Research shows that sitting quietly with your breath can foster both physiological and psychological changes.[1] Breathing is the cornerstone of many other relaxation techniques, as described in chapter 10.

The first step is to notice your breathing patterns. You may be surprised to find that you unconsciously hold your breath during neutral activities, such as while waiting for a web page to load. You may notice times when your breathing speeds up or slows down or habits such as holding in your stomach, which restricts the depth of your breath. You can examine the quality of your breath by placing one hand on your stomach and the other on your upper chest. Observe how each rises and falls. When we are tense, our breath is relatively short and fast and remains in our upper chest. This breathing pattern maintains tension and exerts pressure on the muscles, small bones, and nerves in the upper chest. In contrast, diaphragmatic breathing (or "belly breaths") evokes relaxation and counters the stress response.

To practice diaphragmatic breathing, position yourself comfortably. Inhale slowly and deeply through your nose and practice filling your diaphragm. Notice the hand on your abdomen move outward, while trying to minimize the movement of the hand on your chest. Exhale slowly through your nose or pursed lips—again, note how the hand on your abdomen moves as you exhale. Your breath should feel fairly natural and not forced. If you begin to feel dizzy, ease up; you may be hyperventilating. As needed, change the pace and length of your breaths to find a natural and relaxing rhythm. Start with a modest goal, such as breathing this way for one or more minutes. Notice any changes in the way you feel, particularly whether you feel calmer or more comfortable.

Experiment with slow, deep breathing as a response to mounting pain and to keep your pain at bay. If you find deep breathing brings relief, use it to ease morning pain, to enter sleep at night, or at intervals to enhance your well-being. Breathing exercises require deliberate attention but not a great time commitment or a shift in activities—you're already breathing throughout the entire day! It can be helpful to associate certain moments or conditions with an awareness of your breath, such as training yourself to breathe slowly while at the computer or driving or at the first signs of discomfort. With practice, slow, deep breathing can become more automatic.

Progressive muscle relaxation. This technique trains you to identify muscle tension and induce relaxation by systematically tensing and releasing your muscles. To do this: Close your eyes. Start with the muscles in your face and slowly move down your body (or start with your toes and move up). Squeeze, then release, each muscle or muscle group in a sequential pattern. The typical directions are to tense your muscles tightly for about ten seconds, then release for about twenty seconds before moving on; however, feel free to adapt according to your experience. Take slow, deep breaths and focus on the physical sensation. Tensing your muscles should not incite pain; if it does, then ease up, stop, or skip over certain muscle groups.

You may also gain benefits from abridged sessions and in any situation. For example, you can zero in on specific areas, such as lifting and tensing your shoulders to relieve the tension you may be holding there. Experiment and see what brings relief. If tensing your muscles worsens your symptoms, this technique is not for you. Read on.

Body scan. This technique walks you through an inventory of your muscle tension and then focuses your attention on relaxing tense areas. Many variants exist for this; all involve fostering body awareness, using a technique to soothe or release tension, and practice. Typically, you start "scanning" your muscles from the top down, breathing slowly as you go. When you encounter a tight area, envision relaxation. You can respond by directing a relaxing, warm sensation to the area, along with words such as *calm* or *relax*, or by breathing a feeling of relaxation to that spot. You might relax a tensed forehead, for example, by imagining it as smooth as silk and free of all wrinkles. You might relax your jaw by allowing your mouth to feel neutral, jaw open and tongue resting on the roof of your mouth. You can send softening feelings to your cheeks, your neck, and on down until you reach the soles of your feet. You might imagine pouring a warm, heavy dose of "relaxation" over your head and letting it flow down your body, releasing tension as it goes. With practice, you can train yourself to frequently scan your body for tension, equipped with an effective soothing response. Many free versions of scripts or online videos for body-scan relaxation exercises are available.

You can conduct a body scan anytime and anywhere. The extent you can relax depends, of course, on your circumstances. It is much easier to relax while reclining than standing in a supermarket line; however, you may be in greater need while in line. You might scan your body and focus on the areas with the greatest tension, such as unclenching your jaw or allowing your shoulders and neck to relax.

Postural checklist. Another way to relax your muscles is by assuming a relaxing, supportive posture. My favorite can be done anywhere you are seated:

- Sit in a chair with your back straight and supported, arms gently bent at the elbow, forearms in your lap with your hands palms up, fingers lightly curled, knees bent, and feet on the floor.
- Plant your feet comfortably on the floor with your toes pointing out. Let your knees open about shoulder width.
- Check that you are not slouching, that your head is centered, and that your sides are symmetrical.
- Once in position, shrug your shoulders and gently let them fall. This reduces any tension in your upper body. Close your eyes and begin taking slow, deep breaths. Remain in this position for at least a few minutes to establish a state of relaxation.

If this proves helpful, work this exercise into your day.

Biofeedback. Biofeedback machines can provide an external gauge of bodily sensations and the effects of your efforts to change your internal experience. Through biofeedback, people have learned how to increase the blood flow to their extremities and raise the temperature of their hands. Biofeedback can similarly reveal the effect of strategies to relax painful muscles. Your success in reducing muscle tension may be indicated by descending lines on graphs or a slowing down of flashing lights or beeping sounds. In this way, biofeedback machines act as something of a sixth sense, providing another means of data. The machines monitor your performance as you attempt to improve your skill; when you are off the mark, you continue to try again. Similar to a scale or thermometer, biofeedback machines precisely gauge your experience. Biofeedback can guide you to influence your experience, even aspects that may have seemed beyond your control. Once you master the process, you no longer need the machinery.

Biofeedback can be both affirming and instructive. After suffering from invisible but often excruciating symptoms, I found it incredibly validating to see my pain graphed on a fancy machine in a pain specialist's office. Just as I had experienced it, the machine indicated high levels of distress in one leg and none in the other. The difference between my legs was so striking that the therapist reversed the electrodes to make sure the equipment wasn't malfunctioning. But the graph for my left leg remained flat, while the right one hit the maximum number, validating my perceived experience. The machine also provided confirmation for the stretches and sitting positions that I found to decrease my leg pain. By working with the machine, I could test and improve the effectiveness of my relaxation exercises. I learned additional strategies—a machine connected to my forehead buzzed until I succeeded in fully relaxing my face and achieving a deeper state of relaxation.

Biofeedback has become a fairly common approach for addressing chronic pain and is often used in conjunction with other therapies. Biofeedback equipment ranges considerably, from simple home versions to elaborate machines in professional settings. Trained biofeedback therapists act as coaches, helping to set goals and offering suggestions on how to improve your performance.

Change your facial expression. There's evidence that facial expressions not only signal moods but may affect them as well. Notice that when you feel angry or anxious, your face may tense, your brows knit, and your jaw clench. And when you're smiling, your mouth and the corners of your eyes lift, along with your spirits. It may actually be helpful to supplant scowls and other pained expressions with lighter ones.

The "half smile" is one of the strategies described by psychologist Marsha Linehan, founder of dialectical behavioral therapy (DBT), to change people's experience in the face of distress.[2] This is different from forcing a full-on smile. Instead, start by allowing your face to relax—check your jaw for clenching and the rest of your face for any areas of tension—then gently induce your mouth into the smile of the *Mona Lisa* or the Buddha. The corners of your eyes may follow suit. You can coax and reinforce this facial expression by thinking about something pleasant or amusing. Don't force your face into a broad or otherwise inauthentic grin. Instead, aim for a very small one, with your face relaxed and the sides of your mouth just slightly upturned. Observe the result. Others may also respond appreciatively to your expression, potentially enhancing your experience further.

Laugh! Moving beyond the smile to full-fledged laughter can deliver powerful medicine. Research shows that laughing releases endorphins (the body's feel-good chemicals), relaxes the body, and promotes a sense of well-being. Norman Cousins called attention to the health benefits of laughter in his 1979 memoir, *Anatomy of an Illness*. Cousins, who suffered from a painful spine condition (ankylosing spondylitis), prescribed himself a regimen of watching comedic movies (Marx Brothers movies in particular) and found that ten minutes of belly laughing gave him two hours of drug-free, pain-free sleep.

Laboratory evidence illustrates that a good belly laugh stimulates most of the major systems of the body. It works your muscles and increases your heart rate and circulation, lending support for Norman Cousins's description of laughing out loud as "internal jogging." According to William Fry, a Stanford psychiatrist and a leading expert on humor and health, intense laughter (even when faked) offers a significant cardiovascular workout followed by a relaxation response. Studies also found that laughter significantly reduces levels of stress hormones.[3]

Laughter tends to be social; you're much more likely to laugh with others than by yourself. So, seek out playful people who laugh readily, and be open to joining in. Why not tell family and friends that laughing together may reduce your pain? The idea that laughter can be healthful is as contagious as laughter itself. The concept of "laugh yoga" originated in India in the mid-1990s and spawned laughter clubs throughout the world. These clubs bring people together (often in the early hours) with the intent of generating deep laughter to enhance well-being. They tend to use playful activities, chants, breathing techniques, and feigned laughs, which in a social context can spread uproarious laughter like wildfire. If interested, check your area for existing clubs or view "laughter yoga" videos on the Internet.

Exercise. Other ways to relax your muscles include physical exercises, including yoga or tai chi, particularly when done with mindful attention. For some people, rhythmic exercises such as walking or swimming can also bring relaxation to muscles.

Therapeutic Massage

Another, increasingly common, method to relax your muscles is therapeutic massage. Research shows that massage produces benefits in a variety of musculoskeletal pain problems, such as low back pain, by releasing taut muscles, easing spasms, and increasing circulation.[4] Studies also suggest that massage has positive impacts on well-being more generally by decreasing cortisol ("a stress hormone") and increasing serotonin and dopamine (our "feel-good" hormones).[5] The way you respond to massage or particular techniques, however, is highly individual. Even research that reports significant effects does not report a 100 percent rate of benefit. Certain massage techniques may be a godsend for one but unhelpful or even bothersome to another. Beware of any claims that massage or massage techniques offer a cure beyond temporary relief or relaxation.

Massage types vary from professional massage therapy to self-massage techniques and devices. If you are interested in experimenting with therapeutic massage, evaluate your experience:

- How do you feel while receiving a massage?
- How do you feel over the course of the day or week following a massage?
- How long does any postmassage soreness last?
- How does your experience differ depending upon the specifics of the massage therapy?

Track your experiences carefully so you can evaluate the immediate and longer-term effects of massage or any other method you try. If you find that massage is generally helpful but increases soreness in the short term, you might experiment with strategies for reducing soreness or try a different massage therapist or option.

Massage therapists are professionals. If the idea of massage therapy feels indulgent, consider this: although anyone living with pain deserves pampering, therapeutic massage is much more than that—it's a legitimate treatment. Massage has become part of the preparatory regimen of professional athletes, concert violinists, and other performers whose work demands able muscles. Massage can also allow you to learn more about your body and tune in to its signals.

If the thought of having someone touch your body is disconcerting, keep in mind that practitioners are trained professionals who should respect your modesty and that massage therapy is therapeutic, not sexual. If you still feel apprehensive, start with a chair massage, in which you sit, fully clothed, in a specially designed chair. (You may have seen these chair massages being demonstrated at a local mall.) You might then ease into the more standard table massage. It is up to you what you wear during a massage. Therapists can work around clothes or uncover the part they are working on. Massage should take place in a comfortable and safe environment and generally away from sources of stress. Avoid scheduling an in-home massage, for example, in a chaotic environment or if children will be underfoot.

Build a therapeutic alliance. Effective massage is based on teamwork. As a massage recipient, it's your responsibility to express your preferences and communicate about your experience. You may prefer light touch to promote relaxation or deeper pressure on tight spots. Before the session begins, discuss your goals, specific preferences, any limitations or apprehensions, and what will enhance your comfort. Once the session is under way, you may or may not want to provide detailed directives—an appreciative groan can encourage more of the same, while an "ouch" conveys that a change is in order. Finding a suitable therapist sometimes requires shopping around as you also figure out your preferences.

Your receptivity also affects your experience. When receiving a massage, relax! This may sound silly; after all, isn't massage supposed to be relaxing? However, a relaxation response is not automatic. Plus, not all massage is relaxing; deeper muscle work can be uncomfortable, even painful. Contemplate the factors that promote relaxation for you, such as taking slow, deep breaths or scanning your body for any clenching. Make sure you are sufficiently warm. Ask for extra blankets if desired; some therapists warm the table with a heating pad or hot water bottle, or offer hot stones. If you receive massage in a health club, you might warm up in a hot tub or steam room before your massage or schedule your massage after a cardiovascular workout. Therapists typically play music to enhance relaxation. If you have a beloved recording, bring it. Therapists should follow your cues about talking. If you prefer a silent massage, convey this implicitly (a professional therapist should respect this cue), or explicitly, if necessary. Once you develop a "talking on the table" relationship, it may seem inconsiderate to ask to return to quiet time. However, a professional massage therapist should abide by this without question.

Find a suitable therapist. To select a therapist, begin with trustworthy referrals, such as from support-group members, physicians, friends, or acquaintances with chronic pain. Massage therapists associated with pain clinics, sports medicine, and physical therapy centers are more likely to be trained in therapeutic techniques than those in day spas or vacation retreats, where "fluff and buff" rubdowns may be more common. However, there is no hard-and-fast rule. Most often, you have to see for yourself and hope the investment is a pleasant one.

In the United States, the term *massage therapist* is currently used for those schooled in therapeutic techniques. Any other term, including *massage* by itself, may be a euphemism for an illicit and untrained service—an important distinction to avoid potentially embarrassing situations. I once mistakenly contacted an establishment advertised under "massage" (not "massage therapy"). After an awkward exchange, I realized that the "adult pleasure" they offered wasn't what I was seeking. It makes sense to avoid buildings with papered windows, neon signs, or anything termed a "massage parlor" and look instead for massage therapists in health spas, in therapeutic venues, or through their national association or licensing board. The National Certification Board for Therapeutic Massage and Bodywork (NCBTMB) maintains a searchable online database with a current list of practitioners who are certified in the United States.

Be skeptical of massage therapists who claim they can cure your condition, attempt to diagnose you, or provide medical advice. Some practitioners combine traditional massage therapy with less conventional therapies. Don't be surprised if an otherwise skilled therapist, knowledgeable about anatomy and your pain condition, shares questionable information. Some of the education in licensed massage schools combines scientific with unscientific ideas. For example, massage therapists are taught that massage removes "toxins" from the body and routinely recommend drinking extra water to flush the system—an idea that lacks a scientific basis. Fortunately, drinking water does no harm, beyond the inconvenience of extra trips to the bathroom.

Massage Therapy Techniques

Massage approaches and techniques are numerous, and those under the category of bodywork are vaster still. It is fairly easy to find testimonials for any or all massage techniques (particularly on the Internet). Keep in mind that people can derive benefits from the positive attention or practitioner's manner as much as or even more than from the techniques themselves. This is especially the case for methods that involve minimal or no physical contact, such as "therapeutic touch," Reiki, or "energy work"—methods in which treatment may involve waving a crystal over your body to connect with your "energy fields."

Review the red flags described in chapter 9 and be skeptical of approaches based on unscientific ideas.

A relevant distinction is between lighter massage intended to promote general well-being and deeper work that focuses on specific problem areas. Massage to generate a calming effect generally comes from the Swedish tradition, which emphasizes long strokes and kneading motions to relax the entire body. Gentle massage should feel good in the moment. You can experiment and see how long such effects last for you. Deeper massage typically begins with similar gentle strokes to relax muscles before focusing more specifically on problem areas.

Deeper massage work goes by many names, including "myofascial release," "deep tissue massage," "trigger-point massage," and "connective tissue therapy," among others, with, unfortunately, very little standardization of procedures. Its general aim is to release tight spots in muscles and connective tissue, including trigger points, which often accompany chronic pain. When pressed, trigger points, or taut bands of fibers that form in muscles, send ("trigger") sensations to other parts of the body. Pressure on a spot in your back, for example, may elicit pain in your head, or arm pain may emanate from a muscle spasm in your shoulder. Trigger points often remain hidden until someone makes you aware of them. You may also be surprised by the intensity of the pain in a spot, once activated, that may be far from where you have been experiencing your pain.

The discovery of trigger points and their reproducible pain pathways was made by Dr. Janet Travell, famous for treating President John F. Kennedy. Dr. Travell, along with Dr. David Simons, later published a medical text detailing the relationship between trigger points and the pain they cause in other specific areas of the body. Travell and Simons's discoveries are the basis of the illustrative posters that often hang on the walls of massage therapy and physical therapy rooms.[6] Skillful therapists, schooled in these techniques, can deactivate trigger points by identifying and applying pressure to tight areas in muscle and fascia. However, therapists' ability to do this varies considerably. Keep in mind that while these techniques can be a source of momentary pain or discomfort, the pain should feel good, even relieving. Be sure to communicate with your therapist, and resist enduring anything beyond your comfort zone. The more acquainted you become with any trigger points you may have, the better you can guide therapists to your tight areas.

Incorporating massage into your life. If you find a particular type of massage therapy helpful, consider how best to work it into your schedule. Standing appointments—whether monthly, biweekly, or weekly—provide something to look forward to and allow for cumulative effects. Proactive scheduling for specific times when you anticipate difficulties, such as around travel, work deadlines, and other stressful events, can help head off flare-ups. Or you may reserve massage therapy for flare-ups. When pain is high, you can take comfort that relief is in sight. In that case, it is important to have a therapist who may have openings for such emergencies.

Fitting massage into your budget. A downside of professional massage is the expense. In most cases, it is not covered by health insurance, though exceptions exist. Some insurance policies include massage therapy—check yours. Physical therapists sometimes include massage techniques in their services. Massage therapy is also more likely to be covered as a component of prescribed physical therapy or if the massage therapist works in-house in a physician's office or pain clinic. When budgeting or preparing taxes, consider whether massage for chronic pain can be considered a health-related expense (rather than a luxury). Fees for massage therapy also vary considerably and are not necessarily related to quality. Some therapists offer first-time discounts; inquire about this when scheduling an initial appointment. Fees at gyms or health spas tend to be lower for members, particularly if you prepay for several sessions at a time. Massage chains are becoming more common and often run specials. Check for massage therapy schools in your area. Massage students often need to accrue credit hours toward their degree and are looking for volunteers for (free) massage sessions.

Massage without a professional. If you're lucky enough to have someone who is willing to offer a shoulder rub, instruct him or her on what works for you. Most people without professional massage training lack techniques to preserve their fingers and arms—so expect shorter sessions and request attention to the neediest parts of your body first. It's worth remembering, as well, to preserve balance in your relationship, and not to turn your friend (or partner or relative) into a therapist, massage or otherwise, however good they may be.

You can also develop skills and tools for self- massage. A gentle rub after a shower or during a break from work can be relaxing and restorative. Of course, you need to be careful not to overdo it or hurt one side of your body while attempting to aid the other. You can experiment, too, with very gentle touch, either on the area of pain or elsewhere. A caressing hand or a soft cloth on your cheek and ear, for example, may turn down the amplitude on pain. Experiment, and repeat if helpful.

Massage Devices

As self-massage gains popularity, the marketplace has become awash in contraptions. Over the years, I have amassed a box full, from which I select whatever fits my current need. Massage tools range from simple home remedies, such as lying on carefully placed tennis balls, to reclining in an extravagant lounge chair with a built-in massager. And new devices are continually debuting. Some are marketed to specific niches, such as the latest "trigger point deactivator" or "fibromyalgia poker stick," with names that promise to meet specific needs. In many cases, identical devices that may not be labeled specifically for people with chronic pain are available for a lower price at your local big-box store. Prices vary widely and do not necessarily correlate with a product's helpfulness. Test out promising products and hold on to your receipts. This can allow you to return unsatisfactory products or include satisfactory ones on your taxes as medical expenses.

Among the hundreds of available products, most can be categorized as follows:

Electric massage machines. These devices, sometimes called "shiatsu massagers," have rotating balls that simulate the kneading motion of the hands of a massage therapist. The fancier ones allow you to adjust the pressure, speed, and direction, and some even climb up and down your back. These can be helpful in relaxing tight muscles and working trigger points. These can be freestanding devices you prop up in a chair, or they may be built directly into a specially designed massage chair.

Massage mats. These long, flat mats are meant for you to lie down on or attach to the back of your seat (they often come with a power adapter for use in the car). Features can include pressure, heat, and vibration. These can be effective in offering distraction from pain and providing soothing stimulation.

Pokers. A huge variety of wooden, metal, and plastic shapes are sold as acupressure devices. These devices have no moving parts; they are designed to apply pressure to a specific spot of your body as you lean against the poker. They come in many designs, all intended to apply specific pressure to tight spots. Some are small enough to fit in the palm of your hand, and others are attached to long canes to allow you to reach out-of-the-way areas. These are designed to help deactivate trigger points that often accompany chronic pain conditions.

Rollers. These devices have wooden, metal, or plastic balls to rub over your sore spots. They allow friends to give massages without developing hand fatigue, and they provide sensations you may find relaxing or distracting. Some are intended to be rolled with one hand, some with two, and some are advertised as "hands-free." Others are electrified, offering a variety of vibration speeds and associated sensations.

As you consider the range of massage tools, think about whether you feel capable of gripping a handle and whether a device may be loud, heavy, or cumbersome, as well as the vendor's return policy. As you use these devices, be careful not to overdo it. Too much self-massage, even the most pleasurable, can cause a painful flare-up. In the absence of a professional massage therapist to guide you, use discretion and common sense. As with everything else, start in moderation and track your response.

Chapter 12

Strategies to Shape Your Self-Talk

Let's say that on a day when you feel relatively good, you decide to try an activity you routinely engaged in before developing pain. At first, it feels familiar and fun. You tell yourself with great optimism, "Chronic pain is not going to stop me. I can do this just like I used to!" Later, you disregard physical discomfort with the thought, "I *should* be able to do this!" and press on until the pain becomes too intense to ignore. In light of your earlier enthusiasm and hopefulness, the resultant flare-up feels especially disappointing. Cascades of discouraging thoughts follow:

> "It's too hard. Why bother? I give up."
> "I'll always feel lousy."
> "This stinks. I can't stand it anymore."
> "This pain is destroying my life."

Sound familiar? Let's examine what just happened. Notice how quickly you talked yourself into feeling frustrated, sad, and even hopeless? Negative thoughts can arise quickly and, if left unexamined, can convince us a situation is futile. It is common for people with chronic pain to become overwhelmed with the unpredictability of flare-ups and experience despair. While it is unlikely that any of the above statements reflects the whole picture, negative thoughts can pop up like mushrooms after a rain, making a bad situation worse. You then suffer not only from the physical pain and fatigue but also from the depressing messages you are telling yourself.

Let's say that instead of fighting against or denying the pain as it increases, you approach the activity in a more moderate way, saying to yourself, "I know that when I am optimistic, I'm prone to pushing past my limits. While I may feel frustrated about my limitations, ignoring them makes things worse. Let me take a moment to consider adjustments that might allow me do the activity next time with less risk of a significant flare-up."

Or you might decide to ask yourself whether doing the activity in your customary way is worth the pain. If you decide it is, you can plan for the predicted flare-up: "I know this decision will result in increased pain for three to four days. I'll make sure to keep those days light so I can recuperate."

Or you could remind yourself of your strength and resilience: "While I hate feeling this lousy, I'll know I'll get through this because I always do. And, in the meantime, I will engage in behaviors to increase my comfort."

Notice that these alternatives do not claim the situation is easy. Instead, they put difficulties in context and focus on what remains within your control. Alternative ways of thinking could allow you to stop a downward spiral and consider experiments for next time. Such experiments might include testing the effect of taking medication proactively, limiting the time you spend on the activity (particularly when starting out), taking deliberate rest breaks, or adapting the activity to increase your comfort.

By attuning to what you tell yourself, you can decide to focus on self-talk that helps you generate a more positive and effective coping style. Experiment with basing your self-talk on a knowledgeable and realistic assessment of your situation. You may be thinking:

"But my thoughts just happen—I can't change them"

"I *am* being realistic—chronic pain is awful."

"It doesn't make sense to tell myself something that isn't true."

Although thoughts *are* often automatic, with practice, you *can* change what you say to yourself.

The Power of Self-Talk: Using Data to Transform Your Experience

This process is the crux of cognitive behavioral therapy (CBT), a psychotherapeutic approach with an impressive amount of research showing its effectiveness in improving life with chronic pain. Studies show that by monitoring what we say to ourselves and replacing self-defeating thoughts with more healthful, positive ones, people can significantly improve their well-being.

Everyone is vulnerable to what CBT refers to as "cognitive distortions," such as catastrophizing (one of more than a dozen types of "faulty logic"), in which you escalate or exaggerate the meaning of a minor event or piece of evidence to catastrophic proportions. The power of CBT comes from catching such distortions and correcting them based on evidence. Your personal tracking data play an essential part in this process by enabling you to check emotional reasoning against facts. As described in chapter 18, you can seek the help of a psychotherapist who specializes in CBT. The present chapter describes the process involved in catching and changing negative self-talk so you can also experiment with this on your own:

(1) Practice mindfulness.

The ability to observe what you say to yourself—whether in the moment or in retrospect—involves self-awareness. By turning mindful attention to your thoughts and emotions, you will be in a better position to identify self-talk or associated shifts in your mood or pain level. Be especially attuned to any moments in which you notice your mood turning sour because, more than likely, a negative thought has sprung up. Ask yourself:

- What did I experience just before my mood shifted (or my pain increased)?
- What am I saying to myself about the situation that is making me feel worse?
- How did I respond when I noticed a shift in my mood (or increase in my pain)?
- What am I saying to myself right now?
- How is my breathing? Are my muscles relaxed or clenched?

By slowing down your reaction—such as by taking a few slow, deep breaths—you open up the possibilities to see things differently, which is a necessary part of changing your self-talk.

(2) *Identify automatic thoughts.*

When you start tuning in to your self-talk, you may be surprised by its intensity. Throughout the day, we each experience a barrage of thoughts, often at an unconscious level, that shape our emotions and behaviors. Most often, self-talk occurs as a stream of consciousness without purposive direction. We often respond in seemingly automatic ways to whatever we perceive at that fleeting moment. During any instant, for example, you may be berating or congratulating yourself, fretting about something present or imagined, or deflecting some thoughts while dwelling on others. We are often unaware of the content of what we say to ourselves; yet self-talk affects our attitude, emotions, energy, and behavior. Let's say, for example, that you find yourself feeling angry and bitter shortly after noticing a healthy woman jogging down the street. In the moment between seeing the jogger and the shift in your mood, the following thoughts may have raced through your head: "Look at her. It's not fair. My pain keeps me from being active and carefree like her."

It may well be that you have no idea why you started to feel angry. On a conscious level, you may not even be aware of the message you told yourself in relation to seeing the jogger. We each have a set of mental tapes—based on our history and experience of the world—that provide immediate assessments of a reality that is generally more nuanced and complex. Even if you noticed the thought, it's common to perceive external factors as causing distress—as in, "That jogger put me in a bad mood," when the jogger didn't actually do anything. Your irritation, instead, came from the story of relative injustice that you fed yourself.

Even if you are unaware of the self-talk that may have preceded a significant mood shift, being able to perceive a shift in mood is a great start! When you are aware your mood has changed, rewind your mental tape to pinpoint what you said to yourself. The most dangerous thoughts fall at the ends of a spectrum. Exaggerating the positive can set you up for disappointment, whereas overly negative self-talk can trigger a downward emotional spiral. We each have our "favorite" pessimistic thoughts, such as "I can't stand this," or "I give up," that arise when pain overtakes us, as well as unrealistic optimistic banter that can drive us to overdo it. Be especially mindful of self-talk that is unduly optimistic or negative or contains "should" statements or other judgments.

You can practice checking in with yourself at pivotal moments, such as when you feel particularly good or when you notice an increase in your pain or a shift in mood. By identifying self-talk as "just talk," you diminish its power. Distinguishing thoughts from facts also allows you the distance to view internal banter with a more critical eye.

Become acquainted with your hot-button thoughts. In most cases, negative thoughts travel in bunches and share certain themes, such as an underlying worry that pain will keep you from being happy. Eliminating negative thoughts is an unrealistic goal. Instead, aim to reduce their intensity while increasing the frequency of more positive thoughts. By reminding yourself, "This is the thought that usually gets me upset," you diminish its power. With practice, you can greet recurrent troubling thoughts with, "You again! I know you! You're that thought that pops up when I'm feeling pretty bad and that really messes me up."

Consider assigning labels or nicknames to familiar negative thoughts, such as your "pessimist," "hopeless," or "life generally sucks" thoughts that visit during low spells or your "ignore the facts" thinking that may arise during pain reprieves and cause mayhem. The better acquainted you become with the extremes in your automatic self-talk, the more able you are to disregard or change them. This brings us to the next step.

(3) Analyze the evidence.

Thinking something does not make it true, even when the message feels strong or even overwhelming. Try to step back and calmly formulate specific questions to assess each thought. Ask yourself, "To what extent is this thought supported by data?" Such inquires allow you to table irrational fears until you weigh the evidence. Thoughts at either end of the optimism-pessimism spectrum are typically rooted in emotional reasoning rather than rational deliberation. Bear in mind that your mood can affect your view of the data. Do your best to approach the facts in an unbiased manner.

For example, consider the thought that arose when observing the jogger. Let's assess the validity of the comparison. Does your pain, in fact, keep you from being active? You might instead say, "It is true that I've had to adapt what I do and that pain can make activities more challenging and less pleasant. At the same time, however, I continue to participate in a wide range of activities, including twirling a hula hoop to music." This poses substantial challenges to your initial thought about your inactivity. Next, evaluate the data on whether the jogger is indeed "carefree." You soon realize that you cannot assess the facts, at least not with the superficial data on which the original statement was based. For all you know, the jogger may experience knee or back pain or may have decided to run to relieve emotional suffering. We cannot know other people's experiences simply by observing them, just as our own internal strife remains largely invisible to onlookers. People who observe me smiling and dancing with my large rainbow-colored hula hoop (which I can enjoy for short internals even at my worst) might conclude that I am carefree!

Punching realistic holes into automatic thoughts changes their emotional impact. This entails stepping back, questioning the thoughts, and being intentionally realistic. You may still feel frustrated about the painful flare-up, or you may grieve the fact that you cannot jog the way you did years ago. But these facts are less likely to escalate your emotions in the way your initial snap judgments did.

It is especially powerful to tackle fixed ideas that underlie difficulties. For example, if you feel helpless against the pain, look to your data on your most successful pain-relieving strategies. If you find yourself stuck on the thought "If I cannot control this disease, I am a total failure," locate evidence that demonstrates times you have positively affected your symptoms or seek out other measures of your successes. Use your data to combat negative thoughts and challenge unrealistic, harmful things you may tell yourself.

(4) Generate positive self-talk based on your data.

Once you have shown that specific negative thoughts lack a factual basis, the trick is to replace them with alternative thoughts that are realistic and encourage positive coping. The very same situation can be viewed from multiple perspectives, and you have the ultimate freedom to select your vantage point. Why not select a positive viewpoint and then reframe—or spin—your self-talk in a way that is consistent with the data and resonates with you? This process does not work if you lie to yourself or are unrealistic about the struggles you face. Selecting a positive framework is not about adopting optimistic platitudes, such as "Don't worry! Everything will be fine!" It does no good to sugarcoat difficulties; false hopes only increase your disappointment when life fails to measure up. Nor does it help to exaggerate difficulties; talk that is overly cautious can reduce your motivation and ability to adapt. Instead, strive for self-talk that emphasizes positive aspects in a realistic way.

Context. It is common to generalize from your most immediate emotional state. This partial amnesia makes fluctuations even more difficult. Your tracking tool puts fluctuations in context—and this knowledge is empowering. Armed with such data, you can remind your "down self" during a flare-up that you've been down before, and this, too, will pass. Reflecting on the transitory aspect of your worst times is vital. You can also gain encouragement by reviewing notes from your best days or best moments. If low days are particularly discouraging, make a habit of writing notes to yourself during your best moments to read during your worst, when you could use the supportive pick-me-up and reminder of better times and days.

Comparisons. People often assess their situation through comparison. From an early age, we identify our peer groups and reflect on where we fit in some imagined pecking order. Your perspective, quite literally, determines how you view the world—whether your glass is half full or half empty. Celebrities who refer to other celebrities' sky-high salaries may begrudge a $2 million paycheck, while their prefamous selves would have celebrated a six-figure income! An immigrant who was a successful professional in his home country but now works a backbreaking menial job may feel bitter over his sacrifices or grateful for the future he may offer his children. Perspective depends on the reference group you choose. It is your choice whether to tell yourself something that emphasizes your pride or your disappointment.

It takes only a glimpse of the evening news to remember that no matter how bad you feel, it could be worse. Nobody is immune to bad experiences. Experiment with telling yourself, "Many bad things happen in the world every day; the odds are that some of them will happen to me." Not because of anything that you have done, but because things happen. Keep this in mind as you review your situation. This strategy is not about belittling your circumstances and will not be effective if you berate yourself for struggling. This is not to say that chronic pain is not difficult (it is!), but as you let go of a narrative of self-pity, you may feel better.

Gratefulness. Let's say you sit down for a luscious meal in a beautiful setting and discover your dinner roll is burned. You can decide to let the burned roll ruin the experience, or you can appreciate the view and the bounty of food (and maybe scrape away the burned parts of your roll). Although chronic pain may be dreadful and exhausting, it does not define your entire experience. The surest way to cultivate a negative attitude is focusing on the sources of your discontent and taking the good parts for granted. Whatever challenges you face, your life no doubt includes things to appreciate.

Experiment by consciously considering what you appreciate, and observe the effects this has on your outlook. Look around and remind yourself of the things that bring you pleasure, comfort, and joy. These may be experiences such as being able to step outside and feel the sun on your face; your relationships with the friends and family who have stuck with you; your passions, small pleasures, accomplishments, and sources of comfort; and the many ways that your body *is* working.

So, for example, if you are feeling helpless against the pain, positive self-talk may be: "I recognize that I'm feeling helpless at this moment; however, I also recognize that I'm far from helpless. While this pain is unpleasant, I have many other things in my life I feel grateful about, and slipping into despair over this pain only worsens it. Instead, I will engage in one of the half-dozen things I can do right now to decrease my pain."

(5) Incorporate this process into your life.

As you find yourself successful in observing and altering self-talk to your advantage, consider ways to incorporate this process in your daily life. This involves training yourself to notice the first signs of distress or exaggerated thinking and challenging your thoughts. You also benefit from incorporating helpful self-talk into the way you approach your life. For example, in the morning, you might tell yourself, "I expect to I feel lousy when I wake up, and I know this improves after a hot shower."

Then, continue with deliberate self-talk to note any improvement and to provide positive reinforcement for effective coping: "Yep, I was right! A shower really does help. I'm glad I got up without hesitating."

Treat negative thoughts as signals to encourage positive coping and difficult situations as opportunities to practice self-talk strategies. Viewing your experience as data can itself generate more positive self-talk: "Whatever I experience today will provide important data in my experiment to improve, which I will use in my decisions about the future."

You can't lose with this approach! Throughout your day, use self-talk to remind yourself that you are a work in progress who is continuing to learn and improve. Encourage yourself through tough times by treating them as the important opportunities for experiments that they provide.

Example of Applying Self-Talk

Let's say you are caring for a young child for the afternoon (whether your child or grandchild, the child of a close friend or neighbor, or a paid babysitting job). Staying mindful of your body, you notice your pain rise. The child, too young to comprehend such things, begs to play another physically taxing game, saying: "Please? Please? Please!" What you say to yourself at this point will shape your response and subsequent experience, as illustrated in the table below:

Thought	Process	Likely result
1. It's pathetic that I can't play with this child!	You judge yourself harshly and are at risk of denying your needs.	You continue to play with the child, which results in intense pain. You beat yourself up later for being so pathetic.
2. I know that playing this game will cause a flare-up, but she's only a child!	You are realistic about the consequences of your behavior but feel defeatist.	You play with the child and experience the expected flare-up. You decide you cannot watch this child again, which feels terribly disappointing.
3. I know that playing this game will cause a flare-up, but I believe it is worth it.	You are realistic about the consequences of your behavior and choose to contend with a flare-up.	You play with the child and have the flare-up you predicted but do not experience emotional suffering because you actively chose and predicted this result.
4. If I play this game, I will feel lousy, which does not seem worth it to me. Let me adapt the way we're playing.	You are realistic about the potential consequences and opt for a more flexible approach that will prevent or at least reduce the odds of a flare-up.	You provide the child with several alternative activities, which you can engage in together while lying down. You feel proud of how you handled the situation and do not suffer a flare-up.

In the first scenario, you demonstrate little awareness of your negative self-talk and compare your situation unfavorably with the "shoulds" that pop into your head—what you *should* be doing, what children *should* experience. This leads to a belief that it is your duty to soldier on, which results in a painful flare-up. Judging yourself as "pathetic" for not being able to play with the child, you continue to berate yourself. Plus, if you do not challenge your initial negative thought, it is more likely to intensify and grow. You may compound your suffering by concluding that you are an unfit caregiver (or parent or grandparent), and, if you are feeling especially down, that you are worthless. While this may sound extreme, it is easy to slip down the slope to demoralization. The trick is to notice the first sign of negative thinking—the "this is pathetic" red flag—and combat it with evidence to the contrary before additional negative thoughts influence your mood and behavior.

In the second scenario, you realistically predict the consequences of playing the game, but you fail to see any alternatives. Instead, you treat the situation as beyond your control, and your ensuing flare-up reinforces feelings of helplessness.

In the third scenario, you acknowledge that engaging in the game will incite a flare-up, but you take responsibility for your choice. By identifying your ability to choose a response, you can decide whether to engage in the behavior, despite its consequences, or to search for alternatives. Because you choose to engage with full knowledge, you are ready with self talk to handle the expected flare-up, and it does not feel distressing. You might later tell yourself: "This is the pain I expected, even chose, for myself, which I know will pass." You can decide to choose pain without additional suffering or regret.

The fourth scenario offers the best outcome. This option becomes accessible when you take a step back to consider your assumptions and choices. Most often, there is room for flexibility. In this example, instead of agreeing to play the game, you seek alternatives that can provide satisfaction for the child without added discomfort for you. Figuring out how to do this is easiest with a calm mind. Here are some examples:

- Gently inform the child that you need to rest for a certain amount of time. Children do not need to be able to tell time to absorb this concept. You can explain that you'll be ready after they draw four pictures, listen to six songs on a DVD, watch a television show or video, or finish another specified activity.

- Invite the child to rest during this time too. Make sure to use the break to restore yourself with meditation; slow, deep breaths; lying down with your feet up; or whatever works for you. After this restorative period, you will be in a position to reconsider the child's request.
- Offer the child alternative activities that would allow you physical downtime in a comfy space. You can read a book together, close your eyes and tell a story, or engage in a restful game, such as sending the child in search of items you specify as a sort of scavenger hunt, or other imaginary pursuit.

The key is the ability to combat negative self-talk, such as, "I should be able . . ." or, "A good mother would . . ." with realistic, helpful talk such as, "The child and I will both benefit from my feeling good. It makes sense to consider ways to provide love and attention that allow me to be comfortable too."

This example happens to involve a young child; however, interactions with adults take place in much the same way. We are likely to encounter situations with adults in which we benefit from requesting a time-out or change in conditions or venue. Regardless of people's age or the intimacy of the relationship, it is unrealistic to expect others to read our minds or anticipate our needs. Sometimes the greatest obstacle you may face in making a request is your own negative self-talk. The ability to ask for what you need in order to thrive (or survive) begins with self-awareness and what you tell yourself about your value, your needs, and the consequences of your choices. If you observe yourself feeling helpless in a situation with others, examine your thoughts. More than likely, you are telling yourself something that interferes with positive adaptation to your circumstances.

Revisiting Self-Talk

Let's revisit the scenario in which you pushed yourself too hard on account of enthusiasm over a cherished activity, which resulted in a surprising and demoralizing flare-up and downward spiral of negative statements. One of the beauties of self-talk is that it is never too late to tinker with your narrative. Even when you've started down a negative path, constructive self-talk can supply hope and open up possibilities. No matter how mindful you may be of your self-talk, we all have moments when we find ourselves exceptionally pessimistic. Therefore, it is important to be able to talk yourself back up from dark places.

It is unfortunately common for people in pain to entertain at least one of the negative statements listed at the start of this chapter at some time or other. With practice, you can evaluate defeatist messages and set yourself back on track. Let's consider each in turn, examining how you might go about shifting your vantage point with deliberate self-talk. The first step is to recognize the negative thought as a thought and not a fact, thereby making it malleable.

"It is too hard. Why bother? I give up."

Start by engaging in a dialogue with this thought: "OK, I realize that I am very disappointed. But, whoa! Look how my thoughts moved at warp speed to the dejected idea of 'giving up.' First of all, I am not sure what it means to 'give up.' I know I like this activity and that I am not ready to toss in the towel. I also know from my experience (recorded with my own hand) that I have succeeded in participating in other activities when I have adjusted them. When I apply my mind and my tracking tool to the task, I'll likely figure this out."

By considering your past experiences, you're likely to conclude that you have little data to support giving up. Instead, you'll likely recognize that as you have with other activities, you'll be able to adapt. However, given your current level of frustration and physical pain, you also realize that this is not the time for creative brainstorming and once you feel better, you'll have lots to explore. Or, alternatively, you may focus on what you can do when you experience this sort of "out-of-control" feeling. Then later, when you are feeling comfortable, you can contemplate strategies to test the next time, such as taking medication proactively, limiting the time spent on the activity (particularly when starting out), taking rest breaks at set intervals, and adapting the activity to increase your comfort.

"I always feel lousy!"

When this thought raises its ugly head, remind yourself that when you feel your worst, it's easy to slip into an "I always feel lousy" mentality. This is the time to look to your tracking data for a realistic alternative set of thoughts, such as: "I feel lousy right now, but I also know that I don't always feel this way. In fact, this is the first time in ten days that my pain reached this level. Judging from previous flare-ups, I can predict that this pain will not last more than a few hours, and its aftereffects should completely resolve within days. I can speed up the recovery process by engaging in gentle stretches, water exercise, or massage, or by relaxing in a hot bath. I'll consider which is most feasible for me right now."

When you get stuck in an "awfulizing" mentality, look through your tracking data at the likely fluctuations you experience. It's a common mistake to minimize your better moments when you feel overwhelmed by difficulties, just as you may be prone to distancing yourself from any thoughts about pain at your best (and most invincible). Beware these extremes, since neither is realistic and both can generate difficulties (by exaggerating your suffering or making you vulnerable to disappointment). Use self-talk based on your tracking data to provide context to your experience.

"This stinks. I can't stand it anymore."

This response reflects a substantial leap in logic—from feeling frustrated to concluding that you can no longer tolerate any difficulty. Here you can ask yourself, "What is the evidence that I can't stand it anymore?"

More than likely, your tracking history demonstrates that you have endured harder circumstances. You may then remind yourself, "No matter how awful this feels, I've withstood worse. In fact, I have plenty of evidence that I am a strong and resourceful person, and while I greatly dislike feeling lousy, I'll get through this episode."

By recognizing a situation as unpleasant but survivable, you can turn your attention to ways to improve the moment. In light of this, you could reframe your thoughts as follows: "I recognize that this pain is hard to endure, but if I take advantage of ways to make myself feel better right now, I can decrease the pain."

Notice that this alternative does not claim the situation is easy. Instead, it puts negative feelings in context and accepts the reality of the situation, which then allows the focus to shift to ways to feel better.

"This pain is destroying my life."

Here again, negative emotions have snowballed to gigantic or catastrophic proportions. Self-talk can rein this in by considering the larger picture and reflecting on things you appreciate and are able to do, despite pain. You can consider uplifting alternatives, such as: "The pain is present but does not control my life or have the power to destroy it; only I can do that. There are many other aspects of my life I find rewarding and enriching—I am much more than this medical condition."

Notice that in all these cases, the reframing does not make light of problems. This process emphasizes the places in which you can see yourself as the agent of change. This is powerful.

How Self-Talk Works

Chronic pain is difficult, depressing, and anxiety producing. By identifying destructive self-talk, evaluating it with available data, and replacing it with more positive messages that promote healthful coping, you can achieve three key goals:

Break cycles. When you feel lousy, it is hard to make sense of your experience and find a balanced perspective. It takes additional effort not to heed your automatic thoughts, which are likely to be disproportionately pessimistic. The greater your pain, the more frazzled you may feel, making it additionally difficult to contend with hardships. Deliberate self-talk can interrupt downward cycles and provide sensible, reassuring encouragement and coping strategies to calm your mind and body. These operate in cycles, too; beneficial thoughts, emotions, and behaviors positively reinforce each other.

Relearn. Even the most stable and steadfast of lives can be derailed by chronic pain. Coping requires incredible adaptive skills, which are made easier when accompanied with encouraging self-talk. Informed self-talk can remind you of the power of strategies you have found helpful, particularly when they feel counterintuitive or exhausting or when you are otherwise not inclined to respond in positive ways: "Even though I feel like staying in bed, I know from past experience that dragging myself up and into the shower, especially a long, hot one, will help me feel better. Life will start to look more appealing to me."

Knowing what works and routinely reminding yourself of this is an effective use of self-talk. At your worst, you may struggle most to take action. Use your tracking data to create a voice that can serve as your personal cheerleader.

Increase control. The randomness of chronic pain is particularly demoralizing—one minute you feel OK, and the next, as though you were flattened by a tank or pierced by an arrow. Research shows that people who report that they have little control over their symptoms also report greater pain and fatigue. By staying on top of your thoughts and responses, you can gain a sense of control in your life.

Increase positive emotions. In her book *Positivity*, Barbara Fredrickson presents substantial evidence from decades of research on the far-reaching effects of positive emotions.[1] But rather than trying to eliminate the negative (an unrealistic goal), she reports that change occurs when people succeed in increasing their ratio of positive to negative emotions (ideally, at least three to one). Moreover, she emphasizes that positive emotions are more than "feeling happy"; they also include feelings like serenity, contentment, pleasure, love, comfort, gratitude, and calmness. By shaping your self-talk, you can increase the pleasure in your life and, by extension, your general well-being. Research also suggests that when people experience positive emotions, natural opioid painkillers are released into the system.[2] Positive emotions may offer strong medicine without the risk of side effects!

New Narratives of Self

Sometimes self-talk is not just about getting through difficult moments, but also about creating a new self-narrative. Chronic pain can alter how you see yourself, including your view of your health, heartiness, abilities, and worth. The more tightly you hang on to your old self, however, the more likely you are to emphasize your identity in terms of loss—such as seeing yourself as a failed musician when you can no longer play the piano due to arthritis. Discovering the "new you" is less about letting go of a former self-conception than about integrating the old and new. Reflect on what you value most in your old self and seek to incorporate these aspects in the new you, in the way former athletes remake themselves as coaches or sportscasters. You may find your musician self emerging as you listen and appreciate music, teach or lecture on music, or cultivate your singing voice.

Creating a new self requires flexibility, patience, and creativity. The more your identity was based on a notion of invincibility, the harder change may be to accept. Explore the stories you are telling yourself, noting areas of inflexibility such as, "If I can't do it the old way, I won't do it at all!" or exaggerations about your former abilities—as if you never required sleep or felt bad and were immune to sickness and aging.

Allow yourself to mourn the losses that come with new limits. But, at the same time, keep in mind that you are a complex individual; no one quality, characteristic, or aspect can define you. However reluctantly, you have likely experienced personal growth as a result of your experiences with pain. As you re-create a new, valuable self, reflect on any ways you may have improved upon who you used to be. You might even consider the possibility of a silver lining: "In some ways, believe it or not, living with pain has enriched my life. It has increased my empathy for others who suffer and caused me to slow down and focus on what really matters. (Don't get me wrong—I'd rid myself of pain in a heartbeat if I could.)" As Arthur Frank describes in *The Wounded Storyteller*, as people with illness find meaning in their experiences, they undergo positive transformations. Some common gains include a new appreciation for life, deeper insight and empathy for others, and greater focus on what people value most in life.[3]

Separate "being" from "doing." Part of the difficulty in adapting to your identity is the emphasis on defining who you are by what you do. Yet what makes you "you" is separate from your accomplishments. That Western society tends to emphasize doing over being compounds the difficulties of physical limitations. I have noticed during memorial services, however, that people often reflect more on the personal qualities of the deceased than on their achievements, even when the list is substantial. Were they kind, patient, and loving? Were they an agreeable friend, a devoted parent or partner, a generous listener? Did they make people in their life feel valued? Treat chronic pain as an opportunity to reflect on the kind of person you'd like to be.

Cultivate a Sense of Humor

Humor extends beyond laughing at jokes to an entire life perspective. Finding humor in difficult circumstances is a tremendous strength. Borrowing from Max Eastman, "Humor is the instinct for taking pain playfully." By seeking humor, you can make difficult and painful things lighter, even laughable. Practice telling yourself something funny about your situation, and be open to a comedic view. Part of humor's strength is the willingness to think creatively and to consider different vantage points. This requires mental flexibility as well as comedic distance, which together can reduce the intensity of the situation and shift your perspective. Humor also offers the chance for emotional release, joy, and laughter. Experiment with ways to cultivate a viewpoint that offers these advantages.

Affirmations

Affirmations are pithy, positive statements you can say to yourself in key moments. The trick is to find statements that resonate with you (and do not feel false). Consider aspects of situations that emphasize your strengths, remind you of what you are most grateful for, credit your struggles, instill pride, or place your difficulties into context. Effective affirmations must be something you *believe.* The following may be useful:

> *I can do this.*
> *I am incredibly strong—look what I can endure.*
> *I can focus on the positive in my life.* (and do)
> *Three slow, deep breaths.* (and take them)
> *I managed yesterday, I'll manage today.*
> *I will feel better if I _____.*
> *I know how to help myself.*
> *There is beauty all around me!* (and notice it)
> *It's only pain.*
> *I'll feel better soon.* (and have in mind what you will do)
> *I see outside myself.* (and look around)
> *I have the tools for this.* (and use them)

When you find an affirmation that works for you, use it. Post it where you often look—the refrigerator door, the computer screen, your wallet, the car dashboard, your medicine cabinet, or selected walls. Or collect affirmations on slips of paper, and when you need to boost your psyche, dip into your affirmation jar.

Chapter 13

Strategies to Pace Yourself

Much literature on chronic pain emphasizes the need to "pace your-self." These two little words depict a simple concept yet a formidable challenge. No doubt you are familiar with the problem of "overdoing it"—a concept that's defined in hindsight while you're nursing your pains. People with chronic pain often grapple with a tension between their desire to partici-pate and their need to take sufficient care of themselves. When your capabili-ties can shift day to day, even moment to moment, calculating your optimal balance of rest and activity is challenging. Moreover, what felt good one moment may cause disabling pain the next:

"Sometimes I feel pretty good, and then—boom! I'm knocked on my ear."
"Pace myself? Huh, I'm moving slow as molasses and I still hurt!"

Sound familiar? The uncertainty of chronic pain makes it especially difficult to chart a course that doesn't incite pain but isn't painfully slow. Pushing too hard intensifies pain, causing frustrating setbacks. Yet too much caution risks that you will miss out on activities that can enrich your life. Pacing is not synony-mous with cutting back. It is about making the most of your energy.

Successful pacing comes from observing what has worked for you (and what hasn't) and conducting deliberate experiments to discover just how much is too much, which activities drain, and which rejuvenate. Use your tracking tool to address relevant questions, such as:

- What are my most able periods of the day?
- How long do my best periods last?

- What happens if I continue beyond that time? Do I "pay for it" the rest of the day, or am I able to recover more quickly by engaging in particular activities?
- What happens when I take breaks? Does this produce energetic periods later?
- What kinds of activities allow me to lengthen my more able periods?
- What kind of downtime is most restorative? Are there particular practices that are most restorative?
- How is this affected by the frequency and length of rest periods?

What you learn helps you identify the middle ground between overachieving and underachieving, as well as when to push and when to pamper yourself.

You may discover that something as simple as setting a timer to remind yourself to take a stretching break increases your stamina, or that five minutes of slow, deep breaths in a comfortable position restores your energy or lowers your pain. You may decide to commit to rest breaks before you join friends for the evening or tackle the next project. Or you may find late-night moments of peace to be your most productive times. And you can discover that partaking in certain activities, despite pain and exhaustion, results in satisfaction and greater (not less) energy and comfort. The more you learn about your body's responses, the more confident you become about when to push through the pain and when to pull back on the reins.

But even when you have fairly reliable data on how your body will likely respond, it can still be challenging to pace yourself when it feels counterintuitive. Effective pacing often involves the ability to hold back even when you feel good or great (lest you overdo it), to read and heed early warning signs to slow down (before you "hit the wall"), and to resist your instinct to opt out when you feel lousy (so that inactivity does not exacerbate pain). This chapter provides tips on pacing choices that may feel opposite to your current emotional and physical state.

How to Jump-Start Yourself When You Feel Low

We all have times when we feel like crawling in bed and doing nothing. However, this is never feasible for very long, and it falls short as a strategy for living.

I have yet to hear from anyone who is suffering from chronic pain or depression—two conditions that understandably create a strong urge to lie low—that staying in bed for a full day or more has improved their ability or mood. While recharging your battery is essential, putting up your feet too often worsens how you feel physically and emotionally. The less you do, the less you can do.

Sometimes, like a car with a low battery, we need a way to jump-start our engine. Pain or not, we have things to do and places to go. When pain and exhaustion feel overwhelming, you may benefit from sitting out until you can gather energy. Yet engagement in life can itself improve how you feel. Sometimes you actually gain energy by exerting yourself, as long as you also incorporate well-placed rest breaks.

Peruse your data for times when you were under stress *and* managed to accomplish something special. In retrospect, you may wonder, "How did I do that?" Contemplate the occasions when you have tapped into an inner energy reserve and turned your day around. When we need to, we can rise to herculean heights. I remember well when my children were infants: no matter how drained I felt, a baby's cry never failed to jump-start me into action. Somewhere tucked away is a seemingly endless supply of fuel just in case you really need it. Of course, constantly pushing is neither sustainable nor wise, as it leads to the dreaded downward spiral. Still, it is helpful to remember that you can rally as needed, and this fuel can supply a solid boost.

Experiment with deliberately jump-starting yourself when you are feeling low, then evaluate the result. When similar conditions arise, you will be knowledgeable about the best way to respond. But even when you understand from past experience that a push is just what you need, it can be difficult to get started. Consider the following techniques when you lack that "get up and go" feeling but know from past experience that a jump-start would be beneficial.

External Jump-Starters

Motivation may come more easily when you are prompted by an external source. Immediate obligations, such as a job or young children, may force you into action. If you are employed, you may find that even when mornings greet you with fire or sledgehammers, you somehow find yourself in the shower, dressing for work, and walking out your door. You may be able to rise nearly automatically like a robot (perhaps a rusty one!), without contemplation, when choice is limited and you have little time to dwell on your pains.

I was not surprised to find in a research report that people who stay employed despite chronic pain tend to fare better than those who stop working.[1] Of course, such findings may be biased because, by definition, people who stay employed may be less disabled than those no longer able to work. Still, something else may be in play. Having a reason to push can lift your spirits and remove your focus from aches and pains. (This is not to downplay the difficulties of working when you are in pain—you may have had to contemplate significant changes in the way you work, as will be discussed in chapters 21 and 22.) However, when work conditions are agreeable—such as having flexible hours, a comfortable space, low stress, varied tasks, and accommodation for rest breaks—employment can improve overall functioning.

Unpaid obligations can similarly serve as motivators. These can include volunteer opportunities you may have taken on, an active social schedule, or involvement in valued activities. Taking care of young children, an ill partner, aging parents, or beloved pets can also spur people into action. Involvement with others often shifts focus and energy away from your difficulties. When you take on the role of primary caregiver, be mindful, as described later in chapter 25, that you do not prioritize others' needs to the detriment of your own.

Conversely, when little is expected of you, you are more likely to dwell on aches and pains, which may, in turn, become more disabling. Even when discontinuing work has come as a welcomed change, you may not find the physical relief you anticipated. Reduced work demands may decrease pain but are unlikely to make it disappear. Pain seems to have a property similar to that of smoke trapped in a box: it tends to fill whatever size container we put it in. So even when you feel only half as bad (or twice as good), pain can continue to present challenges. When you face a long stretch of day with nothing planned, pain can have a way of filling up the space. Experiment and see if you feel better during the times when you locate the gumption to engage in something, particularly something that feels meaningful or enjoyable or fosters a sense of accomplishment.

Internal Jump-Starters

Whatever the demands of life, we all face times with limitless options for the day (or week). As the French existential philosopher Jean-Paul Sartre astutely stated, "We are condemned to be free." The more unstructured time we have, then, the more we rely on our own inner drive. With enormous pain and little in the way of plans, it can be a huge struggle to do anything at all.

When my pain first began, I spent months waiting for a pain reprieve, dreaming of the many things I would do as soon as I felt better. I was under the impression that I had sustained an injury that would heal with time. But, unfortunately, waiting only increased my misery. As time went on, I felt worse both physically and emotionally. During that time, I happened upon a news story about a local artist with a chronic pain condition, and her comments made an impression on me. In a quote running next to a photograph of her inspiring sculptures, she confided that she would never create anything if she only worked when she felt good. These words have stayed with me. I took them as a call to find an internal jump-start for my life.

Your Life to Live

Even trite clichés can be powerful to ponder. Try this one: "You only live once." Think about it. This is it. At the end of your life, what is it that you hope to have accomplished? Chronic pain can help you cut to the chase. For any given day, what really matters most to you? What if you had a short time each day when you felt great? How would you spend it? Would you indulge in something pleasurable, be present with someone special, or engage in a meaningful act? Your response may reveal where to focus your energy.

While you may not have a moment when you feel terrific, with planning and determination, we can all have moments when we feel good enough. By jump-starting yourself, you can engage in meaningful endeavors and feel better for it. Moreover, when you are fully engaged, pain really can retreat to a back burner. Test and see what activities provide sufficient distraction or pleasure to send pain in retreat. Plus, as you learn from your experiments, you can increase the time that you feel good.

Altruistic acts. Taking on responsibility for others can be a huge motivator. If you do not have immediate family in need of assistance, consider volunteer opportunities that appeal to you. While it may seem counterintuitive to give when you yourself are struggling, such altruistic acts can operate paradoxically and improve how you feel. We sometimes become so wrapped up in our own private suffering that we become isolated. You may mistakenly think of your suffering as unique or your struggles as inordinate. Moving outside yourself and offering assistance to others in need can broaden your perspective and allow you to forget your own difficulties for a while. Even if an hour a week is as much as you can manage, you may find that volunteer activities provide a powerful, even transformative, experience. They can remind you of the positive things you take for granted and boost your self-esteem by demonstrating that despite limitations, you can contribute in a meaningful way to others.

Envision the act. Instead of fretting about what you can't do, imagine engaging in a desired activity. Lie down or sit in a comfortable position and contemplate how you would begin. For example, if you want to write, use downtime to organize preliminary thoughts. If you want to cook, reflect on the ingredients and recipe. If you have errands to run, envision where you would go. As you do this, consider the optimal conditions for yourself, including the environment that would be most conducive to your comfort. This mental image can help jump-start you into actually doing it. Just as a high diver gains confidence by first visualizing the dive while standing at the edge of the board, picturing yourself successfully completing the task can serve as a jump-start into the task. Contemplation is itself an act of engagement, and when you take this mental step, subsequent steps can build on the momentum and require less energy.

You may be thinking, "But I've tried this. Imagining the activity tends to increase my stress and wear me out, not jump-start me." Instead of allowing yourself to be overwhelmed by the many things you'd like or need to do, narrow your focus to a specific task. Then divide the project into even smaller, more manageable pieces. Focus on starting the task or working on one small piece of it, rather than imagining every aspect needed to finish it. Later, if you have additional energy, you can contemplate the next piece, or you may decide to reflect on your accomplishments thus far.

Taking the first step. As comic and filmmaker Woody Allen once said, "Eighty percent of life is just showing up." Sometimes "just showing up" is hard work. It can involve preparations, transportation, and having to face and interact with others—all difficult tasks when you feel crummy. An alternate strategy to envisioning the task is *not to think* and, instead, start moving toward the first tiny step necessary to get ready. Let's say you are aware that swimming in the morning helps you feel better, but each morning you awake too exhausted to contemplate going to the pool. Rather than dwelling on this impasse, focus only on putting on your swimsuit. This manageable act may provide sufficient momentum to propel you forward. Then, without giving it much thought, take the next step, and put a towel in your gym bag. Continue, step by step, and before you know it, you may find yourself in the water.

Set deadlines. Many of us respond differently when we feel a sense of immediacy. Even when you value a task, event, or activity, it can be easy to postpone when it is not pressing. Therefore, if you want to make sure you follow through—whether for your job, social life, family, or personal pleasure—set a reasonable deadline for the first step. Then, continue to create deadlines for each subsequent part. If a deadline becomes unrealistic, modify it until it becomes achievable. And, each time you meet a deadline, celebrate!

Schedule fun dates. Social plans can feel risky. When you feel lousy, it can be difficult to imagine anything as being pleasurable. Such reluctance, however, prevents you from spending time with the people and things you enjoy. And, as it turns out (especially when you are mindful of your comfort), you are likely to feel better for your efforts. Experiment to discover the activities that improve your well-being.

Early on in my own experiments, I would log my expectations as I set out for an evening with friends, such as by noting, "I do not feel up to this." I soon found that about four times out of five, I had a marvelous time and stayed much later than planned. When it comes to social activity, be selective. Limit your plans, as much as possible, to people and events you thoroughly enjoy. Scheduling plans you can count on for fun provides an effective jump-start. Read your local newspapers (or go online) to find worthy events and mark your calendar. Buy tickets in advance to stay committed. In most cases, you'll be glad you did!

Savor your time. Chronic pain can make you focus on what matters most, careful not to squander your precious time and energy. We each have certain "windows of opportunity" in which we feel our best. Choose carefully how you fill your windows, and savor them. The smaller your windows, the more valuable they become. Tell yourself, "If this is the only thing I do today, I will feel happy." Deliberately plan to make your best periods satisfying. And make deliberate plans that help you savor your recuperative periods as well.

Think long-term. At different points, we tend to reflect on our life thus far. Upon reflection, it may well be that you remember pain and fatigue. However, it is also likely that the days that felt significant despite discomfort stand out in your mind. Ask yourself, "At the end of this week, month, year, or decade, what would it mean to have lived successfully?" Decide what matters most—your relationships, paid work, personal projects—and incorporate these, as you can, into your daily life. Keep the larger picture in sight; at the end of the day (or week or year), you will come out ahead.

Pick the project. Give some thought to the activities that would most compel you into action. Writing to a dear friend, getting up on time for work, tackling a piece of an ongoing project, folding a load of laundry, making headway at work, staying out of bed during the day, throwing a dinner party, or running errands can all represent goals that challenge your abilities and provide feelings of satisfaction. Sometimes it works best to focus on the most important or pressing item and start on it before you run out of steam. Other times, it helps to begin with the easiest one. And when you feel particularly run-down, favorite activities may jump-start you into action. Pick what works for you.

Pain expenditures. From pain springs life. Consider that childbirth involves exquisite pain with a monumental outcome. Judging from the number of people in the world, billions of women must have judged labor pain to be worthwhile. For many of us, intense pain is a daily reality. Just as you think about how you want to spend your time or money, you face the decision of how to allocate your pain. It is your choice what seems worthy of a "pain expenditure." You can face this rationally with a pain budget, just as you would for other expenditures. Elect the activities that would be most worthy of the risk of a pain flare-up. At times, you may decide it is worthwhile to accomplish something, even if it guarantees additional pain. Activities that are "worthy of pain" are sure jump-starts.

Prepare for down periods. When you are at a low point, it can be difficult to imagine things otherwise. Part of this may come from cognitive changes that occur when you are sad or depressed. Pathbreaking research by Barbara Fredrickson and her colleagues in psychology at the University of North Carolina at Chapel Hill shows that negative emotions decrease our ability to think expansively or creatively or to problem solve—making it that much harder to help yourself need help. Devise strategies when you are in decent spirits that you can use when you're not.

Plan after-care. When you can predict that a certain activity or event, such as sitting through a meeting, exercising, or visiting family, will increase pain, be deliberate in planning after-care. An evening out becomes less stressful when you can expect to follow it up with a soothing retreat, such as a hot bath. When facing a particularly demanding week, include a midweek massage or other restorative treat. The promise of pampering makes pain easier to accept. Make the restorative time an integral part of your schedule and not just an option "if I have time." Test the effect of deliberate downtime with your favorite music, curling up in bed with an audiobook, rejuvenating yourself with a heating pad, dunking in a hot tub, or whatever helps sustain you.

Morning movers. Many of us can expect to awake feeling lousy. Mornings are a time of high pain for many pain conditions. Anticipate this and be ready with your morning jump-starts. These may be a daily mantra, such as, "Hot shower, here I come," or keeping effective pain medication at your bedside along with a cup of water.

Contemplative breaks. Whenever you would benefit from contemplation, create a comfortable space for yourself to slow down and reflect. Before embarking on a project, I often curl up in bed or on my hammock and think it through step by step. It may seem counterintuitive to use rest as a way to begin an activity. But contemplative breaks can remove you from the chaotic "frazzled" feeling that often accompanies discomfort. As you feel calmer and can think more clearly, it becomes easier to embark on the next step. Contemplative breaks also let your fantasies reign. Instead of dwelling on what your body is *not* doing, treat rest periods as indulgent moments. In your mental playground, you can practice dance steps (for there will be times you can dance!). You can think through dilemmas and priorities, analyze a recent movie, say prayers, or mentally write a letter to a friend. Experiment with what helps lift your spirits during purposive breaks.

These jump-start strategies overlap and can be used in tandem. With chronic pain, we do not have the luxury of postponing things until we feel great. Most days will have pain—some more, some less. Jump-start strategies help you to engage in life, rather than waiting for an idyllic pain-free moment that may never arrive. Reviewing your tracking sheets also reinforces the value of motivating yourself—particularly when you feel lousy—to engage in behaviors that improve how you feel.

Finish Things before They Finish You

Pacing is all about balance. In addition to being able to jump-start yourself as needed, you also need to be able to slow down to thwart or reduce pain flare-ups. Effective pacing incorporates activity and rest and may allow you, eventually, to do nearly everything you want, albeit at an adjusted pace.

I just can't seem to get enough done! Your well-being is likely to affect your ambition. On bad days, you may be too busy licking wounds to fret about what you are missing, but the better you feel, the more your ambitions can soar. During times when pain is low, you may envision a busy, productive day, only to find partway through it that you feel awful and need to stop. This can be very frustrating. Keep in mind that working toward ambitious plans requires long-term strategies and patience. Over time, I have succeeded (for the most part) in accepting my pace for what it is, while continuing to strive for more. Keep in mind that even the healthiest people struggle to find time to do all the things they want. The trick is to juggle your desires and capabilities. Plus, you can still enjoy and cherish feelings of optimism, however ephemeral, that spring up in your best moments and inspire you toward your dreams. Consider the following strategies when you find that your drive is overwhelming your capabilities.

Adjust the list. At the end of each day or week, if more items remain on your list than you could cross off, rethink your expectations. Decide what you value most and assign it first priority. Then, evaluate the feasibility of the other items—are they above and beyond reasonable expectations? Consider the advice of a ten-year-old who usually accomplishes everything on his daily list: "Use short paper and write big." While there's nothing inherently wrong with striving to do more, it is a problem to find yourself continually frustrated or postponing high-priority tasks while trying to finish less important ones. Devoting even just a few minutes toward your goals every day adds up. Sometimes getting through the day is an appropriate goal in and of itself. On such days, give yourself credit just for getting through it.

Give yourself a break. Experiment to discover when enough is enough, and then factor in break time just as you would activity. Discover whether you do best by taking frequent short breaks or by pushing through the first half of a day and spending the remainder resting on your laurels. Of course, we do not always have control over our schedule. You may be working, taking care of others, or both. But whatever your schedule may be, plan recuperative downtime. As you push yourself, take comfort in knowing you will benefit from stopping, propping up your feet, and giving yourself a break. It is much preferable to take a planned break than to cry out in desperation for a rest. With adequate rest stops, a second or even a third wind may follow.

Cultivate flexibility. Responding to pain, especially unanticipated pain, requires flexibility. Experiment with ways to pace yourself to the fluctuating conditions of the day. Consider the day in increments. As you move through each phase, assess whether you can continue or would benefit more from a recuperative break. Proceed with what you think will bring the best result, and observe what happens. Continue to negotiate your day without either giving up or overdoing. When you feel telltale signs of an imminent flare-up, instead of calling it a day, try an alternative task. Alternating tasks can be sustaining. For example, when your cognitive skills are fading, switch to a mindless physical task. Or, if your body needs a rest, use a hands-free phone to catch up on calls. Try moving around in ways that revitalize tired, achy muscles. When changing gears does not do the trick, give yourself a spontaneous break—without beating yourself up over it.

Have a plan B. Many paths lead to the same goal. If you become fixated on plan A, you may lose sight of any alternatives. It is best to establish a plan B so you can continue to participate even if plan A goes down the tubes. When others are involved, your attitude can be significant. Instead of pouting that your plans didn't work out, simply explain, "I had to take a shortcut, and this worked better for me." In general, it's a good policy to emphasize what you *can* accomplish, rather than dwelling on what you can't. Try to embrace plan B in a positive light by telling yourself, "Good for me for being flexible!" This may generate a better overall feeling than had you remained feeling stuck and frustrated.

Normalize your situation. It is easy to fall victim to wishful thinking and tell yourself, "If only I felt better, this would be easy." While this may well be true, dwelling on it doesn't help. Pain cannot be wished away, and fixating on a fantasy can become disabling. Rather than focusing on the unfairness of chronic pain, try to "normalize" your situation and move on. In other words, tell yourself, "This is normal for me these days—it may be slower than I'd like, but for now, this is how I do things." This attitude allows you to accept your current circumstances and then move forward. The reality of life is that many people have to adapt to a great variety of obstacles and hardships. The more you can treat adaptations as part of life, rather than lamenting their injustices, the happier you will feel. Find a mantra that reinforces this message, such as, "This is what works best for me." Say it and believe it. If you have trouble believing it, try the "fake it 'til you make it" approach—and say it anyway until it helps.

An acquaintance with chronic pain recently shared with me her strategy to program her computer to prompt her to take breaks at intervals for relaxation exercises. While she was clearly proud of her innovation, for a moment, her expression changed as she said dejectedly, "This is what I have to do just to sit at my desk!" We exchanged a "That's life" shrug and smile. While this may not be her preferred way to work, it is what works for now. By accepting this as normal, she is more content, comfortable, and productive as a result.

Letting Things Go

There are times when despite your best efforts, you'll have to let things go. You may have discovered you cannot do it all, at least not without incurring terrible pain. Even when you scale back considerably, the risk of overdoing it never strays too far and can rear its head with speed and tenacity. Also, unforeseen events and circumstances can upend your plans, no matter how effective your pacing strategy. At times, everybody has to face the reality that it is time to let go. Deciding when and what to cut back can be difficult, especially when complicated by emotions such as disappointment, frustration, guilt, and shame. Paradoxically, letting go can be most difficult when we feel relatively well and our limits are less apparent. Often, the hardest part is figuring out when to lighten the load. Once the decision is made, and you accept it, it can bring tremendous relief. Use the following to help sort out when it makes sense to relinquish a valued activity:

How important is this to others? It feels bad to let down people who are counting on you. Yet, in your own dismay, you may exaggerate the impact and loss on others. Rather than guessing how others may feel about the importance of a given activity or task, ask them directly. If you learn that others are less invested than you assumed, it becomes easier to devise alternate plans. This reduces feelings of guilt and lets you reevaluate the importance of the activity to you. However, if you learn that others are invested in the project and want you to stick to the original plan, at least you have concrete feedback to consider. Your next step would be to consider exactly what they want or expect and how adaptable they may be to an alternative plan (and what such a plan might look like). Keep in mind that disappointing others is an inevitable part of life, chronic pain or not! Information about others' needs and desires is a key factor in making sensible decisions. But before negotiating with anyone else, create an environment for yourself that feels comfortable and calm, and contemplate the remaining questions:

What does it mean to me? Identify the meaning you may have attached to the activity or task. Assess the role of the project on your finances, sense of self, or whatever other realm seems relevant. Stay particularly alert to any judgmental beliefs you may have, such as, "If I don't finish this project as planned, I am a failure." This brings us to the next question:

How realistic am I being? Sometimes what we say to ourselves is more judgmental than our circumstances warrant. Check any worrisome thoughts against reality, and evaluate the magnitude of your feelings in relation to what seems realistic. (See chapter 12.)

What costs would be involved? Weigh the costs of carrying out an activity against the costs of forgoing it. What sacrifices would you have to make to accomplish the task in question? Would you have to neglect other pressing activities or relationships? To what extent would you be setting yourself up for a flare-up? Consider the repercussions of a decision not to follow through with the project or activity.

What alternatives are available? Most decisions we face are not all-or-nothing. Try to explore the gray in between. There are many options for socializing with friends, for example, that fall between cooking for thirty and opting for life as a hermit. You might decide to invite over a few friends for drinks and dessert. This would provide the benefit of relaxed conversation and social engagement without overtaxing you. Expand your thinking. Ask yourself if you might be overlooking doable options, such as participating in something for part of the time, requesting assistance, or changing the day or schedule to a more accommodating time.

Can I make this positive? Whenever possible, seek out the silver lining. If you decide to opt out of an activity, explore potential benefits. By freeing your schedule, for example, you may be able to engage in valued self-care, which not only feels good but also increases the odds you will be up for something else soon. Whatever you may be giving up, brainstorm to discover at least one benefit that may not be immediately apparent.

Forgive yourself! With chronic illness comes certain disappointments. But feeling bad about feeling bad only adds to your suffering. Don't be hard on yourself as well. Nobody would choose to feel lousy, and beating yourself up over it only makes you feel worse. Consider, instead, a supportive mantra such as "This is what my body allowed me to do today" or "It is important that I take care of myself." Or you might focus on what you have been able to accomplish: "Good for me. Look what I was able to achieve!" Just as you deserve to celebrate all accomplishments, great and modest, praise yourself when you are able to let something go. Letting go can be difficult. Let yourself experience the relief of a lightened load, the triumph of having come to a decision, and the joy of valuing your well-being enough to give yourself a break.

Aim at something doable.
Chip away at it at regular intervals.
When you need a rest, give yourself a break.
And when you accomplish something, give yourself credit!

I have used all these pacing strategies liberally in my efforts to finish this book. No doubt it would have been much easier for me if I did not contend with pain and could sit for hours at the keyboard. Instead, I adopted a flexible approach, which sometimes involved working in five-minute intervals and other times setting the work aside for days, even months. On other occasions, I was able to lose myself (and my pain) for long stretches in the creative process. Given the challenges, I've celebrated the completion of paragraphs, pages, and chapters. Had it not been for the pain, the project may have been easier, but the accomplishment would not have been as sweet.

Chapter 14

Strategies to Improve Your Sleep

"Sleep on it" is prudent advice when it comes to important decisions. Sleep can dramatically alter your perspective and well-being. Common wisdom holds that an average adult requires approximately eight hours of sleep each night for optimal functioning, slightly less in later years, and more during younger ones. With chronic pain, achieving quality sleep is especially vital but additionally challenging. The relationship between sleep and well-being operates in a cyclical nature: restorative sleep reduces your vulnerability to pain, which allows for better sleep; poor sleep increases pain, which further disrupts sleep. Inadequate sleep also increases people's vulnerability to emotional logic, diminishing their capacity to contend with pain and the difficulties that often arise with it. Yet people with chronic pain are less likely to achieve a solid eight hours, and with pain conditions like rheumatoid arthritis or fibromyalgia, they may awake unrefreshed even when they do. The key is to identify your sleep/rest needs and how to best achieve them. Experimenting to improve your experience with sleep is crucial to improvement.

Establish Bedtime Routines and Rituals

Baby-advice literature brims with suggestions about creating quieting rhythms and routines to lull youngsters to sleep. For nurtured children, the time preceding bed may involve a relaxing routine such as a warm bath, a glass of milk, book reading, and cuddling before an affectionate tucking into bed. Adults, however, may pay less attention to their own winding-down process and simply collapse, exhausted, at the end of the day, hoping for sleep to overtake them.

Unfortunately, this is not always successful. As adults, we have more on our minds, which can prohibit a peaceful transition to sleep. On top of this, physical pains can significantly interfere with comfort and sleep. Adults may benefit from takeaway lessons from the "lullaby industry."

Baby yourself! Think about easing into sleep as a process, and experiment with what helps. It's easier to sleep when you are physically comfortable; even minor pains can interfere. Experiment with ways to develop a sleep-conducive feeling in the hours preceding bed. It may help to avoid mentally challenging or stimulating activities, such as provocative conversations or exercise, and, instead, indulge in a pleasant, relaxing activity, such as a hot bath, gentle stretching, meditation, light reading, or other ways to unwind from your day. Follow this up with relaxing bedtime treats—a hot water bottle or rice bag on your pillow, calming music, sensual touch—and you can turn bedtime into a retreat.

Promote a restful mind. Worry thoughts tend to expand in the later hours. If you suffer from an active mind, explore strategies, rituals, or rules to prevent thoughts from thwarting slumber. Consider the advice to limit your bedroom activities to sleep, relaxation, and intimacy. For example, refrain from talk about work or worrisome topics after an allotted evening hour. If you suffer from a busy mind, it may also help to write out a to-do list or worry list before bedtime. Abstract worries tend to produce more anxiety than concrete ones. The act of recording your thoughts may allow you to release them so they do not float free in your mind, where they can disturb sleep. You can then relax more easily, secure in the knowledge the list will be there in the morning when you are more ready to tackle it. Try other strategies (described in more detail in chapters 10 and 11), such as meditation; slow, deep breaths; self-hypnosis; guided imagery; and progressive muscle relaxation, that you may find helpful in promoting a relaxed body and mind.

Attend to the "tired moment." It is more restful to fall asleep quickly than to lie in bed waiting, watching the clock. Attend to your body's signals. As you engage in your nightly rituals, note when you feel a "tired moment," or urge to sleep. For those taking nighttime medication, this may occur at a predictable interval after you take your pills. Test the timing of medication and entrance into bed to find what works best for a good night's sleep. Plan your evening so you are ready to lie down at the first sign of sleep readiness, rather than squandering this feeling on brushing teeth, changing into sleep clothes, and so on. Experiment and find your optimal bedtime.

Create a restful environment. Treat your bedroom as a sacred environment. Close your eyes and imagine your perfect sleep space—perhaps a comfortable bed in a room that is quiet, dark, and neither too warm nor too cold. Then, compare your ideal with the room where you now sleep, and think about what it would take to bridge the gap between your ideal and your reality. Sometimes you can alter the environment itself. Other times, the most effective approach is to change the way you perceive the environment. Consider:

- *Light.* If you crave darkness, hang darkening blinds to block the light from entering your room, or wear eyeshades so that you perceive the room as dark. Or you may want to "set your clock" each morning by allowing a flood of natural light to enter your window.
- *Sound.* The variation in noise level can be more disruptive to sleep than the sounds themselves. Because in most cases you cannot alter the noise around you—city traffic sounds, a snoring partner, house sounds, or a wooded area that comes alive early in the morning—consider strategies to reduce its disturbing effects, such as wearing earplugs, using a white noise or other sound machine, or running a fan. When possible, test the noise level of appliances while in the store.
- *Temperature.* If you can control your thermostat, maintain the room at a comfortable temperature range. If not, improvise. You might adapt to a cold room with a plush duvet or comforter and to a warm room with crisp cotton linens. Experiment with layering—covers that feel right as you fall asleep may feel too warm as the night goes on.
- *Humidity.* Air that is too dry can interfere with sleep. Saline sprays or Vaseline can soothe nasal passages. Humidifiers and indoor tabletop fountains also work double duty: they alleviate dryness and provide a steady sound to block out random noises.
- *Your dream bed.* Don't be misled by advertisements for "orthopedic" or "medically approved" mattresses (no requirements are needed to use such terms). Before committing to a particular sleep system—whether a water bed, memory foam, or a more traditional bed—conduct sufficient research. Most stores do not allow returns, so make sure it feels right. Certain stores do make an exception to this rule and offer promotions, such as a "one-hundred-day guarantee," in which you can exchange or return your bed for a full refund. When available, this is ideal because it

provides a true test. If the stores in your areas do not offer this, don't be shy about lying down in mattress stores long enough for a realistic test; bring in your favorite pillow if they do not carry similar ones. One store clerk invited me to "nap all afternoon" if it would help my decision. And, if you cannot afford a new bed right now, experiment with low-budget ways to upgrade your current system, such as adding a sheet of eggcrate foam on top and a bed board underneath.

- *Your dream pillow.* Having a pillow that is comfortable and supportive is as important as a good mattress. Pillows range in their filling, shape, intended position, and the way they contour around specific areas. Some are advertised as ergonomic. Some are specifically designed for side sleepers to place between their knees, or under their lower back, or supporting their upper arm. Full-length pillows, often recommended for pregnant women, cradle the body. Some pillows are marketed for jaw pain, low back pain, cervical pain, arthritis, and a variety of other pain conditions. This specificity, however, is no guarantee; experiment to find your ideal arrangement. You may find that you prefer a makeshift placement of several flat pillows positioned just so or a rolled-up towel supporting your neck. Let your data, not the hype, determine what belongs on your bed.
- *Sleep position and location.* The position in which you fall asleep can determine how you feel the next day. I know that I pay dearly when I fall asleep watching television rather than in my now-perfected pillow arrangement. At times, it may take extra effort to position yourself, particularly when you are tired. Experiment to see whether it is worth the effort.

Sleeping with Others

Additional considerations arise when you share your bed. You may have a restless or noisy bed partner, or young children or affectionate pets making their way into your bed.

Sleep partner. If you have a partner who snores, earplugs may be sufficient. Keep in mind that earplugs vary in their effectiveness and comfort; so don't despair if the first pair doesn't suit you. Encouraging your partner to explore the cause of his or her snoring may benefit you both. If you or your partner wake each other, it may be worthwhile to invest in a king-size bed, or push together two twins, to allow closeness and sleep. Weigh what works best for you and the relationship. When feasible, it may be helpful to have a second comfortable place to sleep that you can use as needed.

Young children. During a baby's first few months of life, sleep disruption is inevitable. Parents benefit from following "sleep when the baby sleeps" advice and sharing the burden of care with others, as possible. Fortunately, children outgrow their need for nighttime care. If you are routinely awakened during the night by young children, consult the ample literature on ways to improve their sleep. Children can learn to read a clock at surprisingly young ages—especially digital clocks. Instruct young children on when they are permitted to wake you up (and when they are not!). Create morning rituals that foster independence and keep them safe so you can rest peacefully. For example, stock a lower kitchen cabinet with breakfast foods and instruct them on how to help themselves.

Pets. Animal lovers who want to share their lair with pets face a personal cost-benefit calculation. Determine the extent to which visits from your pets at particular hours enhance or detract from your well-being. If you want to reduce nocturnal visits, explore behavioral training methods. You can also insulate yourself from unwanted noises and limit their access to late-night and early-morning visits.

Awaking during the Night

Nighttime awakenings can undermine sleep quality. If you experience these, investigate the source of your sleep disturbances. You may have to conduct experiments with a host of areas of your life to enhance sleep quality. Consider your sleep environment (noise, temperature, comfort), exercise, pacing, diet (including stimulants and what you last eat before bed), and factors that may affect your stress level.

If awakenings continue to be a problem (and there is a normal increase as you age), your focus may become how to return to sleep as promptly and easily as possible. Medical wisdom tends to advocate getting up and doing something unexciting rather than staying in bed, particularly if you feel anxious. However, for people with chronic pain, it may make more sense to rest if you feel sufficiently comfortable. Experiment with relaxation exercises such as meditation, diaphragmatic breathing, or imagery to foster deep relaxation (described in chapters 10 and 11). If physical discomfort is the reason you awake, address this. For a rare occurrence, a hot shower may do the trick; however, middle-of-the-night showers as a rule would be disruptive. If pain continues to wake you and interfere with your ability to return to sleep, talk with your physician about medication.

Medication for Sleep

Sleep medications are discussed in chapter 17. To help your doctor consider what may be most effective, consider the following:

- Do you have trouble falling asleep?
- When do you tend to get your best sleep?
- How often do you awake during the night?
- When you awake at night, are you able to return to sleep?
    o If yes, how long does this take?
    o What do you typically do when you awake?
    o How do you tend to feel?

This information will help your doctor determine what to recommend.

To Nap or Not to Nap

For most people who suffer from insomnia or sleep trouble, it is generally advised to eliminate daytime naps. The logic is that while skipping a nap may be difficult at first, it's better to reserve nighttime for your best sleep. This advice may be generally helpful, but it is not universal. Some people with chronic pain may find nighttime sleep to be insufficient and require naps or rest breaks at intervals throughout the day. Depending on your schedule, you may benefit from additional downtime. Test your situation, and adjust as appropriate.

Treat Any Sleep Disorders

Finally, consider whether a sleep disorder may be aggravating your symptoms. When you suffer from a chronic condition, it is easy to attribute *everything* to that condition, even when a symptom may reflect something else. Talk with your doctor about any other experiences you may have that interfere with your sleep, such as frequent urination. Two common sleep problems are obstructive sleep apnea and periodic limb movements (or restless leg syndrome). People with sleep apnea tend to snore loudly and have periodic pauses in breathing, followed by a snort as they begin to breathe again. People with restless leg syndrome tend to jerk or kick their legs during the night. In both cases, sufferers may be unaware of any problem until their partner complains. If you have a bedmate, ask about any loud, sudden snores or frequent kicks. If so, talk to your doctor. Treating sleep disorders will improve symptoms of pain, fatigue, and fogginess; moreover, if untreated, sleep apnea can be dangerous.

Chapter 15

Strategies to Exercise More Effectively

"Y ou can have weak muscles that hurt or strong muscles that hurt."
These words—spoken by Dr. Norman Rosen, a physician with
chronic pain himself who was the first doctor to make significant inroads in my
care—have made a lasting impression on me. While exercise may not be curative, it can increase your stamina, strength, and overall well-being. Range-of-
motion, strengthening, and aerobic exercise are advocated for nearly every pain
condition. The Mayo Clinic, for example, encourages strengthening and fitness in people with arthritis to reduce joint pain, improve sleep, combat
fatigue, and enhance self-esteem. The Spondylitis Association of America
advocates exercise for maintaining good posture and flexibility, which can help
lessen the pain of this degenerative spinal condition. Studies also report
decreased pain from appropriate aerobic conditioning in people with lupus,
rheumatoid arthritis, fibromyalgia, and reflex sympathetic dystrophy, among
most other systemic syndromes. Specific exercises can also lessen the frequency
and severity of low back pain, knee pain, sciatica, migraines, jaw pain, and
other regional syndromes. Moreover, exercise increases quality of life by
keeping muscles stronger and more flexible, helping to control weight, and
increasing energy, all of which enable you to be more active. Exercise can also
have a profound positive impact on mental health.

For pain sufferers, however, exercise presents a paradox: despite its significant benefits, exercise can feel impossible when you are exhausted or suffer
from stiff joints, shooting pains in your legs or lower back, or a myriad of other
difficulties that can undermine even the most modest athletic pursuits. Getting
up and moving may feel like the exact opposite of what you should be doing.
Your previous attempts to exercise may have been unsuccessful, resulting in

increased suffering. Perhaps, like me, you fluctuated between pushing too hard and giving up. Yet getting up and moving will help you feel better—if not immediately, then over time. Lack of movement generally makes stiff muscles stiffer and more painful. Plus, atrophied muscles and supportive tissue further increase pain and disability.

How can I exercise while I'm struggling with debilitating pain and exhaustion? Despite the challenges involved, exercise and fitness are possible. The trick is to approach exercise in a deliberate fashion, guided by the data you collect. This chapter describes strategies and options to consider in building a successful exercise program. But before you begin, consult with your physician about any precautions specific to your condition, age, and health. See what you are cleared to try, and then use the suggestions in this chapter and your personal tracking tool to devise a rewarding routine.

Approaching Exercise and Fitness

With chronic pain, exercise can be complicated. Knowing that "exercise matters" does not prepare you for how to proceed. You may have to motivate yourself to try something you fear and, at the same time, remain vigilant in your efforts to avoid overdoing it. With some pain conditions, seemingly negligible exertions can elicit severe reactions. But do not despair. Whatever your circumstances, there is something you *can* do without exacerbating your pain—and doing something far exceeds doing nothing! Furthermore, by determining and then sticking to what works, you will increase your capacity and abilities. The following tips will help you develop, increase, and sustain an exercise program:

Start slow and build up. There's no such thing as too slow. One of the biggest missteps is doing too much too soon. If you have not exercised for some time, your muscles may be weak and easily traumatized. Start small. Use your PAINTRACKING tool to determine what your body tolerates, then gradually increase the duration, frequency, or intensity. If you increase in accordance with your body's responses, you can achieve a challenging and rewarding exercise program.

For eager beavers who want to jump in and test their limits, consider this: A central goal of exercise is sustainability; you want to be able to exercise frequently. It's also more encouraging to increase your exertions than to have to scale them back, repeatedly. Plus, when it comes to adding something to your schedule, a smaller commitment may be easier. We all have reasons we may not be able to commit to a one-hour workout, but how about one minute of movement? No joke. At your worst, a minute a day may be what you can tolerate without increasing your pain, at least at first. Then, if you proceed like the tortoise, slow and steady, you can build up until you achieve a substantial workout.

This "start slow" advice especially pertains to anyone who has not been exercising, has been experiencing prohibitive pain responses to exercise, or has other difficulties achieving a sustainable exercise program. If you are already successfully engaged in an exercise program, keep it up!

No pain, yes gain. Forget the "no pain, no gain" mantra. Pushing through pain or to extreme fatigue is likely to result in flare-ups and end your enthusiasm for exercise. Instead, adjust as needed, noting any discomfort during your workout as well as afterward. Exercise that might cause a tolerable level of post-exertion soreness in someone else may lead to more prolonged and intense pain for chronic pain sufferers. So, take it easy. Pain operates in a cyclical fashion. When workouts make you feel worse, you can keep yourself in a heightened state of pain.

Patience, patience. The pace required to build a sustainable exercise program (without painful flare-ups) requires endurance and faith. Patience can be especially challenging for athletic individuals. When I first read about the helpfulness of exercise, I literally tried to exercise the pain out of my body. While I bounced on a Stairmaster®, endorphins helped me feel invincible. Hours afterward, however, the pain was excruciating. My life became divided between intense workouts and sheer agony, and, not surprisingly, I began to question the helpfulness of exercise and my ability to engage in it. It was not until I cut back to between one and five minutes of exercise that I could exercise without increased pain. Slowly, I worked up to an hour-long workout (which I have maintained for years) without any ill effects by sticking to my tracking data. When I have experienced a setback (such as from run-of-the-mill illnesses and injuries, minor car accidents, pregnancy, or surgery), I have been able to readjust, knowing that with time, I'll be able to resume my more substantial workout.

So, shore up your patience. It may require greater strength and discipline to work within your current abilities than to push ahead. Take pride in your ability to hold the reins and proceed slowly. Your patience will be rewarded with that glorious sweaty level of exertion, without the physical and emotional backlash that comes from overdoing it.

Relax. Tensed muscles tend to be more painful. During exercise, relax your body as much as possible. Some exercise is more conducive to relaxation; swaying to reggae music or moving in the water can loosen muscles and elevate your mood. But whatever you choose, mentally scan your body for places where you may be tensing while exercising. Some common culprits are jaws and shoulders. As you identify tight spots, focus on ways to relax them. While walking or jogging, for example, let your arms swing freely by your side, rather than keeping them rigid or balling your hands into tight fists. When using exercise equipment, use a loose grip whenever possible. If you are taking an exercise class, you may have to do things a little differently. If a tight grip causes pain, you might opt out of segments with barbells or engage in the exercises without weights—or, alternatively, invest in a set of strap-on weights.

Schedule it in. We benefit most from regular exercise. Consider what fits your schedule. This could be a minimal routine you can repeat several times a day wherever you are, or you may prefer scheduled workout days. Exercising first thing in the morning may reduce stiffness and aches; mid-afternoon movement can ward off the doldrums and recharge your battery; exercising in the evening can offer a way to end the day with a boost. When exercise is incorporated into your routine, it becomes easier to maintain.

Understandably, your motivation can plummet when you feel your worst—but don't let bad days derail your program. Review your data to remind yourself of what works. This is especially important when you don't feel like exercising, even when you know it would help. Remind yourself, when you want to choose bed over the gym, of the rejuvenating effect of a twenty-minute visit to the pool. Devise strategies to ease the transition, such as packing your gym bag ahead of time or making plans to exercise with a friend. As you recognize the benefits of your exercise program, awaking in pain can become a signal for exercise rather than a reason to lie low.

Before and after. Even healthy people can develop soreness after exertion. Evaluate your data to determine an acceptable level of soreness and strategies to reduce it. Experiment with warm-up and warm-down routines, the timing of your medication, and soothing postexercise activities. You may discover you feel your best for some period following exercise. Pumping endorphins and loosened muscles may generate a pain reprieve and increased energy. If so, calculate how long this tends to last so that you can take full advantage of this time.

Modify. It's best to ignore typical guidelines about how you *should* exercise and to instead do what is supported by your personal data. Treating exercise instructions as suggestions rather than directives opens up a wide range of activities you can try, such as aerobics, yoga, hiking, Pilates, jogging, biking, and even weight training. Avoid competing with others or some imagined sense of what you *should* be doing. Adapt exercise advice, classes, coaching, and equipment to meet your circumstances, even classes that may be geared to "your category," such as water aerobics for people with arthritis or rehabilitation exercise classes. Physical therapists can help you with modifications and review whether you are doing specific exercises effectively. But pace yourself based on what works for you.

Build a new intuition. When in doubt, heed your records rather than your body when deciding how hard to push or when to hold back. Stiff joints when you begin exercise may seem like a reason to stop, yet you may discover that the stiffness subsides with movement. Aerobic exercise may feel wonderful in the moment but incite a flare-up later that day. This approach will enable you to establish a zone within which you can engage in beneficial exercise, despite initial stiffness or fatigue, while avoiding painful flare-ups. As you internalize information from your records, you develop a new intuition about your body's signs and messages.

Recognize your choices. While starting slowly and adapting to avoid flare-ups is generally effective for chronic pain, it may not fit your priorities. The goal of PAINTRACKING is not to avoid pain, but to be able to make informed choices. It is up to you whether something is worth the pain. You might choose to join friends for a challenging bike ride or play tennis with your sons, regardless of the predictable flare-up that will follow. Use your PAINTRACKING tool to find the balance of activity, exercise, and rest that provides you with the greatest satisfaction. A sustainable exercise schedule for you may be light exercise on a daily basis or two mornings a week of strenuous exercise followed by restorative time, or it may include occasional plans to push harder.

Addressing setbacks. Even the most well-crafted, stable exercise plans will involve setbacks. Exercise is only one factor that affects how you feel, making your response somewhat unpredictable. At times, exercise will deplete you. You may be able to figure out the conditions under which this occurs by reviewing your data. It is important to accept a certain amount of unpredictability. At times, you may require more downtime than expected. This, too, is data; test the effectiveness of your response to unexpected pain. Your approach can keep such events from ruining your day.

Fitness Goals

Whatever your unique personal fitness goals, consider the following: (1) cardiovascular fitness, (2) flexibility, and (3) muscle strength.

Cardiovascular Fitness

Aerobic fitness is universally beneficial: it strengthens your heart, improves blood circulation, enables your organs to work more efficiently, and promotes physical and emotional wellness. This is particularly important for people who live with pain. Abundant research demonstrates that aerobic exercise can decrease pain, improve sleep and stamina, and enhance overall well-being.[1] Part of this comes from stimulating endorphins, the body's natural painkiller. You do not have to be a marathon runner to experience a "runner's high." Engaging in any cardiovascular exercise releases endorphins and other chemicals with morphinelike properties into your bloodstream that relieve pain and elevate your mood.

You achieve cardiovascular fitness by engaging in exercise that works your heart, or is "aerobic." Aerobic exercise does not require that you feel out of breath or winded, or that you push yourself that hard. In fact, the more out of shape you are, the easier it is to raise your heart rate—a consolation when you may have gone some time without exercising. To determine when exercise reaches an aerobic level, monitor your pulse. According to the American College of Sports Medicine, the training effect of aerobic exercise takes place between 60 and 90 percent of your maximum heart rate (calculated as 220 minus your age). So, for example, if you are twenty years old, exercise begins to be aerobic when your pulse reaches 120 beats per minute. (At thirty, it begins at 114; at forty, it begins at 108; at fifty, it begins at 102; and so on.) Experiment and see what it takes for your heart rate to reach 60 percent of your maximum. As your body acclimates to exercise, you'll be able to tolerate greater exertions before you note an increase in your heart rate. This is a sign of increased physical fitness.

What kind of exercise raises your heart rate? Whatever gets you moving! Popular cardiovascular activities for people with pain are water exercise and walking, but don't feel restricted to these. Exercise is a lifelong commitment; select activities you enjoy and look forward to, not dread. Dance, walk, cycle, swim, do yoga, exercise to a video or game, or twirl about in the water. Make your workouts more pleasurable by listening to music or an audiobook or inviting a friend to join you. Try to choose activities that are convenient and involve minimal hassle. As exercise becomes part of your routine, you are more likely to crave it. In the beginning, you may have to "fake it 'til you make it." But over time, you will likely appreciate the way exercise makes you feel, and you'll miss it when you have to skip a workout.

Water exercise. Many people with chronic pain enjoy exercising in water. Its buoyancy alleviates pressure from muscles and joints and allows many movements that would be unthinkable on land. Pool exercise offers a supportive environment for stretching, cardiovascular, range-of-motion, and strengthening exercises, regardless of your balance or fragility. Options include swimming, walking or jogging, and aqua aerobics. Water aerobics classes have become quite popular, and health clubs offer many varieties. Most classes include a warm-up, stretches, and a cool-down phase, along with an aerobic and/or strength-training component. The Arthritis Foundation created a program, offered through many local gyms, that gently activates each muscle group. Don't be deceived by what may look lightweight or by the demographics of participants. Stripped of the harsh effects of gravity's pull, aqua aerobics can seem deceptively easy. However, water provides tremendous resistance. Start modestly and increase as your tracking data advise.

Water fitness classes can be conducted in shallow or deep water (or both) and may be gentle (such as classes designed for people with arthritis or in rehabilitation from surgery or an injury) or fairly intense cardio challenges. In deep water, exercises are typically done with the added buoyancy of a foam "noodle," belt, or other device to keep you afloat; in shallow water, you stand on the pool floor, which provides some weight-bearing benefit. Keep in mind, however, that water exercise is generally not considered weight bearing, which means that it does not help maintain bone density. When possible, alternate between water exercise and weight-bearing land exercise.

Walking. Walking is a weight-bearing exercise that can done anywhere. Don't underestimate its benefits. Walking keeps leg muscles strong, strengthens postural muscles of the stomach and back, and increases endurance. Experiment with walking as a means of transportation; when possible, choose meeting places with friends or colleagues within walking distance. Walking outside can provide an enjoyable respite, particularly if you have access to a nature path, an interesting neighborhood, or a social opportunity with a friend or organized walking group. For colder months, consider joining a gym or even strolling briskly at your local indoor mall.

When walking, experiment with your posture. You may benefit from swinging your arms freely or keeping a tucked-in tummy until it becomes second nature. Tracking your exertions is easy—mark the distance by landmarks, laps around a track, a specialized application on your smartphone, or the numbers on a treadmill. Treadmills offer the bonus of being able to manipulate distance, speed, and incline; some even measure heart rate. You can experiment with incline and pacing and see, for example, whether walking on a steeper incline at a leisurely pace allows you to increase your heart rate without stressing your body. Test what works best for you.

Exercise machines. Aerobic exercise machines simulate activities such as climbing stairs, running (and without the impact), bicycling (in various positions), skiing, and rowing. From a data standpoint, exercise machines allow you to standardize your workout and increase or decrease the intensity at precise intervals. Gyms and health spas stock a variety of equipment, such as a machine that simulates swimming and the elliptical trainer, which simulates jogging with little impact because your feet are firmly planted on ample pedals. After more than a decade in which I was unable to run or jog, I marveled at the sensation of impact-free running. If you are considering investing in an aerobic exercise machine for a home gym, test it out first to make sure you like it enough to use it regularly. No need to end up with a fancy towel rack to remind you of a failed exercise scheme.

Exercise classes. The advantages of class are companionship, a fixed schedule (which you can build into your week), and the motivation that comes from commitment. The selection can be vast. Depending where you live, classes may be available in yoga, African dance, cycling, martial arts, Zumba®, Jazzercise®, kickboxing, and Pilates, among others. You might be thinking, "But I can't do that!" Keep in mind, however, that you can amend as needed. If you would enjoy a particular class, approach it creatively. It can take courage to advocate for yourself in a class and deviate from what others are doing. You may worry about how you appear compared with others or the message this may convey. If you have such concerns, talk with the instructor. Briefly explain that you have a pain condition and need to adapt some exercises or may sit out occasionally. The instructor should not take offense at this, and many instructors will offer helpful alternatives for you to try. If you suffer from a competitive streak, reserve your comparison for yourself from day to day and week to week. Cheer yourself on for what you are able to accomplish!

You can check with relevant organizations, support groups, and medical professionals in your area about exercise classes for people with chronic pain or related problems. Or consider taking a "virtual class" in the comfort of your home by using exercise audiotapes, videos, or simulation games.

Because chronic pains fluctuate dramatically, you may benefit from having more than one type of aerobic exercise. Injuries, flare-ups, and weather conditions can also disrupt your plans. When leg pain interferes with walking, snap on a buoyancy belt and walk laps at the local pool. When you have to miss a workout, look forward to your next one. Cut back as needed, and, by all means, resist the urge to double up for any missed sessions—a surefire recipe for a flare-up.

Flexibility

Tight muscles make for more painful muscles. When people have pain, they often compensate by favoring certain muscles over others, which leads to increased stiffness and restriction. Stretching can lengthen muscles and soft tissues. Stretching can be more than a prelude to a workout; when you experience pain, stretching can offer a fundamental act of kindness to aching muscles. You can also stretch as a way to recuperate during breaks from static activities, such as sitting at the keyboard. Experiment with ways that stretching can reduce your pain, stiffness, stress on joints, limitations of movement, and muscle soreness.

Much information is available on how to stretch. Books and websites demonstrate various stretching routines for specific conditions such as low back pain, TMJ, sciatica, and other painful conditions. There are stretches designed for nearly every part of your body, from your neck and wrists to your ankles. Most gyms have charts illustrating general stretches for general wellness. Talk with your doctor, physical therapist, or other appropriate healthcare team member about stretches that are right for you, including any restrictions you may have, such as following surgery. You can also gain guidance on stretches from professionals such as yoga instructors, physical therapists, and personal trainers. Keep in mind, however, that you know your body, limits, and strengths better than anyone. Consider the following guidelines when stretching:

Stretching should not hurt! If it does, you are pushing too hard. Effective stretching does not require pushing yourself. Stretch only up to the point of mild tension, not pain.

Monitor how your body feels. Stretching tight muscles should feel good, even relieving. Don't stretch farther than is comfortable or force your body into difficult positions, or you are liable to strain or tear a muscle.

Stretch while warm. The best time to increase your flexibility is when your muscles are warm and supple, such as immediately after a hot shower or cardiovascular workout. Cold muscles are more vulnerable to injury.

Move slowly. Stretching should feel gentle, even peaceful. Do not rush. Try to approach a stretch as if you are moving in slow motion. This will ensure that you don't move too fast or in a sudden or jerky manner, which could lead to injury. Stretching is an opportunity to quiet your mind and attend to your breath, as in yoga. You may choose to accompany your stretching with soft music.

Hold the stretch. Move into stretches slowly and avoid bouncing, which can tear muscles. Hold your stretch long enough to allow your muscles and joints to become loose (about twenty seconds). If it feels good, repeat.

Maintain balance. Because muscle groups are interrelated, make sure to stretch related muscles and on alternate sides. If you are stretching your neck to the left, for example, make sure that you also stretch it to the right for approximately the same amount of time.

Range of motion. Incorporate movements that take your joints through their regular range of motion, such as raising your arms over your head or rolling your shoulders forward and back. These gentle exercises can be done as frequently as feels right to you.

Breathe! Be mindful that you are not holding your breath while stretching. To get the most out of a stretch, relax and breathe slowly and diaphragmatically, filling your belly, not your chest. Inhale slowly and deeply before each stretch, then exhale into the stretch. As you exhale, you can allow your stretch to elongate. Then relax, hold the stretch in position, and breathe.

Try this stretch to demonstrate the role of breath. (Do not try this if you have any difficulty standing or are unable to bend your waist, back, or neck.)

- Stand up and bend slightly at your waist. Allow your head and arms to hang down toward your toes, but do not reach for your toes or try to touch them. Just let your arms dangle and your neck relax. This should feel neutral or good. Refrain from any deliberate stretching. You should not experience areas of tightness, such as in your calves. If you do, start over, bending more minimally.
- Take a slow, deep breath, in and out. Allow your belly to inflate and deflate.
- Next, inhale deeply, and then, as you exhale, allow the top half of your body to lower very slightly. This should feel natural, not forced. In fact, you may notice that you are lowering your arms, shoulders, or head somewhat automatically on the exhale.
- Continue to breathe, focusing on your exhale as the time to relax and allow your muscles to stretch. You may notice your shoulders relaxing downward, your head and neck lowering, or your spine gently curving with each exhale.
- Continue until you experience a mild sign of tension in your body. Hold yourself in this position for several breaths. Then, slowly and gently return to standing.

Notice that your exhaled breath (with the help of gravity) seemed to move your body farther into the stretch. By focusing on your breath, proceeding slowly, and gently elongating your stretch as you exhale, you can slowly increase a stretch without hurting yourself.

If you discover positive effects of stretching, consider ways to incorporate it into your routine. Stretching can be done from many positions—seated, lying down, standing, or buoyant in the water—providing multiple options.

- You may welcome early-morning stretches while still in a warm bed or following a hot shower as a way to start off your day more limber.
- You might include stretching as a component of your aerobic workouts or as restorative breaks throughout your day.
- You might decide to take a class that focuses on flexibility and range of motion.

- You may find that specific stretches alleviate or prevent muscle spasms or other significant symptoms.
- Or you may find stretching to be a source of pleasure, even if it does not appear to provide lasting relief.

Before concluding that stretching is unhelpful, consult with a trusted specialist to make sure that you are engaging in the most effective stretches for your particular situation and that your technique is sound.

Muscle Strength

However counterintuitive it may seem, strength training can be very effective in reducing pain. A substantial body of research shows its beneficial effects on low back pain, osteoarthritis, rheumatoid arthritis, fibromyalgia, neck pain, and other painful conditions.[2] Studies on women with neck pain suggest that strength training can result in greater and even more prolonged relief than other forms of exercise.[3] Strong muscles enhance your capabilities and endurance—meaning you can do more with less effort, whether it's climbing stairs, lifting an infant, or toting books or groceries. Strengthening core stabilization muscles decreases musculoskeletal pain by strengthening muscles that support your joints. It also shores up your bones, boosts your stamina, and allows you to keep or increase your muscle mass and strength, which otherwise decrease with age. Muscles that are weak or atrophied are more vulnerable to injury, fatigue, and increased pain.

Yet, when you hurt, strength training may seem unappealing or unrealistic. The theory behind building strength is to overload the musculoskeletal system, which may sound severe when your system already feels overloaded. Living with pain is effortful; you may crave gentleness rather than additional muscle load. Plus, you may think weight training is the domain of able-bodied young men who grunt as they heave enormous barbells with their enormous muscles. However, increasing your strength is not synonymous with "bodybuilding" or "bulking up." You can approach strengthening gradually and progressively in ways that are safe and effective regardless of your age, physique, or health.

Strength-training programs run the gamut from simple setups for home or office use to more elaborate gym-based routines. Options for equipment are similarly vast, including household items (such as soup cans), free weights (small barbells or dumbbells), weight machines for circuit training, strength and tone classes (such as Pilates), products that provide resistance (such as rubbery physical therapy bands), and the resistance from your own body (as in calisthenics) or the water (as in pool exercise). Designing your ideal program depends on your goals; preferences; condition; and any vulnerability you may have, such as inflammation, joint instability, or a surgical history. Make sure to consult with your healthcare professional before embarking on a strengthening program.

The central goals are to devise a routine that targets your most important areas, maximizes your efforts, and follows appropriate form to avoid injury. Guidance from physical therapists can be particularly helpful in getting started. Plus, there's a whole industry to make strength training accessible—use it! Seek guidance from books, trained fitness professionals, or classes where the instructor can check your form as you learn. Make sure that anyone who assists you understands your situation. You may have to explain that you have to proceed more cautiously, with lighter weights or more gradual increases than the "average" person. Do not give in to pressure. No matter how much expertise a trainer may have, set your pace in accordance with your individual data.

In order to create a sustainable program, consider your lifestyle. Are you interested in a program you can do anywhere? Or do you want to incorporate a strength component into your existing cardiovascular workouts at the gym? By working with a physical therapist or other knowledgeable professional, you can devise a personalized routine to strengthen core muscles and the ones that are most essential to your functioning. Strengthening exercises do not require a great time investment but do require regularity. Here are some ideas to consider:

The "minimal gadgetry, in minutes, wherever" workout. Calisthenics —push-ups, abdominal crunches, squats, various arm and leg lifts—require no equipment and can be done anywhere, anytime. Do not underestimate the power of seemingly simple exercises, including some you can do while seated or lying down. You may be surprised by the extent to which certain small movements can recruit your muscles; done properly, for example, pelvic tilts, or gently raising alternate arms and legs while lying facedown, can require significant exertion. As you advance, you might include simple resistance products that can be pulled, stretched, squeezed, or bent. Colorful lightweight elastic tubing or bands, which provide resistance when stretched, are commonly used in physical therapy and are available in most sporting goods stores, along with other resistant exercisers. Consider a schedule that fits yours; this may be a short morning or evening routine, along with your stretches, or a couple times a week following your aerobic exercises. You may also find exercises that fit in with your daily activities—such as leg lifts while at the computer to strengthen the muscles around your knees, or pelvic tilts while at stoplights to strengthen your core. The goal, as with all exercise, is to engage in it often enough to receive the benefits without overdoing it. Use your tracking tool to aid you in this process.

Free weights. Exercises with free weights can help improve your balance and strengthen key muscle groups. Work with an appropriate professional to devise a set of exercises for your needs and goals and to ensure you are using proper form and technique. Most gyms offer a wide array of weights; if you are a member, you can benefit from guidance by fitness staff or from instruction as part of a strengthening class. Be mindful, whether on your own or in class, to avoid weights that are unnecessarily heavy. When you start out, focus on your form and establish your baseline before adding weight. For some exercises, you may find that lifting the weight of your arms or legs is sufficient, especially if you move slowly. As you track your response, add weight (or repetitions) accordingly. Most recommendations on weight lifting advise scheduling a day off in between to allow your muscles to rest and heal. Look to your data to determine your best rhythm.

If you prefer a home system, be creative. Before investing in a set of weights, experiment with household items, such as a bag of rice, water bottles, or cans. As you improve, include additional repetitions, sets, or movements. As the goal is not bodybuilding, you may not need more than a few sizes of weights. If grasping irritates your hands, arms, or neck, try weights that strap on to your arms or legs. These also provide resistance for calisthenic exercises.

Circuit training. Weight machines can feel intimidating if it's your first time, but they are built to be both gentle and comprehensive, and they offer many benefits, including the accomplishment that comes with challenging yourself with something new. Make use of professional guidance to learn the proper way to operate each machine, and consult your doctor to make sure there are no must-avoids on your list. When used properly, weight machines ensure good form and isolate muscle groups. Following a circuit program can ensure balanced attention to muscle groups.

There's no reason to overdo it when you start slow and increase as indicated by your response. When I first tried circuit training, I started without the weight; in other words, I removed the pin from each large weight stack and lifted only the mechanism itself. This allowed me to go through the movements and test how each machine felt—and, later, how I felt—before deciding to add in the first weight. Over time, I built up (without soreness) to as much as forty pounds on some machines and with multiple repetitions (and I'm a fairly small person). Most gyms make tracking your exertions and progress easy by providing and storing personal charts to record your weights and repetitions on each machine. You can then replicate your program or increase or reduce as needed. If you are considering home equipment, experiment to make sure you will remain committed to the process and research the quality and appropriateness of machines for your circumstances.

Strengthening in the pool. Water exercises offer a gentle alternative to land-based calisthenics or weight lifting. The largest constraint is the need for pool access. The benefits include being able to engage in exercises that may be challenging (or impossible) on land and, because the water is soothing and supportive, reduced muscle soreness, stiffness, and risk of injury. Work at your own level, determining the intensity of resistance by the size and speed of your movements. Water-based exercise is especially good for those with joint problems because it allows you to strengthen muscles around painful joints with minimal compression on joints.

You can create a program of movements to strengthen core muscles, extend and flex joints, and increase range of motion. You can strengthen your muscles in a balanced way: for instance, each time you push against the water, you could then pull back in the opposite direction with the opposing muscle pair (e.g., the hamstrings and quadriceps). Water exercises can also improve balance because you need to activate your back and abdominal muscles in order to stay vertical. Strengthening these core muscles can also alleviate low back and other types of pain. Just as in weight training, your muscles contract against the resistance and become stronger with each session. You can increase your exertion without any equipment. Water offers natural resistance—about twelve to fifteen times greater than air.[4] Simply increase repetitions and the number of sets as you would with weights. But if you want even greater intensity, look into equipment designed for pool use, such as webbed gloves, water weights, tubing, and various plastic and foam floats.

One important caveat is to be careful not to overdo it. The buoyancy of water can mask the extent of your exertion. Be mindful of the speed of your movements and the position of your body (including whether your hands are open, cupped, or flat); otherwise, you may unwittingly vary the intensity of your workout.

Some important guidelines to follow in strength training:

Start slowly. As with cardiovascular exercise, there's no such thing as too slowly. Whatever method you choose, the goal is to strengthen your muscles, not to lift as much as possible. Start small and build up as indicated by increasing either the amount of weight or the number of repetitions and sets. If you are just starting out, or returning after a lengthy time, there's no harm in using the "no weight" or "just one" approach, then increasing as indicated by your results.

Use proper form. Learn and master the proper form, posture, and technique to work your muscles in a balanced manner. This allows you to get the most out of your exercise and reduces the risk of injury from an incorrect approach. Be careful against "guarding" or favoring sore muscles; this can lead to unevenness, tension, and postural imbalances, which then put strain on other areas.

Look to professionals. Because of the importance of proper form, work with a qualified fitness instructor or physical therapist for at least a few sessions to make sure your form is correct. (And avoid pushing beyond your comfort zone, regardless of anyone's credentials.)

Heed your body. Strength training should not cause pain (beyond a tolerable level of soreness), whether in the moment or later. While exercising, feeling good can indicate you are exercising properly.

Strive for balance. Ideally, you should include strengthening exercises for each of the major body areas (legs, chest, shoulders, back, arms, and abdominals). The important thing is to strengthen your muscles in a balanced way, including the key muscle groups that work in conjunction with each other.

Breathe. Do not hold your breath while exercising. Try to inhale and exhale slowly to keep your muscles relaxed, comfortable, and supplied with oxygen. You may benefit from exhaling on exertion and inhaling on the less strenuous part of the movement.

Frequency. It is fairly standard to limit strengthening exercises to two to three times a week to allow muscles to recover. If you begin very slowly (such as with a single push-up), you might decide to do it daily or even several times a day. As for increasing intensity, there's no magic number of repetitions that indicates it is time to advance to the next level. Generally, the more weight or resistance you choose, the fewer repetitions are needed, although you may feel better keeping weight and resistance below a certain threshold. Trust your experiments.

Know Your Current Body

Work with the body you have right now, not the one you wish you had or may have had in the past. This allows you to choose exercises that will not incite acute pain. You may have to learn this the hard way, like me. Only after a rocky time in which I continued to push myself beyond my limits did I finally accept the necessity of scaling back and pacing myself. Perhaps you can learn from my mistakes rather than yours. No matter how you begin, you will be able to increase your fitness, strength, and flexibility. At the worst, you will be stronger, in better shape, and look better . . . and still hurt. But more likely, mindful exercise will decrease your pain and increase your abilities. Use your data to inspire the encouraging speech you may need, either to start slowly or to push yourself to lace your walking shoes. Sometimes, the hardest part is getting started. Whatever you decide to do, just do something!

Chapter 16

Collaborating Effectively with Your Doctor

Constructing a Supportive Medical Team

The first step is to find an effective and supportive doctor. Because you will be working as a team, select your teammate carefully. Look to your social networks for recommendations. If your pains have been diagnosed, ask local support group members and facilitators to share their experiences of doctors in your area. National advocacy organizations often compile lists of supportive physicians who focus on your particular condition or disease. See if your organization does—and, if you discover a compassionate doctor who is not included on the list, contribute his or her name to assist others in their search.

What Kind of Doctor Should I See?

Your choice of doctor depends on your situation. While searching for a diagnosis, it makes sense to see a general practitioner (often called "family practice") or general internist rather than a specialist. If you already have a relationship with a family doctor or internist, start there. Then, based on your doctor's findings, you may be referred to any number of specialists. During this process, be mindful of "doctor fatigue," a condition of exhaustion that I've seen described in chat rooms that stems from the experience of meeting too many doctors who do not treat their experiences as legitimate. Try to stick with doctors who were recommended by people you trust.

There are many types of chronic pains—some that are understood, others that are not ("idiopathic pain" refers to pains of unknown origin). But even when you have a diagnosis, it's not always clear what type of doctor you should see. The following practitioners commonly treat chronic pain conditions:

Rheumatologists. Rheumatologists specialize in conditions of the muscles, joints, and bones, which tend to be chronic, such as certain autoimmune diseases, inflammatory diseases, and musculoskeletal pain disorders. These account for more than one hundred different diagnoses, including rheumatoid arthritis, osteoarthritis, lupus, back pain, osteoporosis, and tendonitis. According to the American College of Rheumatology, this specialty is "trained to do the detective work necessary to discover the cause of swelling and pain."[1] Rheumatologists often work using a team approach, either as consultants to other physicians or as managers of a team that may include nurses, physical or occupational therapists, and psychotherapists. Rheumatology is a subspecialty of internal medicine or pediatrics. This means that following medical school, rheumatologists did their medical residency in either general internal medicine or pediatrics, then completed another two to three years of training in rheumatology.

Physiatrists (pronounced "fizz–EYE-a-trists"). According to the Association of Academic Physiatrists, this specialty treats musculoskeletal injuries and pain syndromes and seeks to help people to decrease pain and disability and restore function through rehabilitation.[2] Conditions physiatrists treat range from spinal cord injuries and stroke to arthritis, back pain, fibromyalgia, and tendonitis. Physiatrists often team with a wide range of specialists, including physical therapists, occupational therapists, recreational therapists, rehabilitation nurses, psychologists, social workers, and speech-language pathologists, to promote rehabilitation. Treatments commonly used are exercise, physical therapy, heat or ice, electrical stimulation, medication, steroid injections, trigger-point injections, and spinal epidurals, as well as assistive devices. Becoming a physiatrist involves a minimum of four years of residence in physical medicine and rehabilitation after medical school.

Neurologists. According to the American Academy of Neurology, neurologists have specialized training in diagnosing, treating, and managing disorders of the brain and nervous system.[3] Neurologists are equipped to order and interpret many high-tech diagnostic tests, such as magnetic resonance imaging (MRI); computerized tomography or computer-assisted tomography (CT or CAT scan); transcranial Doppler; neurosonography; electroencephalograms (EEG); electromyogram and other nerve conduction studies; sleep studies; and cerebral spinal fluid analysis (spinal tap or lumbar puncture). Training includes one year of internal medicine after medical school, followed by three years of training in neurology. Many neurologists subspecialize further (requiring additional training) in areas such as pain management, epilepsy, or movement disorders. Neurologists can work with you as a primary care provider, a consultant to your other doctors, or both, depending on the frequency of care required.

Other specialists. If you experience pain in a particular area of the body, especially in the early stages when you are seeking a diagnosis, you might look to the associated specialist—a gynecologist or urologist for pelvic pain, a dentist for jaw pain, or a podiatrist for foot pain. When your symptoms are treated as something of a medical mystery, the most important thing is having a doctor who is skilled in differential diagnosis and will carefully consider your experience. If you can afford it, or your health insurance will cover it, seek out second (and sometimes further) opinions in your search for answers.

Generalists versus Specialists

As you can see, the areas of expertise of rheumatologists, physiatrists, and neurologists overlap. Often, a doctor's specialty is less important than his or her interest in you and your condition. Look beyond the specialty to the specific physician. Some doctors (from any number of specialties), including physician's assistants, take an interest in pain management. Look into any pain clinics in your area. Finding a doctor who is abreast of cutting-edge research and treatments for your condition has advantages, but it is at least as important to find a doctor who treats you with respect and is committed to working with you to find answers. While doctors vary in the extent to which they are up to date on recent advances, they should be willing to seek answers as needed and accept information from patients. Even doctors with no specialized training in your condition can be helpful advocates if they take personal interest in your care.

Evaluating Doctor Visits

What should you expect in a doctor visit? It can be difficult to evaluate doctor visits, and the status difference can make the idea of evaluating doctors feel somewhat inappropriate. Given doctors' training, experience, and expertise, patients sometimes doubt or blame themselves rather than question their doctor's assessment. Plus, it is not always clear what matters most. The goal in chronic pain treatment is to manage symptoms rather than eliminate them. This can make it difficult to assess how well treatment is going.

Yet effective treatment in an area as complex as pain management relies on both the doctor's skillfulness and the strength of the doctor-patient relationship. Improvements come through systematic experimentation with appropriate treatments and a strong working alliance. Consider the following to gauge your potential collaboration:

Is your doctor courteous? Does he or she take you and your symptoms seriously? The best physicians will be considerate and enthusiastic about working with you to find answers and effective treatments. Doctoring well also involves viewing each patient as a unique individual to be supported, even when prescribed treatments do not work as hoped or when additional problems or complications arise. This involves listening nonjudgmentally to your experience and advocating for your interests.

Does your doctor seem interested in your condition? Not all physicians, regardless of their specialty, will be up to date on every condition. One sign of helpful physicians is their willingness to learn more about available treatment approaches, including being open to receiving information from their patients. Comprehensive physicians will also approach your particular symptoms in a systematic way in an attempt to get at the root of the problem, rather than treating each symptom as a separate wildfire. It's also helpful to recognize that chronic pain conditions can be challenging to treat. As appropriate, temper your expectation for consistent, high-quality care with the recognition that doctors are human.

Does your doctor seem thorough? Was a complete history taken? Chronic pain conditions can be fairly complex and poorly understood. For doctors to gain a comprehensive understanding of your experience requires that they take a detailed medical history along with a thorough physical exam. The doctor should inquire about other areas of your life, including your sleep quality, and any other symptoms. Take note of how your doctor considers the experiences you describe. A rigorous physician needs to assume the role of detective to consider the multiple difficulties that often arise with chronic pain. Within the constraints placed on routine office visits, doctors should reserve time to evaluate any changes in your condition, requiring longer visits as needed.

Does your doctor involve you in the treatment plan? Effective treatment will rely on your working together as a team. The doctor should spell out the treatment goals with you and discuss the pros and cons of different treatment options, inviting and valuing your input. If you would like to include family members or other support people in this process, your doctor should likewise welcome their participation.

How does your physician approach trying and evaluating different combinations of medication? Successful chronic pain treatment often includes multiple medications. Because pain is subjective—your doctor only knows how you feel by what you report—it's imperative that your doctor listen to you and select medication based on its promise for relief and your feedback. This often requires patience, as the trial-and-error process of finding optimal medications can be complicated. Whenever you begin a new medication or a change in dose, your doctor should provide necessary information, such as the potential benefits and adverse reactions, the time frame needed to evaluate its effects, and a game plan in case you experience difficulties before your next scheduled appointment. It is your responsibility to follow the prescribed course and communicate any problems that arise, and it is the doctor's role to respond respectfully to your feedback. Treatments that are clearly not helping should be stopped promptly and the plan adjusted accordingly.

Does your doctor take a team approach? Because of the multifaceted effects of chronic pain, many pain specialists work on interdisciplinary teams, including practitioners who offer hands-on and other adaptive therapies. Seeing a doctor in a pain clinic or other team setting holds advantages. However, doctors can also, when appropriate, create a team with other professionals (such as physical therapists or psychotherapists) to assess or treat any persistent difficulties. The team approach may be particularly helpful during early or acute phases. The most important team relationship is the one between you and your doctors.

Guidelines for an Effective Partnership with Your Physician

Unlike the traditional relationship model of an all-knowing doctor and a passive patient, treating chronic pain requires a comfortable working partnership. It's helpful if you can view your doctor as a knowledgeable teammate who is working with you toward the same goal. Finding a compassionate doctor helps. You can also uphold your side of the relationship by following these suggestions:

Be patient, and express your appreciation. It is human to experience frustration, and times may arise when you or your doctor experiences frustration with the outcome of an approach or the slow pace of progress. Keep in mind that frustration with the condition or situation should not translate into frustration with the doctor or patient. Contribute to morale by viewing the larger picture and by expressing appreciation for considerate treatment. Most often, progress is gradual and incremental. Make sure that you share *any* improvements in your comfort, ability, or outlook and that you rejoice when treatments provide benefit.

Communicate clearly and respectfully. Your accurate description of symptoms and side effects forms the basis of your doctor's decisions. This works best when communication is clear and respectful; ideally, it develops over time as you each learn about the other's communication style. Avoid minimizing or exaggerating your experience; it's neither your job to spare your doctor from the news that you have not improved nor to embellish your story with unnecessarily graphic detail. Accurate descriptions and documentation of your abilities and difficulties are vital not only for the doctor who selects treatments but also in the event that you apply for disability compensation (as described in chapter 22). Strive to represent your experience in a succinct and accurate manner.

Communication also benefits from realistic expectations. With uncertain conditions, nobody has all the answers. Doctors, like anyone else, will vary in their willingness to admit they do not know something. Initially, it is your doctor's job to educate you about your condition and treatment options. But it is reasonable to expect that with time, your roles may shift as you become an expert on your personal experience, and your doctor may take on more of a consultant role. Some doctors will be more comfortable than others letting their patients take the lead, which may include their accepting articles and other informative materials from patients. Be assertive—ask your doctor politely, but directly, about the most effective way to work together.

Be up front about medications. Doctors will vary in their comfort and experience prescribing newer medications, stronger medications (particularly opioids), and medications in combination. Patients also fall anywhere on the spectrum between eagerness to try *anything* that might help and apprehension about long-term reliance on medication. It helps to work with a doctor whose approach is congruent with yours. Solicit your doctor's views, and discuss any concerns either of you may have. Finding medications that significantly reduce symptoms can involve modifications based on careful tracking. Neither you nor your physician should throw up hands in defeat if this process takes time, you experience unpleasant side effects, or an advertised medication does not bring hoped-for relief.

Prepare for office visits. Always keep your visits. If you must cancel or change an appointment, do so in a timely fashion. Doctor's offices are like businesses and should run on schedule. (You can also call ahead to find out if your doctor is running on schedule.) It is a good idea to let your doctor, or his or her representative, see a list of your concerns before the visit so he or she can manage the time. Respect the time limits of the office visit and come prepared. The more effectively you convey your experience, the more you can benefit from your doctor's insights. Be ready to provide a quick synopsis, including relevant changes and questions. It helps to record and bring in your pressing questions to make sure you ask them. Find out from your doctor what would be most appropriate to share from your tracking data and the best way to do this. You may want to bring relevant data to your appointment if you anticipate that this would help you answer questions. The better able you are to convey your experience during the office visit, the better your doctor will be able to understand your experience and adjust treatments accordingly. As described below, it may be worthwhile to invest time in creating documents with specific information.

How to Prepare for a First Visit

Find out about the doctor. Once you receive a referral to a doctor (or doctors), see what you can find out. Before scheduling the appointment, you can ask the receptionist or nurse if the doctor has a special interest in your condition. This is especially important for conditions that are rare or considered controversial. Some doctors grant brief phone interviews with prospective patients. If so, you can inquire about his or her familiarity with your diagnosis, interest in working with patients with that condition, or view of particular treatments. Organize your thoughts for a five-minute phone call; that way, even if you talk longer, you have made sure to ask your most pressing questions up front. During the call, listen to the doctor's response (rather than conveying your "story") to learn about his approach. If the doctor is unavailable for a phone consultation—and many are not—you might want to schedule an appointment to get acquainted. This provides an opportunity to evaluate your comfort with the doctor and practice at a time when you are not in crisis or focused on a particular problem—and before you invest significant time and energy or transfer confidential records. Some offices offer "get acquainted" appointments free of charge or for a reduced fee.

Whether you schedule a "get acquainted" visit or more typical first appointment, make sure to inquire about the time allotted for your visit. People with chronic pain often require more than a fifteen-minute appointment. If that is what is offered, consider requesting a longer slot, and be prepared to pay for it.

When scheduling your first appointment, feel free to ask the receptionist to send you patient information and intake forms. Some offices provide these online or by mail, fax, or e-mail. You can then fill out the forms in the comfort of home and with greater accuracy, since you can check your records and prescription bottles. Another strategy to enable you to fill out information accurately and without effort is to create and bring an up-to-date medical résumé.

Create a medical résumé. At first visits, providing a detailed medical history introduces the doctor to you and your experience. Unfortunately, for people with chronic pain, trying to convey all relevant information can be rather involved. You may have seen multiple specialists and tried numerous medications and other treatments, which you find nearly impossible to recall. Plus, recounting potentially depressing facts can be emotionally draining. The process can threaten to transform your identity, in all its beautiful complexity, into "chronic patient." By creating a medical résumé of relevant information, you can come prepared and also avoid the emotional task of recalling and describing your difficulties. Having a ready document also preserves office time for your pressing concerns or questions. Giving a complete medical history can devour the better part of a valuable first visit.

Keep your medical résumé concise. The advice to limit a job résumé to one page also applies here—keep your medical résumé short for easy reading, and highlight what matters most. This eliminates the cumbersome task of having to dig through unnecessary detail. This display of forethought and organization can also contribute to an effective partnership. Simpler versions of a medical résumé can be used for subsequent visits, as described below.

Doctors will vary in the way they treat a medical résumé. Some will welcome such handouts; others may find them off-putting, at least initially. Offer a copy to the doctor with a warm smile, explaining that it helps you remember. Even if the doctor prefers to ask you questions rather than read your summary, having it for reference can help you feel calmer and more assured during the process. If the doctor opts to read your summary, your role becomes to offer clarification as needed. Even if the doctor does not read the résumé, he or she can refer to it at a later time. Include any pressing questions as part of your medical summary, and present them at the start of the visit so the doctor can budget time accordingly. Doctors have to keep to fairly tight schedules, and they appreciate efficiency. As you develop a relationship, you and your doctor may develop a particular format. Providing documentation on your current status in the form of medical résumés can also be useful in the event that you file for a disability claim. Just like your tracking data, your medical résumé documents your conditions and questions at different times, allowing you to note any significant changes.

Consider the following example résumé. However you decide to organize yours, it helps to use headings for easy review.

Example Format of Medical Résumé for First Visit

I.   At the top, make sure to include the **appointment date**, name of the **doctor**, and your identifying information (**name** and **date of birth**). This information ensures that your document will stay meaningful (even if the paper is not filed carefully).

II.   **Objective of visit.** (Limit this to one or two per visit.) Some examples: I want to improve my sleep; I'm looking for a doctor to help reduce my pain and fatigue; I'm planning a pregnancy and want to discuss the safety of my current medication.

III.   **Onset of Symptoms.** Example: February 2007, after car collision.

IV.   **Diagnosis.** (Name and other relevant information.) For example: Fibromyalgia, November 2008, by Juana Feelbetta, MD. Confirmed by Dr. Goodhands (rheumatologist) and Dr. Ayudame (physiatrist).

V.   **Brief History.** (Brief summary.) For example: Prior to the accident, I was a healthy, active, physically fit student. I sustained two broken ribs, bruises, and whiplash from a head-on collision. Pain in my neck, back, and chest continued even after the ribs healed, and it worsened over the following months, spreading to my hips and legs. After physical therapy, and a combination of medications, I have become more functional. However, pain and fatigue continue to be a problem.

VI.   **Surgeries/Hospitalizations.** (Include dates and names of any procedures, along with names of practitioners and hospitals.)

VII.   **Symptoms.** (Give a brief summary of current experience.) Example: I awake feeling like I was hit by a truck. My pain varies from a dull ache to an acute all-over burning pain. My worst problem is my arms—I cannot type or write for more than a minute and have difficulty carrying things. Cold temperatures aggravate my pain. Today's **pain rating** is 7 out of 10.

VIII. **Current Medications.** (Include how you take each, and include any supplements.) Example:
1. 300 mg gabapentin at bedtime
2. 0.5 mg clonazepam at bedtime
3. 5 mg zolpidem at bedtime when cannot sleep (about once a month)
4. Tramadol, 1/2 tablet dose as needed (0–3 tablets daily)
5. 1 multivitamin once daily
6. 1 Omega-3 fish oil capsule (in morning)

IX. **Exercise.** (Include any current exercise.) Example: I walk for 1 hour on treadmill (2 times per week), strengthening exercises with 2-lb. weight 20 minutes (3 times per week); stretch (every a.m. and p.m.)

X. **Other Aids.** (Note which treatments seem to help and which do not.) For example: Massage, hot baths, breathing exercises, relaxation techniques all help symptoms.

Bring other relevant information. In the event that you did not fill out paperwork before your appointment, bring with you whatever information (on paper, in your appointment book, or on your smartphone) that will aid you with intake forms. Make sure you have information such as:

1. Personal information: Social Security number; employer's name and address; insurance information, including group and member number and subscriber's name.
2. Names, phone numbers, and mailing addresses of any doctors whom you would like to receive notes from the office visit.

Maintain a History of Healthcare Professionals

Other documents that can be helpful include a history of doctors you have seen, medications you have tried, and your experiences with these. While the effort to create these documents may seem daunting, the good news is that after your initial investment of piecing together a history, it's simple to update, whether by keeping a file or spreadsheet on the computer or a paper logbook.

Because it is common for people with chronic pain to see many doctors in their search for diagnoses and improvement, the details can start to blur. It may be hard to believe you could forget whether your experience was positive or negative and why, but as time passes, memories fade. Maintaining a list can be helpful for personal reasons, such as reminding yourself of what you have been through and who and what has been helpful. Your current physician may also want to request medical records. In the event that you file for disability insurance, an accurate list of doctors can be very important. Include other practitioners, such as physical therapists, psychotherapists, or massage therapists, for the same reasons.

List of practitioners as of February 2012
(fill in date to keep current)

Name and contact info	Specialty	Dates	Experience and treatment
Bite D. Bullit Newneck, NJ (910) 666-2525	Orthopedist	2007	Thought my symptoms were stress related and would resolve
Juana Feelbetta Badarms, CA (415) 555-2222	Internist, specialty in pain	2008	Diagnosed fibromyalgia
Gotta Moove Badarms, CA (415) 234-8583	Physical therapist	2008	Helped me regain functionality with stretches, heat, strengthening
Abbey Road Mehurt, NC (919) 123-1234	Family medicine	2008	Tried Elavil; referred me to a rheumatologist
Norman Krapkey Mehurt, NC (919) 919-1919	Rheumatologist	2008	1 visit, Doesn't "believe" in fibromyalgia
Imin Goodhands Mehurt, NC (919) 738-3838	Rheumatologist	2008	Helped me find medications (list here) to improve how I feel
Juan Ayudame Dolor, NC (919) 232-4868	Physiatrist	2009–	Helped me create a sustainable exercise program

Track Your Experience with Medications (and Any Other Treatments)

It is enormously beneficial to know which medications you have tried and your responses. While searching for relief, you may have learned to talk like a virtual pharmacist, rattling off prescription medications and classes of drugs. However, a gentle reminder is in order: do not trust your memory. No matter how knowledgeable you may become, it is virtually impossible to recall your experiences with multiple medications. Systematic records can keep you from repeating medications (and sometimes classes of medications) that you have tried with poor response.

Start with your tracking data for your more current information on medications and your responses to them. Do not fret over medications that predate your tracking efforts. Instead, don your investigator's hat and try to re-create your experiences as accurately as you can. Many pharmacists keep lists of all the prescriptions you have had filled with them, and they can provide you with a copy dating back several years. Or you may have kept receipts in your tax file. Your doctor's records should include all the medications prescribed for you while you were a patient there. If you are unable to fill in past detail, focus on the present. Time will pass, your medications will continue to change, and you can accrue these new data. You may find it helpful to compile a document that catalogs your medication, such as:

List of medications tried as of February 2012
(*fill in date to keep current*)

Medication	Dosage	Dates	Benefits	Side Effect
Zolpidem*	0.5 mg (qhs)	2007– present	Knocks me out when I cannot fall asleep	Amnesia (if I stay up)
Amitriptyline	5–20 mg (qam)	3 mos in 2008 Again in 2011	Helped some, but too unpleasant	Groggy and brain-dead until noon
Clonazepam*	0.5 mg (qhs)	2008– present	Helps sleep and pain	Fatigue if used in daytime
Clonidine	0.1 mg (qam)	2008	Unclear	None
Duloxetine	300 mg (qam)	2010 (3 months)	Less morning pain	Irritable, insomnia
Lidocaine injections		2007, 2010	Increased mobility	Some soreness
Methadone	5 mg (qam)	2008–09	Helpful once acclimated	HARD to adjust to—dizzy, nauseated; difficult withdrawal
Gabapentin*	300 mg (bid)	1998– present	Reduces pain	Swollen legs, memory problems, weight gain
NSAIDs (many!)		2007–08	No benefit	Nausea, diarrhea
Paroxetine	30 mg (qam)	1997–98	Reduced pain	Irritability
Oxycodone*	Half dose, as needed	2008– present	Reduces pain	Minimal with low dose
Acetaminophin with codeine	tried twice	2007	Minimal benefit	Vomiting
Tramadol	tried once	2008	Unclear	Dizzy, unsteady
Sertraline	??	2008	Unclear	Nausea

*currently taking

Please note: **These records are fictitious. They are intended as illustration only and not information on actual effects.**

How to Prepare for Subsequent Doctor Visits

Preparing for subsequent visits is much easier. The goal is to provide feedback since the last visit and to communicate your main objective for the current one. Writing down your agenda is invaluable. It is often insufficient to *think* about what you want to say; office visits have time limits, and doctors may have a separate agenda. Create a *short* document—one copy for you and one for your doctor (which can also go in your records)—with three pieces of information:

1. Your current **Objective** or **Questions**. What do you want from the appointment? Make sure to let your doctor know this up front. For example: I am still feeling groggy during the day and want to discuss my options.

2. Your current **Assessment**. Let your doctor know how you have been doing and, in particular, about any changes. (This is important for your treatment as well as your medical records.) Example: My pain level has improved, but I continue to be tired.

   Details: Most days I require an afternoon nap (2–3 hours). On days with a full schedule, I feel so exhausted that I can barely get out of bed, and sometimes I sleep the entire day. My pain continues to spike if I use my arms (such as trying to type, doing too much exercise [more than 30 minutes], and from cold drafts, bright lights, and tension). At these times, my pain is about 7/10. Otherwise, it averages about 4 or 5/10.

3. Your current **Treatment** regimen. Although your doctor has records of your medication, it can be helpful to keep information handy on everything you are doing to feel better. If you have more than one physician on your healthcare team (e.g., you see an internist for most of your care, an occasional specialist, and a psychologist for symptoms of depression), these records can keep your entire team informed. For medications that are prescribed "as needed," report to your doctor on how you are taking them and your response. Include any other therapies as well.

Example:

40 mg duloxetine (morning)—helping pain, but feel jittery

2 mg clonazepam (bedtime)—sleeping better, but foggy-headed into the day

Water aerobics 30 minutes, 2–3/week—helpful

Massage therapy 40 minutes, twice /month—helps with pain, but $$.

This practice saves a tremendous amount of time during the visit and increases the likelihood that you will have your needs addressed. Handing your questions to your doctor before the visit begins allows you both to make the most effective use of the time together. You may also find it easier to be straightforward in writing—less worry, for example, that describing (continued) symptoms will come off as complaining. Your doctor can quickly glean the relevant information about your current situation and goals for the visit. Written documents will likely be included in your chart, either directly or through your doctor's notes for that visit, leaving a valuable paper trail.

When to Seek a New Doctor

It is unfortunate that this topic is necessary; however, I have accumulated stories over the years from people with chronic pains, some diagnosed, some not, who have been mistreated, even by physicians who specialize in chronic pain. It is particularly disheartening to hear from individuals who, in search of validation and help, encounter ridicule or disbelief or are blamed for their own suffering. In my own search for compassionate care, I have received inappropriate, belittling responses from a handful of physicians. Thankfully, in my case, these were the exceptions, not the rule.

It can be helpful to bear in mind the root of doctor insensitivity. Try to imagine being a doctor who trained for years to match symptoms with diagnoses and prescribe treatments to reduce suffering. In walks someone with a confusing array of symptoms that do not respond to treatment. The person appears to be in acute distress, despite your best efforts. Even the best-intentioned physician may struggle with this. It may not come as a surprise that the medical literature has referred to chronic pain patients as "a chronic challenge," "difficult," and "extremely frustrating." Also, depending on the diagnosis (or lack thereof), a subset of practitioners may doubt the reality of pains they cannot see, instead attributing chronic complaints to malingering or the exaggeration of typical aches and pains.

Combine this problem with the medical profession's history of undertreating chronic pain: There is long-standing, albeit decreasing, bias against treating chronic pain with strong medications. While strong medications are now prescribed more routinely for acute postoperative pain or to alleviate suffering in the final stages of terminal illness, they are much less frequently used for severe pain that is chronic but not terminal. Although this bias may arise from a genuine concern to "cause no harm," the unintended consequence is that individuals do not receive needed pain relief. Part of doctors' reluctance to prescribe controlled substances also stems from policies intended to discourage drug abuse and addiction.

Treating chronic pain can be a difficult, challenging, and frustrating task for doctors. Some may attempt to relieve their frustration by seeking a target to blame—and, unfortunately, this sometimes falls on the patient. I believe that most doctors want to provide meaningful diagnoses that yield effective treatment. In the face of difficult-to-treat chronic pains, even the most gifted physicians may feel inadequate. Eager to see evidence of their effectiveness, physicians may become frustrated when patients return with additional complaints and adverse reactions to prescribed medications.

While frustration may be understandable, every patient deserves the doctor's dedication and respect. The following red flags signal inappropriate or unhelpful behaviors. If you encounter any of these flags, you might want to seek a more supportive physician. The comments supplied as illustrations all come from real-life encounters with physicians.

Red Flags: Warnings That It May Be Time to Seek Help Elsewhere

Comments That Suggest Disbelief in the Extent of Your Suffering

"You can't have a pain that goes from *here* to *here* to *there*!"
"Look at you! You cannot possibly hurt as much as you say!"

"I get backaches from time to time. Just live with it."

"Everybody has aches and pains. I don't feel so great when I wake up either."

If, after your best efforts to communicate your experience, your physician persists in treating you like a hypochondriac, treat yourself to a new doctor. Living with pain is difficult. We all deserve doctors who take our experience seriously.

Statements about Not "Believing" Your Symptoms

"You just need a nice long vacation. You'll feel fine."

"I am not one of those doctors who believe in [*your condition*]."

"I can't find anything wrong, so tell me, what's really going on?"

Pain is not like Santa Claus or the Tooth Fairy: there's no room for disbelief. Do not waste your time, energy, or resources arguing that your experience is real. This is different from having a doctor who does not know what is causing the pain or lacks experience treating your condition.

Exhaustion: The Throwing Up of Hands

"Nothing I do works for you! I am out of ideas."

Consider it a gift when doctors let you know they are feeling inadequate; at least this is an honest response. Your response in such cases depends on your relationship and available options. Don't automatically assume you are being fired as a patient! Take a moment to reflect on your next step. If you are otherwise happy with your doctor—if you find him or her otherwise respectful, smart, patient, and genuinely interested in your well-being—consider offering a pep talk or articles that you have found helpful. Otherwise, you might ask for a referral to someone your doctor thinks might be more appropriate. Acknowledge the effort your physician has expended, and express your appreciation. If, on the other hand, you have not been satisfied with your doctor, take his or her confession as a sign that it is indeed time to move on.

Anger or Impatience at Your "Failing" to Improve

> "Look, I put you on medication that is supposed to help—what else can I do?"
> "I don't know what's wrong with you. You complain about every medicine I've tried."

It is one thing to experience frustration but another to take it out on a patient. If it seems you have reached the end of a productive relationship, consider parting ways.

Inappropriate Implication That Your Symptoms Are All in Your Head

> "I've tested for everything, and every test comes back normal—there is nothing medically wrong with you."
> "What's wrong? I have not seen anyone so down about how they feel."
> "You must be having romantic troubles."
> "Were you molested as a child?"

While it is valuable that your physician considers all aspects of your life, this should not be in a way that discounts your physical ailments. If you have explained that your psychological distress is due to the chronic challenges of pain, your doctor should respect this. Psychotherapy can be very helpful in coping with challenges of chronic pain, but only as a complement to (and not a substitute for) appropriate medical care.

Reluctance (or Refusal) to Work with You on Pain-Management Medication

> "You need to stop your pain medication so you don't become dependent on it."
> "After a motorcycle accident, I took narcotics for a while, and then I decreased them until I didn't need any. If you do the same thing, your pain will disappear."
> "You will have pain for a long time, so I don't think it's a good idea to medicate it."

"I am uncomfortable prescribing pain medications for this kind of thing."

"I'm afraid that you'll sell these medications on the street."

"The medications you have been taking for pain are probably creating pain intolerance—I'm against prescribing them."

There may be good reasons that your doctor prefers a particular kind of medication or is against combining certain others. Conscientious physicians will explain their thinking and, if asked, provide literature on the subject. However, it's another story when a doctor refuses to consider a wide range of medications (including opioids), particularly if you have had positive experiences with such medications in the past.

Responding to Red Flags

One red flag by itself may not provide sufficient grounds to leave your physician. As a first step, evaluate your overall care. Does the red-flag incident seem out of character, or is it part of a larger pattern of mistreatment? Moreover, sometimes alternatives to your current doctor are limited—particularly if you live in a small town or have a restrictive insurance policy.

Before deciding to leave a physician, try to address the problem. Be up front with your doctor. You each have the right to expect the other to be a committed teammate. Doctors often lament about "noncompliant patients" who shirk their responsibilities by not taking medication as prescribed, not following recommendations for diet and exercise, or other transgressions. Often, such patients have reasons for noncompliance (such as serious side effects or the cost of medication) that need to be brought to light and addressed. We should make the same allowances for physicians.

Consider what you would like from your doctor. Keep your response polite and direct. It helps to maintain a calm voice—cool off if necessary before approaching your doctor—and use "I statements" rather than pointing fingers. For example, you might say, "I feel saddened by your comments. I am doing the best I can and really appreciate your working with me." Doctors are human, too, so consider offering an empathetic comment: "I'll bet treating chronic pain can be frustrating for you, too!" Or try humor. Start by saying, in a joking manner, that "people in pain can sure be a pain!" before asserting your concern.

If your differences persist, however, let your doctor know that you'd hoped to work together but will be looking elsewhere. Inquire whether he or she can refer you to someone who may be better suited to you.

Chapter 17

Strategies to Make Sense of Prescription Medications

Medications are often essential in chronic-pain management. Finding what works, however, can be challenging. Even when specific medications are promoted for your condition, what you respond to best is likely to be uniquely tailored to your needs. This process likely involves experimenting with multiple medications at different dosages and comparing their results. Experimenting with medications in this way can feel overwhelming because of their sheer number, the uncertainty of your responses, and the time commitment involved. However, doctors who work in the "pain trenches" will tell you this process is invaluable. Without it, you risk taking one or more ineffective medications and potentially missing out on a superior treatment.

PAINTRACKING is essential in this process. Through tracking and communicating this information with your doctor, you can discover what provides the greatest net gain. This chapter will help you become more knowledgeable about the medications typically prescribed for chronic pain conditions and how to approach them in a reasoned way. It concludes with some promising new research on treating pain. Some tips:

Be realistic. It is easy to look with hope to medication, particularly when new ones enter the market at such a rapid rate. The higher your hopes, however, the more frustrated you will feel if this or that medicine fails to deliver wished-for results. It helps if you keep expectations realistic and stock up on patience. Convey to your doctor that you do not expect a "magic pill" (although wouldn't that be nice?) but want to reduce your most irritating or debilitating symptoms. This can remind you both that your worthwhile search together may be a lengthy one.

Explore your beliefs. Share your beliefs about medications with your

221

healthcare professionals, and inquire about theirs. Doctors vary in their comfort levels for prescribing strong painkillers. Your comfort may depend on your views regarding long-term use, pain level, and tolerance of side effects. To collaborate effectively, it helps if you and your doctor are on the same page.

Discuss the process. The multiple pain specialists who reviewed drafts of this chapter differed on many points, but all agreed that treatment must involve close collaboration with patients—and great patience. Talk with your doctor about the approach he or she will use in selecting and evaluating medications, and note his or her willingness to work closely with you in this process. The test period for many medications should be measured in days, not weeks or months. Your doctor should provide information about each medication, including potential adverse effects, with clear instructions about what to do or whom to call if a medication makes you feel awful. This is very different from prescribing a medication or medications and then checking back with you in three months.

Be familiar with polypharmacy. While a single pain medication sometimes turns out to provide great relief to chronic pains, at other times, superior pain relief comes from a combination of medications, otherwise known as polypharmacy. Low doses of multiple medications can offer unique benefits over a larger dose of one medication. However, the difficulties of this approach are its demands. Some doctors shy away from polypharmacy because it is more complex and requires careful titration. Prescribing several medications at one time makes it very difficult to discern the effects of any. For this reason, it may be preferable to start with one medication and then add or change based on your response. However, your doctor may have reason to prescribe several medications from the start. Whether starting with one or multiple medications, it is impossible to do well without very careful tracking and communication. Talk with your doctor about how he or she will work with you to evaluate the effects of each, including their interactions.

Stay informed. When starting a new treatment or undergoing a change in dosage, ask what you should expect, including the typical intensity and duration of common side effects and how to treat them. Make sure you understand how to evaluate a medication, including the number of days required for you to form a conclusion about its effectiveness, and what to do if you wish to discontinue the trial. Never stop using prescribed medications without consulting your physician first: some need to be discontinued gradually and under careful supervision. If side effects are intolerable or you are otherwise unhappy with a medication, waiting until your next doctor's appointment is counterproductive. Establish a strategy with your doctor for such eventualities. Before leaving the office, make sure you address the following questions:

Questions to ask your doctor when trying a new medication:

1. How long should it take to evaluate the effect of this medication?
2. Will this medication take effect with the first dose, or does it need to build up in my system (and if so, what is the expected time frame)?
3. What side effects might I experience?
4. How long should it take for side effects to subside?
5. What should I do if I begin to feel uncomfortable with this medication?
6. What is the best way to communicate with you during this trial period if I need assistance?

Be mindful of timing. Trying new medications can be an emotional experience, and not knowing how your body will respond can produce anxiety. Plus, you may be grappling with your hopes for improvement and your worries about side effects. Whenever feasible, try to schedule changes in medication during periods of low stress and high stability (e.g., your normal workweek—and not when you *or your doctor* will be traveling). This allows you to evaluate the effects more reliably and respond to any problems that may arise.

Assess side effects. Every medication, even aspirin, has possible side effects. At times, the list of potential problems can seem daunting. Remember, however, that drug companies are required by law to include all reactions people have had while taking a particular drug (even those reactions that may be due to other causes). Ask your doctor about common side effects and how to assess them. Some are expected to pass, or may be treatable, while others are not. Let your doctor know if you have reacted poorly to particular medications in the past.

What matters is what *you* actually experience. Use your tracking tool to note daytime drowsiness, constipation, dry mouth, agitation, weight gain, cognitive problems, or other side effects, as well as the success of strategies to minimize these. Assess, too, whether any remaining adverse effects are worth the benefits. Keep in mind that the potential for interaction effects increases with multiple medications. Make sure your doctor is fully informed of everything you are taking or considering, including vitamins, supplements, and over-the-counter (OTC) treatments.

Find the lowest dose that works. Medications are sometimes prescribed in standard one-size-fits-all doses. Yet each of us may respond differently. An optimal dosage is just high enough to alleviate symptoms and low enough to minimize unpleasant side effects. Some medications require time to build up in your system. Your doctor might begin conservatively with a low (or moderate) dose, slowly increasing your dose until you note intolerable side effects, a lack of additional benefit, or both. Larger doses typically come with more pronounced side effects, which can lead you to reject otherwise helpful treatments prematurely. Starting with a dose that is higher than needed can also mask the possibility that less would be as good or better.

When pain is severe, however, you may not want to start with a low dose. Your doctor may decide, instead, to start with a high dose and, if it looks promising, titrate it downward to minimize side effects. Your starting dose is something to negotiate with your physician. People eager for relief and less concerned about particular potential adverse reactions may reap greater benefits by starting with a fairly potent dose, while people who are more vulnerable to unpleasant side effects may profit from starting low and increasing very gradually.

If you are particularly sensitive to medications, or find an otherwise helpful medication difficult to tolerate, be inquisitive about lower doses that may be available. Even the most knowledgeable physicians may be unaware of lower than standard doses for certain medications. Do not be afraid to ask your doctor directly, consult with your pharmacist, or research available dosages online. For example, Neurontin® (the generic is gabapentin) is typically prescribed in 300 mg capsules for nerve pain; doctors may be unaware that it is available in 100 mg capsules. This information would provide more flexibility in your treatment. If your doctor prescribes the same dose in smaller increments (for example, 600 mg as 100 mg six times a day, rather than as 300 mg twice a day), you can test the effects of taking lower doses more frequently or taking less overall (such as 500 mg rather than 600 mg). This may be a costlier method at first because of the likely price difference between doses. But if you arrive at a lower, better-tolerated dose that is effective, it is a long-term savings. Compounding pharmacies also offer individualized alternatives. Because compounding pharmacists mix ingredients to the unique specifications of each patient, this option tends to be expensive—but, depending on your circumstances and calculations, may be worth it.

Divide doses appropriately. For medications that do not come in lower doses, alternatives often exist. Sometimes this requires creativity. Talk with your doctor. Medications may be available as capsules, tablets, and oral solutions, which increases your options. (Compounding pharmacists can also change the form of a drug, such as from a solid pill to a liquid.) The dose size of liquid medicines is easiest to regulate. When safe and appropriate, tablets can also be divided. Note that many pills come scored (that is, with a line across the center for easier division), and pharmacies sell pill cutters for this purpose. If a halved pill has a jagged edge, take it with care or wrap it in a small piece of bread to save your throat from a scratch. Capsules can also be divided. One method is to dissolve a capsule's contents in a neutral liquid in a measuring cup; then, pour your dose, and store the remainder in the refrigerator for your next dose. Make sure to mix or shake well immediately before your next dose. Of course, you should exercise safety and use appropriate labels and seals, especially if you share your refrigerator with children. Keep in mind that some medications should never be divided, such as extended-release formulations, designed to dissolve farther along in the digestive tract. Others degrade quickly when exposed to air or humidity. If your doctor approves dividing doses, you have additional ways to test what works for you, and the potential cost savings can be beneficial as well.

Financial considerations. Medications can be prohibitively expensive, particularly when you are uninsured or underinsured or have a prescription plan with a substantial co-payment. Consider the following questions when trying to keep your medications affordable:

How new is the medication? Newer medications, marketed under brand names, are protected by patents, which prevent other companies from offering equivalent products and driving down the price. Pharmaceutical companies have a vested interest in extending their patents to recoup their costs for research and development and increase their profits.[1] Patent protection typically lasts twenty years, sometimes longer. For consumers, it is largely a question of weighing the appeal of novel medications against their cost. Talk with your doctor about the potential benefits of newer medications compared to older ones that may have similar properties or effects but cost substantially less. If you opt to try a newer medication, allow the cost to motivate you to evaluate your experience even more carefully.

Is a generic available? After a certain number of years, the original manufacturer no longer maintains exclusive rights to its formula. Other companies are then allowed to copy and market drugs under the simplified chemical name or by another brand name. This competition significantly lowers prices. Generic products have to undergo testing to demonstrate whether they are biologically equivalent to the original drug, which presumably results in the same therapeutic value.[2] By law, generics are required to include the identical active ingredients but not necessarily the same inert ones (such as dyes, coatings, and binders). Controversy has long raged over the extent to which generics offer the same effectiveness as brand-name drugs. Much of this is fueled by the original manufacturers seeking to maintain some competitive advantage.[3] Sometimes doctors prescribe a brand name because it is simpler or has a catchier name or because they may have been influenced by the onslaught of advertising by pharmaceutical companies; other times, they may select brand names for desired properties, such as the belief that a particular extended-release medication dispenses more reliably into your system. Always ask about generic equivalents first.

In the United States, policies vary about whether you, as the patient, may request a generic at the pharmacy or whether your doctor needs to authorize such substitutions. In some states, generic substitutions are automatic (unless a doctor explicitly specifies no substitutions). If you are interested in receiving a generic equivalent for your more expensive medications, make sure to mention this to your doctor and/or pharmacist.

Is there a more cost-effective dose? Another way to reduce cost is by checking into the per-dose cost. Sometimes the price of a higher-dose medication is marginal—in other words, a thirty-day supply of a particular medication may be nearly the same, regardless of whether it is for thirty days of 50 mg pills or 100 mg pills. If this is the case, it may be worthwhile to ask your doctor about any feasible options. For example, if you are taking 1 mg a day, your doctor may be comfortable prescribing half of a 2 mg tablet daily, which would enable your prescription to last twice as long. For those paying out of pocket, the savings can be substantial. Your doctor, however, may have good reason not to do this for certain medications.

Are there legitimate discounts? Retail prices for medications can vary widely. Many large pharmacies list retail prices online, allowing you to comparison shop. The retail price of generic medications is sometimes lower than a standard insurance copayment. Some big-box stores with pharmacies publish a list of generic medications that they sell for as little as a few dollars for a month's supply, with steeper discounts for three-month supplies. Even if you have insurance, check with your pharmacist about the cost if you pay retail. You may be surprised to find that you sometimes save money by *not* using your insurance.

You can also find substantial variation among nongeneric medication. Cost variation is especially dramatic online. See for yourself by entering "low cost" or "discounted" and "prescription medications" into your search engine—you will find yourself in a sea of offers, many of which sound too good to be true and likely are. Many of these companies operate from abroad under a different set of rules or may be unregulated—or, worse yet, out-and-out scams. At the same time, many legitimate options exist for obtaining medications at a discounted price. Talk with your doctor or pharmacist, and look for reputable organizations that offer reduced prescription costs. Nearly all pharmaceutical companies have patient-assistance programs for those who find the cost of a medication prohibitive and whose financial circumstances make it difficult, if not impossible, to pay for a prescription. You can find information on these programs by searching the drug company and then talking with your doctor.

Addiction and abuse: separate fuss from facts. The topic of drug abuse and addiction in the treatment of chronic pain has received much attention. News stories on specific medications, such as OxyContin® (extended-release oxycodone), or celebrities' struggles with painkillers have highlighted the dangers of opioids in particular. Until recently, fearing the potential for drug abuse, doctors have tended to avoid prescribing opioids for nonterminal chronic pain. This had the unfortunate result of denying treatment to many who would have benefited greatly.

By the 1990s, however, this view was significantly challenged by doctors specializing in pain treatment, along with pharmaceutical companies that manufacture opioid medications. Together, they promoted the efficacy of these drugs and the idea that risk of abuse and addiction among people with chronic pain is minimal. Publications emerged highlighting the low risk among pain patients.[4] In the mid-1990s, for example, the *Journal of Pain and Symptom*

Management devoted a three-part series to countering what the editor described as the unwarranted rejection of opioids in the treatment of chronic pain in nonterminal illnesses. He explained that the favorable experience of opioid use in the long-term management of cancer pain demonstrated opioids' effectiveness for other types of chronic pain.[5]

Understand the central concepts. Part of the difficulty and biases that arise around the use of strong medication comes from confusion among the central concepts: physical dependence, abuse, addiction, and tolerance. Unfortunately, the use of these terms is inconsistent within the lay, medical, and psychiatric communities. Yet these distinctions are crucial for evaluating the risks associated with particular medications in the treatment of chronic conditions.

Let's start with *physical dependence*. This refers to the fact that if you suddenly stop taking a medication, you will experience withdrawal. This can happen even when a medication is taken exactly as prescribed. Symptoms of withdrawal are unpleasant, vary depending on the substance, and can last days or even weeks. By itself, physical dependence is not necessarily problematic. Think of coffee drinkers who enjoy a regular morning brew and experience headaches should they skip their customary cup—this is physical dependence. People with diabetes are physically dependent on insulin, a prescription medication necessary for their health. Problems of physical dependence can be thought of as something that happens *after you stop taking a drug*, rather than a problem associated with use of the drug itself. Withdrawal symptoms can be minimized and sometimes prevented by reducing the dose of medication gradually over weeks or months rather than stopping "cold turkey." Many symptoms of withdrawal can also be treated by other prescription medications.

Abuse, in contrast, pertains to *behaviors* around the use of a medication or other substance. According to the *Diagnostic and Statistical Manual of Mental Disorders*, fourth edition, or DSM-IV (the diagnostic manual for mental health professionals published by the American Psychiatric Association), abuse exists when significant impairment or distress occurs in response to the use of the medication. In other words, recurrent use of a substance would lead to problems like failure to fulfill major work, school, or family obligations; physically hazardous behavior or legal problems; or persistent social or interpersonal problems such as fighting. This is an interesting paradox for people with chronic pain, who generally look to medications as a means to *reduce* their problems in living.

Addiction involves behavioral difficulties as in abuse, often coupled with physical dependence, *plus* compulsive use that may be accompanied by strong cravings and efforts to obtain more and more of the drug. This concept is often confused with physical dependence, despite the significant differences. Part of this is due to the confusion and inconsistent use of terms by laypeople and by health and mental health professionals alike. Addiction is sometimes referred to as "psychological dependence" or "substance abuse disorder" or "substance dependence" or just "dependence." However, the concept of physical dependence (explained above as something that happens when you *stop* a drug) is distinct from addiction, which is about *the way in which you take a drug*.

The DSM-IV (which unfortunately uses the term "substance dependence" for the diagnosis of addiction) describes it as a clinically significant impairment or distress that occurs on account of the use of a substance. Impairments may include being unable to reduce or control use; spending considerable time and energy trying to obtain the medication (such as visiting multiple doctors and driving long distances) or recovering from its effects; having to give up or reduce important social, occupational, or recreational activities; or continuing to use the medication despite knowledge of persistent or recurrent problems caused or worsened by the use of medication. To put it simply, addiction is compulsive use despite harm.

Tolerance just means that you have to increase the dosage to get the same effects you did earlier. This can go with addiction, physical dependence, or neither.

Use medications responsibly. The goal is to be open to medications that offer promise without making yourself vulnerable to problems or allowing your (or your doctor's) undue fears to result in undertreatment of your pain. This relies on being honest with your doctor and yourself about the role of medication in your life. A variety of organizations offer "watch lists" to assess whether you or someone you know may be addicted to or abusing medication. These lists tend to be derivatives of DSM-IV diagnostic criteria for medication, alcohol, and street drugs. Consider the following questions to assess your risk for addiction or abuse.

Assessing your risk for addiction or abuse:

1. Do you have a personal or family history of problems with alcohol and/or other substances? (vulnerability)
2. Are you increasing your dose to achieve the same effect? (tolerance)
3. Are you using or increasing your medication for reasons other than pain management, such as the high it creates? (abuse)
4. Are you experiencing problems in your life around the use of this medication? (abuse and/or addiction)

Is there a risk for substance addiction or abuse? An effective approach strives for a reasonable balance that neither discounts nor exaggerates potential problems. Talk openly with your doctor, including about any personal or family history of abuse or addiction. Together, evaluate your reasons for any apprehension about using certain classes of medication. Then, commit to a plan in which, whatever medications you take, you will carefully monitor your intake and response. If you are at risk for abuse or addiction, it helps to work with a supportive physician and counselor to assist with decisions about medications and risk-lowering strategies.

Are you increasing your dosage? Understand that it is common to develop a tolerance to medications as your body adjusts to them. Your tracking tool can be essential here to keep you and your healthcare provider abreast of your use and its effectiveness, so bring this information to doctor visits. Keep in mind that increases in dose are sometimes medically necessary; you may require greater amounts on account of worsening symptoms. At other times, however, developing a tolerance to a medication reduces effectiveness, increasing both the amount you need and the risk of side effects and other problems. If you observe over time that you require greater doses to achieve the same relief, report this to your doctor. There are numerous strategies your doctor can help you use to keep your dose at low but clinically effective levels, such as prescribing an ancillary medication, instituting a temporary "drug holiday" or dose reduction, and/or rotating the specific medication used.[6]

Are there other reasons for craving the medication? Be mindful of the reasons you give yourself when reaching for your prescription bottle. If you observe that you are looking to medication for reasons other than pain relief, attend to this red flag. You may be depressed and self-medicating to escape. It can be especially challenging to recognize trends you would rather not see or acknowledge. Be on the lookout for data that track any significant changes. Overusing or abusing medication can lead to many harmful consequences.

Are there problems in your life? Be sure to note any times when your medication seems to be causing problems in your life. These are important to address, whether they stem from addiction or abuse or they arise because a medication is otherwise inappropriate for you. Also, ask others if they have noticed changes in your behavior or appearance. Repeated abuse can lead to disabling social, emotional, financial, and health consequences. If you experience problems associated with the use of your medication, confide in your doctor and be open to seeking help from an appropriate professional or other resource.

Are you obtaining your medication as prescribed? You should be receiving all of your medication from one doctor, or, if you see multiple doctors, make sure they are aware of everything being prescribed to you for pain. Doctors are on the lookout for "drug-seeking" behavior and will be justifiably suspicious if you are keeping information about your prescription medications from them. One caveat: when pain is undertreated, people may appear to be drug seeking in their efforts to obtain adequate pain relief. Such "pseudo-addiction" is distinguishable from addiction in that the behaviors no longer continue when pain is effectively treated.

Beware of drug interactions. Be sure to discuss *all* relevant interaction effects with your doctor. Any medication can have serious side effects and should be used with caution and discussed with your physician. When you take more than one medication, they multiply, rather than just add to, each other's effects. Medications can also lose potency from consumption of something as innocuous as grapefruit juice. Alcohol can significantly increase the sedating qualities of many medications, which can be a lethal combination. Be up front with your doctor about your use of alcohol, and ask directly about the safety of alcohol with all medications you have been prescribed. This also applies to street drugs. Unfortunately, people with chronic pain sometimes turn to illegal drugs to self-medicate when pain is undertreated. Prescription medications, unlike street drugs, have been tested for safety and effectiveness, and their production is regulated. Street drugs carry many risks, and they do not come with a list of "side effects" to monitor. If you are using street drugs in an effort to quell pain, seek help from a trusted professional or program.

Pain-treatment agreement. Many physicians and medical clinics require patients to sign a treatment contract, particularly when opioids are prescribed. If approached constructively, contracts offer valuable opportunities to improve communication and document your shared understanding. Agreements can include side effects and drug interactions to note, therapeutic goals, and roles and expectations for both patient and physician. If your doctor introduces a contract as part of treatment, see that your own concerns are included as well. The document should reflect a shared understanding that emerges from collaboration and not serve as a substitute for discussion.

Medications commonly used in pain management. You deserve to know about anything going into your body—so know your medications. This will help you to understand your experience and potential alternatives as you or your physician become interested in new approaches. Many pain-management medications are prescribed "off label"—that is, they are medications originally created for one purpose but found to be helpful for symptoms not included in the original approval process. In the United States, for a medication to be marketed explicitly for a particular condition, a pharmaceutical company must submit it to an expensive and labor-intensive Food and Drug Administration (FDA) process to test its safety and effectiveness for that use. Yet, through clinical wisdom and non-FDA clinical trials, many medications are discovered to hold benefits for other maladies. Off-label uses are legal and sometimes more common than the original use. The limiting factor is that drug companies cannot advertise off-label uses. As chronic pain receives greater attention, expect to see more medications introduced for treating pain, such as pregabalin and duloxetine, the first drugs explicitly promoted for fibromyalgia and related pain conditions. The success of their marketing has paved the way for pharmaceutical companies, eager to capitalize on the now-recognized market of chronic pain, to submit FDA applications.

Existing medicines to treat pain are numerous and growing, making it virtually impossible to know about them all. In what follows, I group common medications into four categories: (1) antidepressants, (2) "chill pills," (3) sleep aids, and (4) analgesics (or pain relievers). These categories provide a broad framework for viewing medications you and your doctor may be considering.

Some caveats: The list is neither exhaustive nor mutually exclusive. The categories can be grouped differently or subdivided, and some medications do not fit neatly into any. Plus, many more medications exist than those I mention. For an extensive, updated list of existing medications, check a current *Physician's Desk Reference* (PDR) or other reliable source.[7]

1. Antidepressants

I'm in pain, not depressed! Why do I need an antidepressant? It may seem off-putting, inappropriate, or downright insulting for a doctor to suggest treating pain with antidepressants. However, this suggestion likely represents an off-label use rather than your physician's belief that your pain is psychological. As your doctor or pharmacist can explain, antidepressants have multiple uses, which include treating pain. They are called antidepressants because they were first tested and approved for the treatment of clinical depression. Doses for pain treatment are often significantly lower than those used for depression.

Tricyclic Antidepressants (TCA)

This category has been around for years and has developed a substantial track record for multiple pain conditions. The advantages of tricyclic antidepressants are their relatively low cost, due to the availability of generic versions, and the decades of research on their effects and safety. TCAs are commonly prescribed for pain conditions, including the burning pain that accompanies nerve trauma.

Examples of tricyclic antidepressants

Brand Name	Generic
Desyrel®	trazodone
Elavil®	amitriptyline
Norpramin®	desipramine
Pamelor®	nortriptyline
Sinequan®	doxepin
Tofranil®	imipramine

Among the most common is Elavil (amitriptyline), one of the oldest and most studied in its class. If you start with amitriptyline and respond poorly, don't assume TCAs are not for you. Your doctor may suggest you try out another medication within this class. Newer TCAs have fewer side effects. Unfortunately, taking TCAs involves patience—it can take several weeks before you experience relief. Typically, you begin with a low dose and increase slowly until you reach a dose that seems effective but has negligible side effects. Discuss a realistic timetable with your doctor for evaluating the effectiveness of any TCA prescribed for you, and ask what you can expect at different dosages.

For some, TCAs provide substantial improvements in both sleep and pain relief. Low doses have been shown to raise endorphins to "normal levels" in people with chronic pain, although how this works is not fully understood. TCAs enhance the concentration of two brain neurotransmitter chemicals—norepinephrine and serotonin—at nerve junctions and synapses. One line of thought is that they offer painkilling properties by dampening pain signals or suppressing the fight-or-flight response hypothesized to be activated in some pain conditions. Or they may help by promoting deep-level sleep. Because of their sleep-enhancing properties, TCAs are often taken around bedtime—earlier if you have trouble falling asleep, later if you have trouble staying asleep.

The downside of TCAs is potentially their side effects, which can include blurred vision, dry mouth, constipation, sedation, weight gain, difficulty urinating, cardiovascular effects (e.g., hypertension, postural hypotension, arrhythmias), and falling down (in older adults), all of which may be reduced with lower dosages. Dry mouth and sedation are common. You can experiment with strategies to contend with dry mouth, such as keeping water handy, a glass of chipped ice at your bedside, or sugar-free candies in your pocket. Weight gain from these medications can be considerable—and is as difficult to lose as if put on the "natural way." Sedation, which can range from grogginess to a hangover, may be vexing. If you sleep well but remain overly tired, discuss with your doctor such options as adjusting the dose, changing the time you take it, or adding a stimulating medication in the morning (e.g., an SSRI—see below). For some, a short afternoon nap, if feasible, can manage fatigue. In others, TCAs cause paradoxical reactions such as a rapid heartbeat or anxiety rather than relaxation. If the side effects remain intolerable after an adequate trial period (typically six to eight weeks at therapeutic dosage), TCAs may not be for you.

Trazodone is not a TCA; I included it here to keep it from being orphaned within the antidepressants. It is prescribed similarly to a TCA but operates differently and has fewer adverse side effects. Its most common effect, sedation, makes it popular as a sleep treatment.

Selective Serotonin Reuptake Inhibitors (SSRIs)

Selective serotonin reuptake inhibitors are a newer generation of antidepressants, probably best known by media attention to Prozac®. Unlike TCAs, which affect a range of brain functions, SSRIs focus specifically on serotonin, our natural feel-good chemical, by increasing the time it remains available to the nerve receptors. Because of the complex way our bodies function, we cannot simply increase serotonin production with a "serotonin pill." If your body perceives excess serotonin, it automatically manufactures less—regardless of your overall serotonin level. To sidestep this automatic feedback loop, SSRIs block the receptors that absorb ("uptake") the serotonin from our system— hence, their name.

Examples of selective serotonin reuptake inhibitors

Brand Name	*Generic*
Celexa®	citalopram
Lexapro®	escitalopram
Paxil®	paroxetine
Prozac®	fluoxetine
Zoloft®	sertraline

By keeping serotonin available longer, SSRIs have the potential to decrease pain, combat fatigue, and increase energy. Studies of SSRIs, however, have not yielded compelling results on pain treatment. However, doctors may consider combining an SSRI with another medication as part of their experiments to provide effective relief (and at less expense than some newer medications). As with the TCAs, SSRIs require patience: doses tend to start low and increase gradually, so evaluating the full effect of an SSRI can take several weeks. People who respond poorly to one SSRI may respond favorably to another. As for side effects, the most common are a caffeinelike high (which may dissipate) and sexual dysfunction, ranging from decreased libido to impotence. The effect of SSRIs on sleep quality is inconclusive.

Examples of mixed reuptake inhibitors

Brand Name	Generic
Cymbalta®	duloxetine
Effexor®	venlafaxine
Savella®	milnacipran
Wellbutrin®	bupropion

Additional antidepressants include different types of mixed reuptake inhibitors. Serotonin-norepinephrine reuptake inhibitors (SNRIs), such as duloxetine and milnacipran, increase the availability of serotonin as well as norepinephrine, a neurotransmitter that reduces nerve pain. They are commonly prescribed for conditions such as diabetes, rheumatoid arthritis, and lupus, when nerve pain or damage is involved. Some have been FDA approved for the treatment of arthritis pain and fibromyalgia. Bupropion is a unique norepinephrine-dopamine reuptake inhibitor that works to extend the length of time dopamine remains available. Mixed reuptake inhibitors hold promise because they combine benefits of two antidepressant agents with a lower incidence of side effects—the most common being nausea, loss of appetite, dry mouth, anxiety, agitation, headache, and insomnia. These work in a similar fashion to TCAs but are more activating than sedating.

2. "Chill Pills"

A large array of medications, from multiple classes, share certain properties in the treatment of chronic pain, which include dampening pain perceptions and increasing sedation. For lack of a technical overarching category, I refer to these as "chill pills." This category is based on how these medications may feel rather than shared characteristics. Medical doctors and pharmacists are unlikely to support my inclusion of certain medications in this section because of their diversity. This grouping includes anxiolytics (to relieve anxiety), muscle relaxants, central nervous system depressants, and some neurotransmitters—each operating through very different mechanisms. But despite their dissimilarities, this grouping may be meaningful from the patient side, as you may find these medications can provide the feeling of turning down the thermostat of internal pain and agitation.

Vast differences exist in these medications' duration of effects, length of time they remain in the system, sedating quality, potential side effects, and risks of physical dependence. Most of these medications do not need to build up in your system for you to feel their effects, so you should be able to evaluate their effectiveness fairly quickly. Their main side effects are fatigue and mental fogginess. Because of their sedative quality, they are often (but not always) prescribed to be taken at night.

Benzodiazepines are a classic category of "chill pills" and have anxiolytic, anticonvulsive, and muscle-relaxant properties. The most famous of this type is Valium®, introduced in 1963 and later dubbed "Mother's Little Helper" by the rock group the Rolling Stones for its widespread use (and abuse) by women coping with the stress of home and family.

Examples of benzodiazepines

Brand Name	Generic
Ativan®	lorazepam
Klonopin®	clonazepam
Valium®	diazepam
Xanax®	alprozolam

Numerous other benzodiazepines have since been introduced. The main difference among them is their half-life, the length of time it takes until half of the peak effects of a medication have cleared your system.

Side effects of benzodiazepines in the dosage range used for the treatment of insomnia or anxiety can cause memory deficits, particularly with acquiring new information and "episodic" memory, which includes remembering details of recent events. In some users, this class of medications can cause depression.[8] Another consideration with benzodiazepines is their tendency to create physical dependence; users may develop tolerance and withdrawal symptoms when discontinuing the medication. Addiction and abuse are also risks. Be particularly mindful of such medications if you are vulnerable to alcoholism. For these reasons, some doctors are reluctant to prescribe benzodiazepines for long-term use. Talk with your doctor about what this may mean for you. As with any medication, track the effect of your dose over time, and if you note a decline in effectiveness or a need for a dose increase, report this to your doctor. If you choose to discontinue benzodiazepines for any reason, work carefully with your doctor to taper down slowly; otherwise, you can experience unpleasant and even dangerous withdrawal symptoms. Benzodiazepines vary significantly in the length of time they stay in your system—as you are tapering, your doctor may have you switch to a medication with a shorter half-life.

The following list includes medications that work in very different ways to help dial back pain.

Other "chill pills"

Brand Name	Generic
Flexeril®	cyclobenzaprine
Lyrica®	pregabalin
Norflex®	orphenadrine
Neurontin®	gabapentin
Robaxin®	methocarbamol
Skelaxin®	metaxalone
Zanaflex®	tizanidine

Some are referred to as "muscle relaxants," even though they work on the brain and not the muscles directly. Muscle relaxants were first introduced following animal studies that showed animals no longer panicked when threatened but were still perfectly capable of defending themselves when attacked. The main side effects are dizziness, drowsiness, and sedation. Because of the diversity in this very broad categorization of mechanisms, your doctor may suggest you try different ones. Much depends on your individual reaction. If you respond optimally, you can get *calm* but *not dopey* at the right dose.

Another category included above is anticonvulsants or antiseizure medications. Pregabalin, the first FDA-approved medication for fibromyalgia and related conditions, is similar in structure and effects to its older cousin gabapentin (now an inexpensive generic). These can be frontline treatments for specific pain conditions or used as adjunct therapies. These anticonvulsants operate by affecting the chemicals in the brain that send pain signals across the nervous system. Studies reveal their effectiveness for pain conditions, and neuropathic pain in particular, but keep in mind that your own tracking data provide the most significant test of personal effectiveness. Among the side effects of these medications are weight gain (which can be substantial), fatigue, swelling of hands and feet, and memory problems, typically in the form of word and name recall.

3. Sleep Aids

Sleep problems are common with chronic pain, and poor sleep exacerbates pain. Chapter 14 describes behavioral strategies to improve sleep, which are first-line treatments for sleep problems. If such treatments prove to be inadequate, reducing pain with low levels of TCAs, muscle relaxants, anticonvulsants, or analgesics can help. If sleep problems persist, your doctor might include sleep aids as part of your pain-management strategy.

Examples of sleep aids (in order of strength)

Generic	*Brand Name (to fall asleep)*	*Brand Name (to stay asleep)*	*Type of medication*
diphenhydramine	Benadryl®	——	OTC
zoleplon	Sonata®	——	Non benzodiazepine
zolpidem	Ambien®	Ambien CR®	Non benzodiazepine
ramelteon	Rozerem®	——	Non benzodiazepine
eszopiclone	Lunesta®	Lunesta®	Non benzodiazepine
triazolam	Halcion®	——	Benzodiazepine
temazepam	Restoril®	Restoril®	Benzodiazepine
clonazepam	Klonopin®	Klonopin®	Benzodiazepine

Prescription sleeping pills can help you fall asleep more easily, stay asleep longer, or both. The above table orders medications by their strength. The older sleeping pills are benzodiazepines, which may cause daytime fatigue and physical dependence. As described earlier, benzodiazepines can also alleviate pain. If your doctor considers a benzodiazepine, your options vary considerably. Consider the difference in half-life, for example, among triazolam (two to five hours), temazepam (eight to twelve hours), and clonazepam (sixteen to fifty hours), which are all considered sleep aids. The newer nonbenzodiazepine sleep aids, in contrast, specifically target brain receptors involved in sleep, rather than more generally depressing the central nervous system. These sleep aids are designed to help with sleep, not pain.

Medications to initiate sleep. For the occasional night of tossing and turning, your doctor may recommend an OTC sleep aid. The most common ones combine a mild pain reliever with an antihistamine (such as diphenhydramine, found in Benadryl), as in Tylenol PM® or its equivalent. These are not indicated for long-term use. Your pharmacist can help you navigate such OTC products for occasional use. Consult with your doctor as you would for prescription medications if you are considering an OTC sleep aid, especially if taking other medications. Bear in mind that some people experience a paradoxical effect from antihistamines and can feel alert and agitated rather than drowsy. This effect can increase with age.

Sleep medications like Ambien (zolpidem) and Sonata (zaleplon) are designed to assist with falling asleep and not interfere with deep sleep patterns. Sonata has the shortest half-life of all the sleep aids (between thirty and sixty minutes), allowing it to be a last-resort bedside treatment for times when the night wears on. (You might also talk with your doctor about the possibility of dividing doses of Ambien for the same use—but not Ambien CR, or any other extended-release medication, which should not be divided.) Rozerem is the first in a new class of medications designed to target the body's sleep-wake cycle. It acts on the melatonin receptors, which regulate our circadian rhythms, and can be used long term without risk of dependence. Lunesta has the longest half-life of the newer sleep aids (about six hours). It can help you fall asleep quickly and also improves sleep quality overall. Halcion, or other benzodiazepines with a similarly short half-life, can also be used for problems falling asleep.

Medications to maintain sleep. If you suffer from frequent awakenings, discuss your options with your doctor. Longer-acting benzodiazepines or sedating antidepressants, such as trazodone, can be useful (as mentioned earlier), particularly if they reduce your daytime pain. Sometimes combining a shorter-acting sleep aid with another medication enhances sleep quality. Otherwise, your doctor may consider long-acting sleep aids, such as extended-release zolpidem (Ambien CR) or Lunesta, described earlier, which reduce the frequency and length of nighttime awakenings. Look for new extended-release sleep aids on the market, perhaps as our population ages into sleep difficulties. One such medication, Circadin®, approved in Europe and currently undergoing clinical trials for the US market, releases melatonin to restore sleep cycles in those age fifty-five or above. An advantage of Circadin is its lack of side effects or potential for dependence.

Precautions. Whenever you use sleep aids, whether OTC or prescription varieties, finish your evening activities and plan for ample time (seven or eight hours) to stay in bed. A serious risk with sedating medication is the potential for behaviors that could be potentially embarrassing or dangerous. People have engaged in activities such as "sleep driving" on hypnotic medications and had no memory the next day. Take precautions to stay safe: Take your pill when comfortably in bed. Disregard urges to pick up the phone, engage in projects, or, worse, leave the house or operate machinery. Make sure to alert anyone you live with of this possible hazard.

Always take the medication as prescribed. Extended-release medications should not be broken, divided, or crushed, since this would interfere with their dispensing mechanisms. Many sleep medications, when used regularly, cause physical dependence and should not be stopped suddenly. Drinking alcohol while taking sleep medications, including OTC varieties, is considered dangerous and discouraged. Talk with your doctor about your need to avoid or limit alcohol given your specific situation and medication. And stay abreast of the effects of sleep aids so you can adjust them as needed with your doctor.

Herbal remedies. Some herbs may foster sleep. Valerian root may be helpful. Its worst property may be its foul odor—something to keep in mind if you are deciding among pill, drop, and tea forms. Melatonin may help establish good sleep cycles by "resetting your internal clock." If you are interested in trying these or other herbal remedies, discuss them with your doctor. You can also find comprehensive, updated, evidence-based information on supplements and herbs online at Natural Medicines Comprehensive Database, although it is membership only.

4. Analgesics (a.k.a. Pain Relievers or Painkillers)

Unlike the medications used off label to treat pain, analgesics are specifically intended to relieve pain. Although none is likely to provide the dramatic effect illustrated in television ads for over-the-counter pain medications, they play a significant role in reducing pain intensity. Many pain sufferers report that analgesics "take the edge off," which can mean the difference between functioning and not. Analgesics operate through specific receptors in the central nervous system and can be administered orally, transdermally (through a patch on the skin), or intrathecally (through an injection in the space around the spinal cord).

Whenever you are given anything "for pain," inquire what class of medication it is. Analgesics range from mild over-the-counter varieties to strong opioids. The mildest are nonprescription medications such as aspirin, acetaminophen (Tylenol), and ibuprofen (Advil®/Motrin®). While these can be effective in treating mild to moderate pain, they are constrained by a strength threshold that limits their power. More intense pain requires stronger medications. Taking larger than recommended dosages of OTC analgesics brings no additional pain relief and can be dangerous. Do not assume that because no prescription is required, OTC medications are completely safe. According to reports published by the Federal Drug Administration, the overuse of acetaminophen is the leading cause of liver failure in the United States. Another potential problem with using pain medication is the possibility of developing medication-overuse headaches, which can occur with *any* type of analgesic, and opioid-induced hyperalgesia, a condition in which the use of opioids increases sensitivity to pain.[9]

Anti-Inflammatory Medications

Some analgesics function through their anti-inflammatory properties. These medications range from over-the-counter to prescription-strength varieties, including steroids. They combine pain-relieving and anti-inflammatory effects and are helpful for pain conditions involving swelling around joints or muscles, such as rheumatoid arthritis, tendonitis, osteoarthritis, and musculoskeletal conditions like low back pain.

Nonsteroidal anti-inflammatory drugs (NSAIDs). Many nonsteroidal anti-inflammatory drugs are available without a prescription and can be effective in treating mild osteoarthritis and muscle pain. They are used as backup when breakthrough pain is not adequately treated by a stronger medication. The analgesic effects of NSAIDs work within a few hours, but a week or longer before the full anti-inflammatory benefits are realized.

Examples of nonsteroidal anti-inflammatory drugs

Brand Name	Generic
Advil/Motrin®	ibuprofen
Aleve®	naproxen
Celebrex®	celecoxib
Daypro®	oxaprozin
Lodine®	etodolac
Mobic®	meloxicam
Orudis®	ketoprofen
Relafen®	nabumetone

Side effects of all NSAIDs include gastrointestinal problems, such as stomach irritation, ulcers, liver damage, and potentially fatal internal bleeding. They have been shown to cause heart failure and elevate blood pressure, due to their fluid-retaining properties. The hazards of regular use are greatest in older adults, people with a history of ulcers or other bleeding complications, and people who drink alcohol regularly. Some prescription NSAIDs, particularly celecoxib, are gentler on the system but carry the same set of risks. To monitor side effects, your doctor may regularly test your blood. Compounding pharmacists can offer specialized NSAIDs that may reduce irritation and other side effects.

NSAIDs work by blocking the production of prostaglandins, chemicals that transmit messages of pain and swelling in inflammatory conditions. Prostaglandins are made of two different enzymes (referred to as COX-1 and COX-2). A newer form of prescription NSAID (e.g., Celebrex) affects COX-2 enzymes only, lowering the risk of stomach injuries, but, unfortunately, it has been found to be riskier for individuals with certain heart conditions. Some of these medications are no longer sold because of concerns about their side effects.[10] Newer ways to deliver NSAIDs apply the medication directly to a joint or soft tissue, such as with a gel or a patch. Talk with your doctor about the appropriateness of using NSAIDs for inflammatory pains and about the type and dose that would be best suited to you. Because not all NSAIDs are the same and their effects vary from person to person, your doctor may have you try different ones before reaching a conclusion about this class of medication.

Corticosteroids. Corticosteroids are strong anti-inflammatory drugs that control severe swelling and pain in conditions that involve inflammation, such as arthritis, lupus, multiple sclerosis, and inflammatory bowel disease. Dozens are available today. Also referred to as steroids, corticosteroids are distinct from anabolic steroids, which are notorious for their abuse by some athletes. Corticosteroids are designed to mimic cortisone, a naturally occurring hormone that reduces pain and inflammation and increases mobility in joints and tissues. When prescribed in doses that exceed your body's usual level of cortisone, they suppress inflammation. They also can help control the destructive process in autoimmune conditions. Corticosteroids sometimes help with pain crises, but they are hardly ever used for long-term treatment because of their potentially fatal adverse effects. Possible side effects of short-term use include fluid retention, increased blood pressure, significant mood swings, and weight gain. Adverse effects that do not resolve or become bothersome merit immediate attention. Risks increase with longer-term use and can include cataracts, diabetes, ulcers, brittle bones, and thinning skin. Long-term therapy is usually reserved for severe cases of inflammatory disease, and then, because side effects accumulate with use, it is generally advised to limit doses.

Examples of corticosteroids

Brand Name	Generic
Cortone Acetate®	cortisone
———	prednisone
Medrol®	methylprednisoline

Corticosteroids are used most often as injections directly into the painful tissue, such as a particular joint, muscle, bursa, or tendon. Steroid injections to the spine (epidural injections) have long been used to relieve low back pain and neck pain caused by disc disease or pinched nerves. Injections can be particularly helpful during early or acute phases by allowing you to engage in exercise and other therapeutic behaviors to lessen pain. Systemic injections are sometimes used when multiple joints are affected, as in rheumatoid arthritis. Injections administer high doses at the affected site without system-wide side effects. However, injections should be used sparingly to prevent cartilage damage or other local effects. If your pain involves inflammation, discuss options with your doctor.

Opioid-Derived Analgesics (Narcotics)

Opioids—derived from natural or artificial forms of opium—are frontline treatments for severe pain after weaker medications have proved inadequate. Many people, including medical professionals, refer to opioids and narcotics interchangeably. The term *narcotic* is used by law enforcement agencies to denote not only opioids but also various other drugs that are illegal. Because of the connection to street drugs, I will refer to this class of medications only as opioids.

It is important to understand that the use of opioids for chronic pain (in the absence of cancer) is controversial. Many believe that these drugs should be used as a last resort. If you have had inadequate pain relief from other classes of medications, talk with your doctor about what opioids may hold for you. This class of medications is not limited by a pain ceiling; higher doses bring greater relief. Limits in dose emerge instead from negative side effects (such as nausea, constipation, dizziness, and sedation) and medical biases against this class of medication. Highly publicized accounts of drug abuse and misuse may have jeopardized legitimate use of opioids in pain treatment. But, as described earlier, *most* people who take pain medication as directed do not become addicted, even with long-term use. At times, doctors may feel the risks outweigh the benefits. This does not necessarily mean the doctor is ill informed. Inquire about your doctor's reasoning.

Doctors typically take a stepwise approach in prescribing opioids, slowly increasing the potency of the medication until the desired effect is achieved. Because your response largely guides treatment, be careful to record all changes in doses, symptoms, and other reactions. The aim is to achieve optimal pain control with minimal side effects. People vary in the extent to which they develop tolerance; some can maintain adequate relief at low to moderate doses for extended periods. If you note a decrease in the pain-relieving properties, report this to your doctor.

Examples of opioids

Generic Opioid	Brand Name	Brand Name (short acting, with acetaminophen)	Brand Name (extended release)
buprenorphine patch	———	———	Butrans®
fentanyl patch	———	———	Duragesic®
hydrocodone	———	Vicodin®	Vicodin ER®
hydromorphone	Dilaudid®	———	Exalgo®
methadone	Dolophine®	———	
morphine sulfate	(morphine)	———	MS Contin®
oxycodone	Roxicodone®	Percocet®	Oxycontin®
oxymorphone	———	Percocet®	Opana ER®
tramadol	Ultram®	Ultracet®	Ultram ER®

Opioids attach to opioid receptors on nerve cells and interrupt pain signals traveling to the brain by imitating the body's own endorphins. They differ in their strength, duration of action, side effects, routes of administration, and newness. Many opioids are available in generic form. The most common, hydrocodone, is in hundreds of brand-name and generic products. The above table includes the generic name of the active ingredient as well as examples of brand names associated with different forms. Opioids are available in both short- and long-acting forms.

Many short-acting medications, such as Vicodin and Percocet, combine a nonopioid agent (such as acetaminophen or aspirin) with an opioid (such as oxycodone or hydrocodone). If you are taking a pure opioid form, make sure to talk with your doctor about the effects of supplementing with a nonopioid analgesic, such as Tylenol or Advil, which can amplify such drugs' potency. Short-acting medications can be taken as needed, providing three to six hours of pain relief and allowing you to adjust to your current needs or anticipated pain triggers.

Some on this list work slightly differently. Methadone is an often-underutilized pain reliever. Given its long history, it is available as a low-cost generic, and considerable research testifies to its safety and effectiveness. Work closely with your doctor if you are considering methadone because it has a long half-life and cumulative effect (it builds up in your system over time), which means it can take some time for the drug's initial side effects to diminish. Tramadol inhibits pain by increasing serotonin and norepinephrine in the spinal cord, which activate an opioid receptor in the central nervous system. Physicians may be more comfortable prescribing this medication because it is not technically an opioid—it just acts like one.

Short-acting analgesics are a good option when pain varies substantially. Your tracking tool is invaluable for assessing how to best use as-needed medications so you have just enough for relief but not "too little, too late." Once pain builds, it is more difficult to interrupt, yet people sometimes save stronger painkillers for when they "really need them," particularly if they don't like taking strong medications or their doctor is reluctant to prescribe opioids for daily use.

For more continuous pain, however, short-acting opioids can create something of a roller coaster ride between doses. If your pain is fairly constant, talk with your doctor. Strategies may include taking short-acting medications more frequently in divided doses to keep a more steady amount in your system. Or long-acting opioids are specifically intended for this, as in the extended-release (ER) options listed in the above chart. Doctors sometimes begin with shorter-acting drugs to determine your optimal dose before switching to a long-acting equivalent. Oral ER medications, such as Oxycontin or Ultram ER, are intended to provide a steady dose of pain relief, thereby eliminating the peaks and valleys of overtreating and undertreating. Methadone, while not available in an ER formula, has a long half-life, requiring less frequent doses (and at a low cost compared to ER medications). Transdermal medications release their drug through a patch on the skin. Duragesic, for example, delivers fentanyl into body fats, slowly releasing it into the bloodstream. Many patches are available in generic form.

Topical Treatments

Other nonopioid pain-relieving patches are available, such as Lidoderm®, which numbs the area with a local anesthetic (lidocaine). Anesthetics can also be delivered through ointments, such as EMLA cream, absorbed through your skin. Other topical treatments include OTC products like Capzasin® and Zostrix®, which use capsaicin, the ingredient associated with the burning sensation in chili peppers. (Make sure to keep this product away from your eyes and other sensitive areas.) Capsaicin is thought to reduce pain by interrupting the transmission of pain messages. Topical treatments work best when you have specific painful areas, and they are most effective on joints close to the skin's surface, such as hands and knees. Capsaicin-containing preparations are available without a prescription, and NSAID-containing ones are beginning to appear as well. Applying hot and cold can also relieve pain (as described in chapter 11).

Injections

For some people, injections provide temporary or more sustained pain relief. Trigger-point injections can relieve pain and increase range of motion, and they are sometimes used for symptoms of fibromyalgia, tension headaches, or myofascial pain syndromes that do not respond to other treatments. Injections can contain saline (simply to break up muscle spasms), an anesthetic (to numb the area), a steroid (to reduce inflammation), or some combination.

Nerve Blocks

Nerve blocks affect the specific nerves involved in the pain. They are regularly used to treat back and neck pain caused by nerve damage or compression, such as herniated discs or spinal stenosis. Local blocks inject anesthetics into the space around the affected nerve—as in Novocaine® during dental surgery or an epidural during childbirth—to relieve chronic nerve pain, such as spinal compression or damage. Neurolytic blocks use chemicals or other agents to damage certain areas of the nerve pathway to relieve severe chronic pain, as in complex regional pain syndromes. Surgical nerve blocks similarly damage or cut certain areas of the nerve to provide a permanent effect. This is typically reserved for severe pain that can accompany cancer, trigeminal neuralgia (a nerve disorder that causes intense facial pain), or other neuropathic pain. The risks of these procedures can include nerve damage (which could lead to muscle paralysis, weakness, or numbness) and, in rare cases, increased pain due to nerve irritation. In discussing options with your doctor, make sure you understand the risks, the potential gains, and what to expect immediately following any procedure.

Implanted Devices

Many pain medications work in the spinal cord, where pain signals travel. With oral medications, providing sufficient amounts to the spinal cord often requires saturating the rest of the body, which causes system-wide side effects. An alternative method involves injecting the medication into the spinal column (intrathecally), which requires a tiny fraction of the dose for potent pain relief. Intrathecal delivery is often done with a surgically implanted pump and catheter, which brings the medicine into the spinal column. The pump holds the medicine, which is adjusted by the wearer using a remote electronic device and is refilled in the doctor's office about every one to four months. Morphine pumps are common. But other medications can be used intrathecally, and new ones continue to enter the market. Among these can be found ziconotide (Prialt®), a new class of medication that is neither opioid nor anti-inflammatory. While ziconotide carries serious side effects, including memory loss and confusion, researchers are actively searching for ways to target specific pain receptors.

Another implanted device for pain relief is a spinal cord–simulation implant, which transmits low-level electrical signals to the spinal cord or specific nerves to block pain signals from reaching the brain. Discuss with your doctor the appropriateness of any of these options, which may require referral to a specialist or a pain or spine center.

Looking to the Future

Pharmaceutical companies and university labs are currently conducting research to improve methods of pain control. A significant limitation of existing strategies is that they tend to affect the whole system, making it difficult to deliver adequate pain relief without also causing unpleasant or prohibitive side effects. Advances in the scientific understanding of the cells and molecules that transmit pain signals are covered in a 2006 review article in *Scientific American* that describes promising new approaches for chronic pain that has been poorly controlled with existing therapies.[11] The fruits of this research are coming down the pike. Among the most exciting new lines of research are:

A drug to "unlearn" chronic pain. Studies have shown that chronic pain occurs through a sensitization of the central nervous system to ongoing pain signals. A new drug, referred to by code name NB001, shows promise for chronic neuropathic pain in animal trials by helping neurons "unlearn" their hypersensitivity to incoming pain signals.[12] Developed by a team of researchers at the University of Toronto led by Dr. Min Zhuo, NB001 works by blocking a particular enzyme (AC1) produced in spinal cord and brain neurons during nerve injury. Zhuo's team has found AC1 to be central to the process in which the system comes to expect pain signals and strengthens the pain-perception pathway.

Testing revealed that NB001 was as effective at a dose ten to fifty times lower than was currently used in existing first-line treatments for neuropathic pain. Because NB001 specifically targets isolated brain regions, it does not affect the heart, liver, kidney, or other organs outside of the central nervous system (CNS). More research is needed on possible negative effects within the CNS, which could include cognition or memory. Lab tests on mice show significant reductions in chronic pain, while leaving responses to acute pain and memory intact (in other words, the mice did not forget earlier painful stimuli).[13] Zhuo's lab is finishing the animal testing required for an FDA clinical trial application and will partner with a pharmaceutical company to develop a medication for its patented formula.

A promising protein. Research on PAP (or prostatic acid phosphatase), spearheaded by Dr. Mark Zylka and his colleagues in the Department of Cell and Molecular Physiology at University of North Carolina at Chapel Hill, has discovered dramatic analgesic effects of PAP, a natural substance that, like insulin, is found in the body (in pain-sensing neurons) and can be manufactured and injected into the body. Using animal models, Dr. Zylka's group found PAP to be eight times more potent than morphine—one injection inhibits pain for many days and successfully suppresses chronic inflammatory pain.[14] They have also discovered important prophylactic effects, such as injecting PAP prior to causing nerve injury or inflammation may offer long-term relief from the pain that would normally follow. This may translate into the use of PAP to prevent postoperative pain as well as postsurgical chronic pain syndromes. Equally significant, PAP appears to offer pain relief without producing any of the side effects of existing pain medications. Instead of targeting opioid or central nervous system receptors, PAP targets adenosine receptors that work directly with the dorsal root ganglia in part of the spinal cord that relays pain signals.

This research, at this point, has shown definite results in lab mice. The researchers are now in the process of moving toward clinical trials in humans. They predict that PAP will work the same way in humans; administering an injection of PAP would bring tremendous pain relief, particularly for local and regional chronic pain syndromes. They have also teamed with the Center for Integrative Chemical Biology and Drug Discovery at UNC to create an oral compound that would reduce pain via this same adenosine receptor pathway. The center, headed by Dr. Stephen Frye, the former worldwide head of discovery medicinal chemistry at GlaxoSmithKline, is devoted to translating basic research into new medications to help patients. According to Dr. Frye, we must increasingly look to university centers for the development of new medicines, rather than relying on large pharmaceutical companies to do this.[15] This collaboration is promising for the development of a pain reliever that is much more potent than existing ones without their unpleasant side effects.

A discovery on acupuncture. Until recently, research on acupuncture has not yielded definite results. Part of the difficulty in testing comes from the difficulties in creating a double-blind research design, the gold standard for scientific evaluation. A recent paper published in *Nature and Neuroscience* found positive evidence of pain relief in mice, which are not vulnerable to placebo effect.[16] According to Dr. Zylka, the mechanism this team uncovered in its research on the effects of acupuncture may mirror the effect of the PAP protein. This provides information not only for greater scientific understanding of the mechanisms behind acupuncture but also for additional research on ways to apply these mechanisms through other means.[17]

Gene therapy for pain control. Gene therapy has become a vibrant area of research for the treatment of pain. Instead of delivering a particular medication, researchers are delivering genes that are specifically altered to produce a pain-relieving effect. The genes are altered by adding something called a *vector* to the blueprint of specific cells, often introduced by an incapacitated virus, which allows information to infect the DNA of specific cells (but doesn't multiply further). The new genes can then produce an opioid or anti-inflammatory effect that selectively targets the peripheral nervous system involved with pain perception. This novel approach, which does not rely on new medications being discovered, greatly expands options for pain treatments. Researchers can use gene transfer to produce naturally occurring transmitters that can block pain transmission without side effects. This is being pursued at different labs, each using distinct vectors, which would target specific sites rather than flood the entire body.

This approach is well established in lab animals. Dr. Andreas Beutler and his colleagues at the Mayo Clinic demonstrated pain control in animals without side effects or other worrisome findings; their next step will be to test for safety on cancer patients who suffer with severe pain.[18] Dr. David Fink and his colleagues at the University of Michigan have just completed clinical safety trials in humans with another gene therapy for pain treatment after studying its effects for more than a decade in animals. The next phase of research will involve a large clinical trial involving a control group. This therapy holds great promise for relieving regional pain problems, such as pain caused by joint or nerve damage or cancer.

Too many promising possibilities to mention them all. Other notables include research on blocking sodium channels—pores in the cell membranes that generate an electric current by selectively emitting charged particles—which has shown a reversal of nerve injury–induced behavior in animals and significant reductions in neuropathic pain in humans.[19] Research on TRPVI (an "ion channel" in pain-sensing neurons), which is activated by capsaicin (the chemical responsible for the heat in chili peppers), has also generated interest in the way temperature and pain sensitization are integrated. Various drugs are in clinical trials on this substance.[20]

The good news is that many research units are looking into new avenues to target chronic pain, and we can expect new treatment options in future years. Many promising research streams, however, do not result in the hoped-for remedy—at least, not right away. The ratio of research to effective treatments is low; however, the number of promising approaches increases these odds. Basic scientific research to develop new approaches is also affected by funding streams. Pharmaceutical companies typically become involved *after* a strategy has been proven effective. You can contribute to the advancement of novel approaches by making philanthropic donations to research institutions whose work you find most promising and by seeking opportunities to volunteer as a research subject when appropriate.

For information on existing medications, see the following web resources: Mayo Clinic, WebMD, PubMed Health, and Medline-Plus. These free and reliable websites, which provided much of the information in this chapter, allow you to look up medications by name or to search by topic area.

Chapter 18

Strategies for Working with Mental Health Professionals

I'm in pain, not crazy. Why would I seek therapy? Many people living with chronic pain have been treated as if their symptoms were psychological in origin. Unfortunately, this ill-informed response can discourage people with pain from seeking help from mental health professionals. Yet living day in and day out with pain creates psychological hardships. Chronic pain is exhausting—it can challenge your coping skills, threaten your sense of self, and affect every aspect of your life. Receiving assistance from someone in the mental healthcare field can help you manage and improve the areas of your life that are affected by pain.

Potential Benefits of Consulting a Mental Health Professional

A safe place to vent. The psychotherapist's office offers a space to describe your experience and express frustrations. At the least, you can enjoy a guilt-free opportunity to tell it like it is, which may reduce urges to unload on your friends and family. Sharing the details of your suffering on a regular basis with the people in your life carries risks. Even the most sympathetic listener can develop compassion fatigue from too-frequent reports of distress. In addition, given the invisible nature of pain, you may not always receive the validation you seek. At times, when you crave a sympathetic ear, you may instead receive unsolicited advice. Mental health professionals are trained to listen, validate, and assist—and living with chronic pain creates plenty of need for these functions. It does not matter how weary you feel during therapy because you are not required to perform—the time is exclusively devoted to you and enhancing your life. When you are facing life uncertainties, being able to count on having someone listen to you on a regular basis can be invaluable.

Learn pain-relief strategies. Many therapists offer tools to help you dial back your pain thermostat. They can teach you how to tune in to your body, slow down, and enter a deep state of relaxation. Consider seeking a therapist who uses hypnosis, guided imagery, biofeedback, diaphragmatic breathing, meditation, mindfulness-based stress reduction, or other techniques that can decrease pain. Therapists who specialize in chronic pain are more likely to have expertise in these treatments. Reviewing your situation with a therapist can also provide insights into the conditions under which you tend to feel better (and worse). You can paintrack together, devising experiments and interpreting their results, then implementing changes in your behavior and self-talk to increase your comfort and capabilities.

Develop more effective coping strategies. Your ability to contend with problems is compromised when you feel vulnerable or overwhelmed by pain. Even the most "mentally healthy" individuals would struggle with day-in, day-out pain and exhaustion. Coping successfully requires an effective repertoire of positive strategies. Unfortunately, when people are under strain, such strategies can be harder to access, and go-to responses such as denial, avoidance, and pity may not be the most beneficial ones. Therapy can help you reflect constructively on your situation, identify your choices, and evaluate what does and does not seem to be working. A good therapist can offer techniques to help you with the struggles that commonly arise with chronic pain, including grief and loss, relationship difficulties, anxiety and depression, and challenging adjustments. Through this process, you can discover your strengths, identify obstacles impeding your progress, and develop increasingly effective coping strategies.

Increase constructive self-talk. Much of the way we feel comes from what we say to ourselves. Chronic pain often pervades every aspect of life— your work, your relationships and roles with family and friends, and, often, your feelings about yourself. Therapists can help you examine your self-talk and reshape the stories you tell yourself about your situation. A growing body of research demonstrates that positive thinking significantly affects people's physiological experience, including their perception of pain. As described in chapter 12, when people experience distress, they are more prone to pessimistic thinking, such as escalating the meaning of a negative experience or perception to catastrophic proportions. The way you view and react to your circumstances can act as a self-fulfilling prophecy. Consider the difference between treating a painful flare-up as a sign your life is over, versus seeing it as a setback you can handle. Therapy can help you replace self-defeating thoughts and behaviors with more productive ones. Cultivating a realistic and positive understanding of your ability to contend with challenging situations allows you to persevere, even flourish.

Validate your experience. Many people with chronic pain do not feel understood. It may be that they fear being honest with the people they want to protect. Or they may feel others cannot relate to their experience, despite everyone's best efforts. Therapy offers an opportunity to be understood. Therapists are trained to listen and understand your experience through your unique vantage point. Group therapy offers another valuable way to feel understood. It can be especially powerful to receive support, empathy, and feedback from people who are going through similar struggles.

Improve your relationships. Chronic illness introduces stress into relationships. If you are part of a couple, pain poses challenges for you both. Like you, your partner likely experiences a strong mix of emotions, which may include sympathy, fear, anger, denial, frustration, or despair. Partners may feel confused by the vacillating abilities they observe and be unsure when to comfort or push. They may feel exhausted with their partner's struggles and guilty about this reaction. "Well" partners may feel uncomfortable sharing their own daily struggles or successes out of fear about the implicit comparisons. Couples may face potential relationship imbalances, substantial questions about their roles, and worries about the difficulties, including financial strain, that can arise with disability.

This turmoil makes open and effective communication more vital. Effective sharing can unite and strengthen couples. Ironically, however, chronic pain complicates couples' ability to express their feelings and desires. Emotions are often charged, and partners may feel uncomfortable raising topics that feel off-limits. Out of a desire not to burden the other, people may avoid sharing the depth of their struggles. Emotion related to chronic pain can be like the proverbial elephant in the room—its presence is enormous, yet you fear to acknowledge it.

Attending therapy as a couple helps people broach sensitive issues and learn to support each other in the process. At a minimum, therapy commits a specific time to focusing on the relationship. Couples therapists differ in approach, but all seek to facilitate communication, identify interpersonal patterns, and help improve those patterns that are working less well. Some therapists teach specific methods for raising and reacting to difficult topics, such as the ways chronic pain affects the relationship. Many assign between-session homework, such as practicing a communication skill or scheduling fun. Therapists also provide education when appropriate.

Attending therapy as a family offers another avenue for changing the impact of chronic pain on those closest to you. Working with a family therapist can help allay fears, increase collaboration, and provide an opportunity to understand and validate each other's experiences. Each family member may carry secret stories that would benefit from exposure. Young children, for example, may internalize what they observe and mistakenly conclude that what their parent feels is somehow their fault. Family therapy also ensures a set time for the family, and homework similarly provides opportunities to engage in new skills together. Therapists can also assist with specific issues, such as how to parent despite pain or bring up touchy topics concerning worries or difficulties within the family. Family members may also benefit from individual therapy to work through their own sadness, anxiety, grief, anger, fear, helplessness, or other reactions.

Work through difficult emotions. Chronic pain is not a life sentence to misery. Just because it might make sense that you feel anxious or depressed about your pain does not mean these feelings are inevitable. Left untreated, strong negative emotions, such as despair, fear, hopelessness, and guilt, can lead to a downward spiral, fueling both emotional and physical suffering. Depression is often associated with chronic pain; however, therapy can help dispel depression, whatever its cause. Therapy can also offer strategies to diminish anxiety that may arise from or be exacerbated by the uncertainties of living with pain. Chronic pain is difficult. Contending with strong negative emotions on top of the physical pain creates suffering. If you were already experiencing depression or anxiety before developing pain, that's even more reason to seek help. Also, if chronic pain has elicited a shift in your outlook, consider therapy as a way to improve your attitude and engagement in life.

Help you reprioritize. Chronic pain may have shifted your career path, other roles, or plans. Having to reprioritize life choices can be incredibly difficult. You may be struggling with weighty questions, such as whether and how you might be able to become a parent, continue in your studies, or support your family, given your current pain. A therapist can help you problem solve about concrete issues and identify emotion-based reasoning that may be getting in the way. Being able to reprioritize effectively can involve difficult decisions, grief work, flexible thinking, and adaptive strategies. The support of a professional can help you through this process.

Help with grief and acceptance. Therapy can help you mourn health-related losses just as you would other significant losses. Living well with chronic illness often requires a grieving process that leads eventually to greater acceptance. This does not mean you like the situation or will stop trying to improve. On the contrary, acceptance is about acknowledging what is, rather than tormenting yourself with how you wish things were. Through greater acceptance, you can move forward with your life, better equipped to care for yourself, adapt, and improve. When you accept that you will sometimes feel sadness, even anger or self-pity, you are less likely to react to these emotions in a way that makes them worse. You can concentrate instead on ways to shorten these periods and make them fewer and farther between.

Evaluate and treat depression. Chronic pain can lead to clinical depression. It is well documented that people with chronic pain develop depression at higher rates than the general population, and the reasons are many: the pain itself; poor sleep; the often lengthy and frustrating process of receiving a diagnosis; inappropriate or ineffective treatment; the seeming randomness of painful flare-ups; grief over losses; lack of support; and additional stressors that accompany chronic pain, including financial, family, and other life problems. Yet depression is not an inevitable aspect of chronic pain. It is, therefore, very important that if you are suffering from depression or any other mental health conditions, these are properly diagnosed and treated.

Address emotional triggers. It is common for people with chronic pain to experience a surge in pain in response to negative emotions. Pain may rise, for example, when people start to feel angry or irritated. This process can occur very quickly, and without deliberate awareness, the association with the cause may be missed. Therapy can help people understand the relationships among thoughts, feelings, and physical comfort. Learning to identify emotional triggers is especially important for people who have suffered from childhood adversity, trauma, or invalidating environments, all of which result in greater emotional vulnerability. An emotional trigger can be a thing as seemingly benign as a word, sight, or sound, if it holds associations with something diffi-cult. Through therapy, people can identify their triggers and learn strategies to stop them from flooding the body with pain. Therapy also offers a place for trauma survivors to heal from the interrelated struggles involved with emo-tional and physical suffering. One strategy may be to reconnect with the body and self in a positive way. Improvement may involve rethinking current living circumstances that are highly triggering.

The Beware List: When Depression Becomes a Problem of Its Own

Everyone experiences sadness. Transitory blue periods are part of the human condition and are normal and expected during times of hardship. Depression, however, is a more persistent sadness that interferes with your ability to engage in and enjoy life, therefore warranting serious attention. No one is immune to depression. It affects people of all ages, social classes, and cultures.

Undiagnosed depression in people with chronic pain also reduces their ability to manage the pain. Negativistic thinking and emotions interfere with the use of effective coping strategies, decrease motivation, and increase the risk of isolation. This, in turn, creates a downward spiral in which depression leads to greater pain, which further fuels the depression.

The criteria for clinical depression are spelled out in the *Diagnostic and Statistical Manual of Mental Disorders* (DSM), the veritable diagnostic bible for mental health professionals. The DSM works like a flowchart or an à la carte menu. To receive a diagnosis of clinical depression, individuals must expe-rience five (or more) of the symptoms listed below, with at least one being "depressed mood" or the loss of pleasure in activities formerly enjoyed.

Symptoms of Depression
(Adapted from DSM-IV[1])

(1) Depressed mood.

(2) Markedly diminished interest or pleasure in all, or almost all, activities, such as eating, exercise, and social and sexual interactions.

(3) Significant weight loss when not dieting or weight gain (e.g., a change of more than 5 percent of body weight in a month) or noticeable change in appetite.

(4) Noticeable change in sleeping patterns, such as fitful sleep, inability to sleep, early-morning awakening, or sleeping too much.

(5) Feelings of extreme restlessness or of being slowed down, to the extent that others can observe this change.

(6) Fatigue or loss of energy nearly every day.

(7) Feelings of worthlessness, hopelessness, or excessive or inappropriate guilt (which may be delusional) nearly every day (not merely self-reproach or guilt about being sick).

(8) Diminished ability to think or concentrate; indecisiveness.

(9) Recurrent thoughts of death and suicide; wishing to die.

Caveats: The symptoms must not be due to

- medication or a medical condition (such as hypothyroidism), or
- bereavement that occurs after the loss of a loved one.

You may notice substantial overlap of the symptoms of depression and chronic pain itself: pain can diminish pleasure, interfere with concentration, and cause sleep difficulty and fatigue as well as changes in eating patterns (e.g., pain can complicate food preparation, and medications can cause weight gain). It may even seem that *anyone* with chronic pain would meet these criteria. However, there are important distinctions.

Clinical Depression: Four Red Flags

The following red flags signal that you are dealing with more than just the expected ups and downs that come from living with pain.

Symptom severity. Pay careful attention to the most serious of the symptoms: feelings of worthlessness or helplessness, or recurrent thoughts of death or suicide. If you experience any of these, seek out a qualified mental health professional. Unfortunately, in the midst of despair, it's challenging to muster the energy to request help, and others' offers of assistance may seem pointless. Yet depression is treatable—you do not have to feel hopeless and miserable, even in the face of pain.

Symptom pervasiveness. Use your tracking data to monitor the *extent* to which you experience sadness, loss of pleasure, or decreased interest in activities. If you feel this way most of the time, on most days (for at least a two-week period), heed this flag! Without assistance, depressed individuals can lose interest in the world around them, undergo serious behavior changes, and become unable to function—all of which would likely increase physical pain as well!

Symptom change. Use your tracking data to identify *changes* in your symptoms or experiences, such as shifts in your cognitive abilities, sleep patterns, or motivation. For example, while you may report fatigue on a daily basis, it's noteworthy if you're staying in bed longer and feeling less motivated. Among possible behavioral changes, be particularly wary of changes in consumption patterns of alcohol or drugs, as this may indicate an attempt to self-medicate depressive symptoms.

Prolonged grief. The DSM-IV does not label symptoms as clinical depression when they occur within two months of the death of a loved one. This caveat may apply well to the grief that accompanies chronic pain—it may similarly make sense to give yourself a couple months to grieve your significant losses (see chapter 26). However, if you find yourself struggling to emerge from your grief and reengage with life, seek out resources and help.

These red flags are intended to help people recognize when they are in dangerous waters. But it is not your job to self-diagnose; if you feel sad and wonder if you might benefit from professional help, chances are you would.

Unfortunately, there are many reasons people are reluctant to seek help for depression. Stigma still persists around mental health issues, and some people may feel shame or guilt over their suffering. Additionally, admitting mental health difficulties can feel risky if you have been treated as if your pain was all in your head and have had to struggle to receive a medical diagnosis for your pain symptoms. Some people may worry that admitting to *any* depressed feelings may undermine their credibility. Moreover, it is easy to miss or deny depression when you *expect* to feel lousy: "Of course I feel down—I hurt all the time!" Well-intentioned friends and family may reinforce this: "Of course you are depressed—look what you are going through!" While such comments may feel supportive, they interfere with seeking help.

Depression is a treatable condition, and relieving depression will help you cope better and improve your ability to manage your pain. Treatments may include antidepressant medication, counseling by a mental health professional, participation in group therapy, self-help techniques, or, likely, a combination of these. While chronic pain is not cheery, it does not condemn you to a life bereft of hope. If you are in despair, take action. Treating depression enables you to contemplate a richer, fuller life.

Selecting a Therapist

When contemplating therapy, ask yourself what you most want to achieve. You may seek treatment for feelings of depression or anxiety or to learn strategies to reduce your pain, communicate more effectively with family, feel less alone, process your grief, discover a new career path, or advocate for yourself in healthcare settings. Identifying your primary goal helps you look for a therapist with experience and expertise in that area.

There are many different types of therapists, specialties, and approaches. Finding a therapist who is right for you may involve shopping around. Because the therapeutic process is built on trust, it is essential that you find a therapist with whom you feel comfortable and can build a working alliance. This may be a tall order if you are apprehensive about therapy. Look to your networks. If you are active in a faith-based community and find the idea of therapy uncomfortable, you may want to investigate the availability of a pastoral counselor or the equivalent in your religious tradition. Seek counsel from people you trust for suggestions, such as members of support groups or your doctor. Online referral databases offer another way to research therapists. You can often view a therapist's professional profile, treatment philosophy, and areas of expertise. When shopping for a psychotherapist or group, ask questions.

Some questions to ask a prospective therapist:

1. What is your experience working with people with chronic pain? (If experienced, what tools does he or she use? If not, assess his or her comfort level with chronic pain.)
2. What is your training? (Feel free to ask about educational background and license.)
3. What is your theoretical orientation? (Feel free to ask for reading materials that will familiarize you with the therapist's approach and help you better understand his or her viewpoint.)
4. Are your services covered by my insurance? (Also, check with your insurance carrier about co-payment and the length of coverage.) What are your fees?
5. After an initial meeting and presentation of problem, what is a realistic length of time in which to expect to see some progress?

Experience with pain? You may want to inquire about a clinician's experience and approach in working with individuals with chronic pain. Some therapists specialize in chronic pain and incorporate tools such as meditation, hypnosis, biofeedback, and guided imagery into their practice. The importance of their familiarity with pain depends on your goals. If you want someone who specializes in pain relief, consider therapists who are connected to a pain clinic, or get recommendations from your doctor or medical center. Ask potential therapists about the specific tools they use to help with pain. Even a therapist with no special training in chronic pain may use tools such as hypnosis that could be used for pain relief.

If you're primarily concerned about a professional's ability to understand you, raise this concern with potential therapists. Feel free to ask direct questions, such as whether the therapist has any idea what it is like to live with chronic pain. Your improvement depends on your comfort with a therapist—and his or her reaction to straightforward questions can provide telling data. I remember grilling therapists, early on in my search for relief, about their experience with severe pain. At that time, I found my experience so hard to fathom that I couldn't believe anyone, even a trained professional, could comprehend its depth. None of my therapists had personal experience with chronic pain. However, I recall with great fondness my very productive work with one young woman who demonstrated in a hundred small ways just how clearly she grasped my reality.

Therapists are trained in helping people reduce suffering and increase their understanding and quality of life. Ask any potential therapists to explain how they will work with you to address your specific goals. Most important is that you can work together and learn, as needed, from each other. Therapists may be willing to read a book or other relevant resource that you recommend to increase their understanding of your experience.

Training? *Therapy* and *psychotherapy* are general terms for mental healthcare. All licensed psychotherapists are required to uphold confidentiality (unless you divulge a plan to harm yourself or someone else), undergo formal training, and participate in continuing education, and they are subject to the rules and standards of a licensing board of the state that licenses them. Practitioners in this field are many. Licensed clinical social workers currently provide the majority of psychotherapy in the United States. Other therapists include psychologists, licensed professional counselors, marriage and family therapists, pastoral counselors, and psychiatrists—although psychiatrists tend now to provide more drug therapy than talk therapy. Traditionally, individual therapy takes place in a weekly fifty-minute session at a therapist's office, but other options exist, including phone sessions, in-home services, and, more recently and controversially, services through the Internet.

Be aware that people without appropriate training may put out a shingle and are not regulated by any state law or agency. All licensed therapists are required to display their credentials in their primary place of work and to answer questions about their qualifications. If you have concerns, contact the relevant licensing board. Most offer online databases so you can check the status of a therapist's license.

A variety of peer counselors also exist. Some receive training from organizations such as churches; others rely on their own school of hard knocks. Unlike licensed therapists, peer counselors do not have formal training, credentials, liability insurance, or the surveillance of professional regulatory boards. The main advantages of seeing a peer counselor may be their afford-ability (service can be free of charge) and their informality, if you are uncom-fortable seeing a mental health professional.

Life coaches and career counselors may be appropriate if your main interest is in navigating a difficult career or life juncture but prefer not to delve into any other issues. The titles "career counselor" and "life coach" are not gov-erned by professional bodies and can mean different things. Some using these titles are licensed professional therapists who have chosen to specialize in career counseling or life coaching, but others enter through informal channels; feel free to inquire about professional status and licensure.

Theoretical orientation? Psychotherapists—whether social workers, psy-chologists, counselors, or psychiatrists—differ in their theoretical orientations. Some emphasize the connections between childhood experiences and present problems; others focus on the here and now, while still others examine con-nections between thoughts, feelings, and behaviors and teach coping skills. Many will report that they are "eclectic," meaning they draw from many dif-ferent therapeutic approaches. When considering a therapist, inquire about his or her theoretical orientation and feel free to ask for reading materials, if desired. If a therapist reports an eclectic approach, you can ask about the main orientation(s) underlying the approach. The more familiar you are with the assumptions and strategies that guide the approach, the better you can evaluate its fit with your life. Too many approaches exist to describe all of them here; instead, I focus on a few that are better known and/or considered particularly helpful with pain:

Psychodynamic psychotherapy.[2] This insight-oriented approach is what people often imagine when thinking about therapy. It works by discovering the impact of often-unconscious thoughts and behaviors on present behavior. Its theoretical orientation comes from psychoanalysis, which is a much more intensive therapy. However, in psychodynamic therapy, you typically sit in a chair (rather than lie on a couch), and the frequency and length of treatment is less intense (weekly sessions for a year, on average, rather than multiple sessions each week for multiple years). This approach can be especially helpful in illu-minating the reasons for the ways you respond to difficulties. You may come to understand, for example, how your role in your family of origin has made it especially difficult to ask for help, or how the meaning you have attached to achievement or suffering is affecting your ability to adapt. How you contend with chronic pain will likely bring up prior difficulties, their meaning, and how you handled them. Much like children often act younger than their years when they feel unwell, we may similarly regress as we feel dependent on others due to chronic pain. During sessions, you will likely have "aha" moments, in which you gain poignant insights about your thoughts and behaviors. The mechanism for change in this approach comes from uncovering and understanding these connections. When you understand *why* you perceive things as you do, you are better able to make desired changes.

Cognitive behavioral therapy (CBT).[3] CBT, likely the most researched approach to chronic pain management, has been shown to be effective in studies across a wide variety of pain conditions. As described in chapter 12, its premise is that you can improve your experience through your response, an approach that dovetails well with PAINTRACKING. CBT therapists teach strategies for monitoring self-talk and for replacing distorted thoughts and self-defeating behaviors with more healthful ones. Any of us can fall prey to "cognitive distortions," and CBT details more than a dozen ways in which our logic can be faulty, such as "catastrophizing," in which we escalate the meaning of a minor event or piece of evidence to outrageous proportions, or "overgeneralization," which refers to mistakenly concluding that an occasional occurrence is the rule. CBT can also involve behavioral strategies, including guided visual imagery, diaphragmatic breathing, meditation, and other relaxation techniques to decrease muscle tension, reduce emotional distress, and divert attention away from pain. Some studies of CBT report problems with compliance, which makes sense if study participants living with pain were required to fill out elaborate worksheets to track, understand, and change their thoughts and behaviors.[4] This is the reason it makes sense to keep simple, relevant tracking data, which can then be used with a CBT therapist.

Dialectical behavioral therapy (DBT).[5] Dialectical behavioral therapy incorporates CBT principles and aspects of Zen Buddhism, with a particular focus on mindfulness (see chapter 10) and acceptance. At its core is the powerful stance that we can *simultaneously* accept our present circumstances and work to improve them. The goal of DBT is to build a "life that is worth living."[6] DBT was created to assist people who were chronically suicidal; however, it has since been applied successfully to help other populations. Its strength for people with chronic pain is its focus on four relevant areas:

(1) Core mindfulness skills build a nonjudgmental awareness of your experience, which helps you accept what is and work toward improvement.

(2) Interpersonal-effectiveness skills help you advocate for your needs without guilt or apology, validate others' experiences, and contend with other relationship challenges that can arise around chronic pain.

(3) Emotion-regulation skills help you identify your emotions without being engulfed by them and decrease your vulnerability to emotional suffering.

(4) Distress-tolerance skills help you get through crisis moments with distraction, self-soothing, strategies to enhance your experience of the present moment, and acceptance.

DBT-oriented therapy helps you tailor these skills to your circumstances. DBT skills are typically taught in skills groups, which also provide the opportunity to gain from other people's experiences and support.

Mindfulness-based stress reduction (MBSR).[7] As described in chapter 10, MBSR, started by Jon Kabat-Zinn, uses mindful meditation to improve the experience of patients with chronic illness, including chronic pain. Offshoot MBSR programs have proliferated worldwide; if you're interested, look for a program through your local hospital or online. As in DBT, a central tenet of MBSR is that pain only becomes suffering through your response to it; you can learn to change your perceptions of pain and thus diminish suffering. MBSR classes help you influence your perception of pain.

Family counseling. Because the effects of pain are far reaching, you may want to consider including your partner or intergenerational family members. Family therapy comes from many different traditions, all linked by the common assumption that anything that affects one member of an intimate system affects all members. Similarly, therapeutic changes affect all members as well. Family therapy can include sharing education on your pain condition, improving communication, addressing interpersonal patterns that can perpetuate problems (without placing blame), and other strategies to increase the functioning of the whole unit.

Group therapy. Group therapy offers a powerful way to feel less alone in your suffering and provides opportunities to give and receive support. Groups can be time limited (e.g., eight to ten sessions) or longer term (a year or more) and either "close-ended" (all members start at the same time) or "open-ended" (membership can change over time). Some groups allow you to attend sporadically; others require more of a commitment. Therapy groups can be led by professionals or laypeople. A group's effectiveness relies on the ability of its facilitator to create a therapeutic environment. Peer-led groups can be helpful, but not if they feel unsafe or degrade into griping sessions. Many different types of groups exist and can be categorized broadly as:

- Skills groups that teach specific techniques, such as CBT, DBT, meditation, or MBSR, and provide the opportunity to learn and practice skills with others. Group members may or may not share the same health conditions. Facilitators are typically licensed therapists.
- Psycho-educational groups that combine social support, counseling, and information about specific health conditions. They are usually led by individuals who are knowledgeable about the condition, and they are often held in or advertised by medical centers.
- Insight-oriented or process groups that focus on the interactions of group members as a way to gain insight about each person's relationships with others. These more traditional "therapy groups" are led by mental health professionals.
- Experiential groups that offer opportunities to explore and heal through art, drama, horticulture, or other creative outlets.
- Support groups that are led by either professionals or peers. Their aim is to provide validation and share coping strategies with others with similar experiences. These can be particularly beneficial when group members instill hope through role modeling of successful coping.

Fees? The cost of therapy varies considerably, in part based on whether you have health insurance and the extent of its coverage. Larger cities are likely to have higher rates, in general, but a broader range of services. Possibilities include services offered through public agencies, nonprofit groups, or faith-based organizations. Some therapists in private practice offer low-cost or sliding-fee options, and some communities provide free services for people who qualify. If you are unable to afford weekly sessions, consider meeting less frequently. Group therapy generally costs less than one-on-one sessions. As you are figuring out what you can afford, don't shortchange yourself. If you are suffering, it may be well worth it to focus on ways to improve your life.

Length of therapy? This depends on your goals and the therapeutic approach you choose. Brief therapy may be adequate for specific problems. However, changing long-standing patterns takes time. Your goals may also change during the process, particularly as you uncover areas of your life that you can further improve. Talk with your therapist about a plan for checking in at intervals to monitor and evaluate your progress. Therapies that may have shorter durations include career counseling; life coaching; or therapy focusing on a particular skill, such as biofeedback or hypnosis.

Closing Note

Embracing a treatment that emphasizes your own role in your pain can feel scary. It takes courage to face your challenges and to take responsibility for how you feel. Even when you lack control over your situation, it is your choice how you respond, which, in turn, influences how you feel. As you know from your tracking data, some of the variation in your pain comes from your choices. A primary goal in both therapy and PAINTRACKING is to figure out the consequences of your choices so you can choose to improve each moment the best that you can. This requires a commitment to participating and being open to change. The work and the benefits of therapy come from implementing insights in your daily life.

Studies have shown that the positive results from therapy come at least as much from the "therapeutic alliance" as they do from the type of therapy you choose. In other words, what may matter most is a solid, trusting relationship with the therapist. Effective therapists share fundamental qualities: they treat the individual as a whole person and not as a diagnosis or case, listen respectfully and nonjudgmentally, stay attuned to your cues (when to push and when to be patient), and work with the factors that are within your control while recognizing those that are not.

When evaluating your experience with mental health professionals, consider the extent to which you feel allied in your commitment to improve. If something feels lacking in the relationship, raise this as an issue to discuss with your therapist. Working through any discomfort or conflicts with your therapist can deepen the relationship and shed light on similar dilemmas you may experience with others outside of therapy. However, if discussing your unease does not resolve it, seek therapy elsewhere. Therapy should provide a safe place to explore issues that would be difficult or even taboo in other contexts.

Part 3

Pain-Living

Chapter 19

Taking Care of Your Home

"There's no place like home." These compelling words, repeated by Dorothy in the classic film *The Wizard of Oz*, transport her back from her Oz adventures to her bed, where familiar and caring faces greet her. For people living with chronic pain, having a soothing and restorative refuge awaiting you can help you through the day—or any journey. Take what you learn from your experiments and tracking and review your living environment for maximum comfort.

The right bed. If you make one significant furniture purchase, make it a bed. As your data likely attest, the quality of your nights affects the quality of your days. Sleeping on a mattress that is too soft or unsupportive can exacerbate pain. Revisit chapter 14 for pointers on shopping for mattresses and other considerations in creating restorative sleep conditions.

Seating. Assess your needs, and strive to equip your place with seating that will enhance your well-being. Consider your seating arrangement when it comes to relaxing, eating meals, and conducting work. If you can invest in multiple chairs, consider:

1. A cozy place. To what extent do you have a place where you can comfortably read, watch TV, socialize, or just relax? This might be a couch, recliner, futon, or pillow mountain.
2. Your dining chair. Make sure you have a place where you can be comfortable enough to enjoy a meal.
3. Your desk chair. If you spend time at a desk or computer station, assess the benefits of a chair in which you are sufficiently supported and able to concentrate.

At the very least, make sure you have one perfect place at home to sit. Sometimes you can transform existing seating with pillows, cushions, and a well-placed ottoman or footrest (or phone book). Think creatively. Chairs intended for other uses may work well as dining chairs or work chairs. Even large inflatable balls (commonly used in physical therapy, exercise, or childbirth) may be perfect seating if they suit you. You may remember John Mahoney's character Marty on the television sitcom *Frasier*, whose beloved, worn chair clashed with his son's stylish, modern décor. Despite squabbles with his son, Marty hung on to his chair. Put your comfort first—this is likely to contribute positively to your family environment. If you decide to purchase a new chair, invest in the search. Like Goldilocks, you may have to sit in multiple chairs before finding the one that's just right. Even when it is "love at first sit," try the chair at your best and worst to make sure it continues to provide comfort. Look into the return policies in the event the chair turns out to be less than you had hoped.

A friendly environment. When you discover the environmental conditions that help you feel your best, incorporate them into your living environment. If you share your place with others, this may involve negotiation and compromise. For example, if your partner prefers the thermostat on the arctic side, you might consider a space heater for your designated "warm zone." If you have housemates who generate high volume, keep earplugs or a headset handy. If you are sensitive to bright lights, look into softer alternatives, such as indirect lighting or dimmer switches. Involving family members in the problem-solving phase can be mutually beneficial; often, people want to help but may not know how. Explain the benefits to your well-being of finding solutions.

A special room. Writer Virginia Woolf observed that in order to write, a woman required a "room of her own" (and some money). With chronic pain, a room of one's own can offer a salubrious refuge from the rest of the world, especially in bustling households. Consider ways to create a space to chill out, listen to music, meditate, engage in self-hypnosis, or practice other forms of self-care that reduce your pain. Design the room to feel peaceful and comfortable. If you cannot achieve a peaceful room, create a peaceful corner for yourself. Or, if you have outside space and desirable weather, consider a hammock or comfortable outdoor seating for a peaceful retreat.

If you live with others, help them respect your privacy when you retreat to your space. You might hang some version of a "Do not disturb" sign, with light-hearted words such as "Healing in session," "Meditation under way," "Mom's time out," or whatever feels appropriate. Or just let others know you need thirty minutes of uninterrupted "chill time." Reassure family members that break time means you will feel better and therefore be more available later— and see that you are. Others, too, may appreciate the benefit of a quiet escape from time to time.

Telephones. Grasping a phone in your hand or between your shoulder and head can wreak havoc on your neck, shoulders, and arms. A wide variety of headsets are available for traditional, cordless, and cell phones, leaving no reason to suffer from the old-fashioned handheld phone. Experiment with options, and assess each for comfort and quality. (Keep receipts.) You can join the ranks of popular singers, business executives, and telephone solicitors and free your arms for other tasks (including stretching or even exercising while talking). Headset phones are vital for the workplace as well (see chapter 21).

Your wardrobe. Dress comfortably. Depending on your pain condition, tight clothes may become increasingly uncomfortable as the day progresses. When selecting clothes, try them on when you're not feeling your best. If staying warm is a challenge because your muscles do not tolerate the weight of a coat or heavy clothing, experiment with layers of lightweight materials. Silk undergarments add warmth and comfort between you and your favorite clothing. Soft, lightweight fleece clothing can be very warm as well as fashionable. Velvet is especially cozy without weighing too heavily on sensitive spots. Cold temperatures can increase muscle tension and, therefore, pain. Before stepping out, zip up and generate a reserve of warmth, such as by drinking a hot beverage or warming your hands in the sink. Warm gloves, socks, boots, hats, and scarves provide significant warmth without adding weight or discomfort.

Minimizing the Pain of Housework

Whatever your personal philosophy on housework, a certain amount is unavoidable. This may involve lowering standards, rethinking your household organization, redistributing the workload among household members, hiring out, or bartering with others. You may have friends who would take on certain chores in exchange for things that wouldn't tax your system.

Evaluate your standards. Observe what you may be telling yourself about how things should be or the symbolic meaning you may place on different aspects of home maintenance. Creating order in your home may create a feeling of order in your life, which would make efficient methods a higher priority. Housework's importance also varies with the extent to which your identity is tied to particular activities, such as cooking meals. If you are judging your household appearance according to a myth about what it means to be a "good partner" or "good parent," assess your self-talk for destructive beliefs (chapter 12). Whatever your situation, consider strategies to reduce the time, effort, and pain spent on such tasks so you can free yourself for other pursuits.

Reorganize for ease. Picture the entrance into your house. Do you (or others) leave a trail of disorder as you enter the house? If so, try to eliminate the number of steps involved. Designate containers, such as small baskets, as collection points for keys, unsorted mail, sunglasses, or other mobile odds and ends. Hooks or a coat tree just inside the door offer a practical solution when hanging a coat becomes an effort. Hooks in the kitchen, too, can simplify reaching for pots and pans (and can be arranged with a stylish flair). If you live with others, enlist their help in creating systems to reduce trouble spots. Investing in such systems can greatly reduce the time and effort used in picking up or searching for missing items.

Simplify closets. It may be worth the investment to reorganize closets as well. Some ideas: Keep your most used items in easy reach. If raising your arms incites pain, reserve lower shelves for high-use items. If it hurts to reach above chest level, use a step stool to raise yourself up instead. Whenever possible, cull your closets. Roomier closets are easier to navigate. If you have things you can no longer use on account of your pain condition, consider donating or selling them. It took me several years before I decided to give away my weighty sweaters, jackets, and form-fitting tops that all ignited pain within minutes of my putting them on. My clothes closets now contain only what I can wear, making it easy to find what I want.

Simplify laundry. Experiment with strategies to minimize the effort, such as deliberately reducing laundry needs. Wear easy-to-care-for clothes that hold up in the washer and dryer and do not require ironing. Buy an identical dozen of your favorite socks, eliminating the need to rummage for pairs. By dressing in layers, you can wear outer garments multiple times, reducing laundry demands, which is especially important if your laundry room involves a hike. Strive for a system that eliminates intermediary steps. Some examples: Bring hangers to the laundry room to slip them into shirts right out of the dryer.

Assign baskets for categories of prewashed laundry, such as by laundry type (whites, delicates, etc.) to eliminate the need to sort dirty laundry into piles at washing time, or by person or room (kids, adults, towels, etc.) to eliminate the need to sort clean laundry before putting it away. Family members can also be responsible for their own baskets. Consider innovations to limit the need to carry laundry, such as pushing a duffel bag of dirties down the stairwell or, when possible, locating the washer and dryer close to the bedrooms.

Floor fun? Experiment with strategies to reduce discomfort involved in cleaning the floor, such as approaching your floors in manageable segments. Be mindful of your posture and your grip on cleaning equipment. When you feel rushed, you are more likely to tense your muscles. Instead, be deliberate in your ergonomic stance: relax, hold the handle gently, and move smoothly. Experiment with incorporating stretches and dance steps into your movements, transforming cleaning into gentle, fun exercise. You might even mop the floor by skating on damp, soapy cloths. Avoid lugging around heavy equipment; if you have a multilevel home, you may find it worthwhile to equip each floor with a lightweight vacuum that you can store and retrieve as needed.

Adapt Your Cooking

Whether you are a one-minute chef or a garden-to-table gourmand, chronic pain does not have to be a reason to relinquish cooking as part of your life (unless this is your wish!).

Think outside the box, or at least off the kitchen counter. Chopping and other preparatory work can be done seated in a comfortable space with your feet up, and listening to music, if you'd like. If it hurts to stand in the kitchen, then don't (or, at least, do it less).

Stay mindful of your position. Pay attention to how you hold and lift items. A tight grasp increases muscle tension. Look for kitchen tools with oversized and rubberized comfort handles. Practice a hold that is just tight enough to keep things off the floor but does not incite pain. Focusing on your breath can help you keep your body more relaxed.

Minimize carrying. Invest in serving trays, and carry them low and close to your body. Using trays reduces hand and arm pain by reducing the number of plates, cups, and other small items you have to grip, and training yourself to carry low and close to your body also minimizes back pains. Before lifting anything substantial, consider your options. A tray on wheels makes transfers even easier.

Minimize heavy lifting. Contemplate your options. Boiling water for pasta, for example, does not mean you have to fill a large pot with water and then carry it to the stove. You might, instead, reverse the order: set the pot on the stove, then bring the water in a manageable-sized pitcher. Or you might slide the pot of water across your counter to the stove, rather than carrying or lifting it. Some deluxe stoves even come with a water or boiling water tap. For the times when you decide to carry something, use both hands and, as much as is practical, hug the item toward your body.

Use bare hands. If gripping cooking implements is painful, consider cooking by hand—literally. Mix ingredients with your bare hands. The human hand is the most versatile and useful implement there is.

Use as few pots as possible. The fewer pots you use, the fewer there are to wash. Look into one-pot recipes. Invest in an all-purpose pan that can go from refrigerator to stove top to oven and back.

Use machines. Kitchen implements and gadgets now exist for virtually any task related to food preparation. Consider tasks you value but struggle to do, and research available gadgets. These can vary from a simple flat rubber grip to help open the most stubborn of jar lids, to elaborate slicers and cookers, which can allow you to create dishes that would otherwise be labor intensive.

Use ingredient shortcuts. You can make fresh, homemade meals with preprepared ingredients. Consider tossing frozen or canned ingredients into your soup or casserole along with fresh counterparts or raiding the supermarket salad bar for the exact amount of chopped celery, pepper, or onion. Stores are stocking larger and more developed sections of ready-to-cook ingredients, such as sliced mushrooms, cleaned and shelled prawns, preassembled shish kebabs for the grill, and sacks of sumptuous stew vegetables. These often cost more; weigh the financial costs against the physical ones involved in being your own sous chef.

Use prepared meals. The quality of prepared meals has also been increasing. There is much to experiment with, from precooked, frozen dinners to ready-to-cook varieties available at large supermarket chains and specialty boutiques, as well as the growing hybrid of restaurant/market. A growing industry also offers precut and premeasured ingredients that you can mix and match, on site, into a week's worth of ready-to-cook meals.

Ask for Help

When we need it most, asking for help can be the hardest, even—or especially— asking those closest to you (see chapters 23 and 24, on relationships). You may be reluctant to admit to certain limitations, whether to others or to yourself. Through experimentation, you can determine when such pride aids you and when it becomes destructive. Pushing yourself beyond your limit means you will require greater help later on. Keep in mind, too, that everyone needs help sometimes. When it comes to seeking assistance, focus on three things: (1) your goals, (2) the person you are asking, and (3) the request itself.

Your goals. Start by determining what you are trying to accomplish. At times, your goal may be to carry groceries by yourself and revel in the accomplishment. Other times, your goal may be to get the groceries into your house without throwing out your back. Once you identify the goal, consider your best options.

Others. Assess the extent to which others are equipped to assist you. This depends on their physical health and schedule as well as the timing of the request. If you have suffered with pain for a long time, it may be difficult to remember what certain tasks felt like without pain. Try to evaluate your request from the viewpoint of the other person. Most people will eagerly lend a hand for a request they consider to be easy, provided they have time. However, it is unreasonable to expect that others will *always* be available or willing to help.

The request. If you want help, ask for it. It's unreasonable to expect anyone (no matter how close you may be) to intuit when you might need help, especially if your capabilities and wellness fluctuate regularly. Others may even worry their unsolicited assistance might be considered intrusive or out of place. So ask!

Try to time your request for when the other person appears available and receptive (not busy or preoccupied). Communicate clearly what you want and why; it's easier for others to respond to specific requests than to vague complaints. Saying, "Would you mind carrying these bags upstairs? My arms are really bothering me today," is better than stating, "It's so hard for me to shop these days" (without making a request). Express requests in a way that helps others feel appreciated—and without expectation, guilt, or pressure. When others do not grant your request, have a plan B handy, such as inquiring if they may be available at a later time or doing part of the task yourself. For example, someone who does not have time to carry in all the groceries may be able to bring in the cold foods and other perishables. Show appreciation for any assistance and gracious acceptance when others are not in the position to assist. It would be unfair to think that just because you had the courage to ask, or because you are having a particularly bad day, others are obliged to do whatever you need.

Involve Partners or Spouses

Ideally, partners or spouses work together as a team, reducing the burden of work. Under ideal circumstances, two is better than one, and through teamwork, more can be accomplished with less expenditure. At the same time, most couples tend to develop specialties in their division of labor, and one member of the couple may shoulder a larger part. When that person develops sore shoulders or is otherwise hindered by chronic pain, the divisions can become more challenging. When it comes to housework, gender differences are common, as deftly illustrated by sociologist Arlie Hochschild in her book *The Second Shift*. Drawing from observation and interviews, she describes how even in the most egalitarian of households, working women often face a "second shift" of domestic work when they return home. Women living with chronic pain may face a greater challenge in creating domestic balance. For men with chronic pain, asking for help with physical tasks or admitting to what feels like a weakness can be unsettling. Men are at risk of pushing through pain rather than relinquishing their "male" role.

This becomes further complicated when one partner is no longer working due to disability. It is easy to assume that because you are at home, you will become more of a homemaker. You may pick up additional responsibilities, such as cooking, cleaning, and other caregiving duties. Sacrifices in income may mean that you pitch in whenever you can, especially if your partner has taken on supplementary work to offset your lost wages. If and when you are up for additional tasks, great! It may be practical to do as much as you can (although make sure to experiment to find the most effective ways to pitch in without increasing pain). But here's the caveat: You are home because you feel too lousy to work. This feels awful enough. Do not succumb to guilt, whether self-induced or from other projected ideas of how you should be spending your day. Assumptions can cause much trouble for you and those in your life. As you transition to a new—and, likely, ever-changing—role, talk openly about how this affects everyone involved and how you can work as a team. Elicit their support.

Couples who can rewrite these rules to fit their current circumstances will fare the best in this journey. As is described in chapter 24, clear communication is key. Acknowledging limitations and setting boundaries is much more effective than overdoing it and becoming demoralized with the resultant pain. Before chronic pain entered the relationship, decisions about household chores may have been implicit. Chronic pain may make it more important to have deliberate discussions. Take time to communicate about expectations. Then prioritize together, adjusting tasks to make them more manageable and considering when it makes sense to seek outside assistance.

In some ways, this dilemma is akin to the quandary faced by healthy stay-at-home parents, who may be expected to keep house while looking after young children. Living with pain and caring for young children are both difficult jobs—having both is harder still. (See chapter 25 for tips on this double whammy.)

Engage Children

The extent to which families engage their children in daily or weekly chores varies. Consider your values and preferred strategies for involving children in chores. Decide what constitutes age-appropriate housework, focusing on tasks that will reduce your stress and strain. Young children can create messes in no time flat. Evaluate your house for trouble spots—places you are cleaning up repeatedly—and create a system to reduce this problem. This may involve accessible storage bins and the expectation that your child will use them. Find creative ways to engage children by making cleanup into a game. Limit the number of toys available to young hands to one or two, and rotate toys from a place out of sight and reach. (Children can delight in the appearance of novel toys and old favorites while you delight in the uncluttered floor.)

Toddlers and preschoolers are eager to imitate grown-up behaviors; you can harness this enthusiasm. Finding small tasks not only boosts children's confidence, but it also reinforces the idea that "everyone pitches in." Encourage any special interest or creativity: you may have a promising chef in your household. As they age, continue to praise their contributions, and increase responsibilities as seems compatible with their abilities and your child-rearing philosophy. Consider the mastery of housework skills just as you would any other lesson you impart to your children to prepare them for independence. Children will more eagerly take on additional responsibilities when these are framed as an extension of your trust and confidence in them, rather than as an unpleasant task.

As children age, emphasize the cooperative element with your most matter-of-fact voice; avoid imparting guilt. You can treat pitching in as expected behavior while expressing gratitude for their contributions: "I really appreciate how thoroughly you cleaned the kitchen this evening—that was very helpful of you." Treat cleaning up after meals as part of the event—each member of the family, for example, carries dishes to the sink or dishwasher. Teach children to deposit dirty laundry in the appropriate place, turned right-side out. If you explain that you will be washing only the clothes you find in the appropriate bins, they will quickly learn the importance of making sure they deliver their favorite clothing to the proper place.

You can decide to make chore time more fun for everyone by turning on music and engaging in a family cleanup dance. Keep in mind that young children do not see housework as drudgery—until they learn that from us. When this secret leaks out, it may be time to consider a system that distributes and rewards contributions. For the areas in which you encounter resistance, you may have to up the ante. But, as a former dolphin trainer describes in *Don't Shoot the Dog!* positive reinforcement works best when doled out in tiny, bite-size pieces—think a hearty "Thank you!" rather than a trip to Disney World for putting puzzle pieces back into their box. Children, like dolphins, will perform best when their desired behaviors are followed by a tiny "biscuit."[1] Consider ways to reward your child's extra effort with a special activity, such as allowing him or her to choose the dinner menu or spend additional time on a favorite distraction, or use tokens they can cash in for (modest) prized items or freedoms. During my children's Pokémon® phase, they sought out chores so they could rack up points to earn a small collectible plastic figurine (which I had bought in bulk on eBay). To shape behavior, keep incentives modest. Once the behavior becomes habit, occasional and heartfelt words of appreciation may be sufficient to sustain it. No need to break the bank for thanks.

It is unrealistic to expect that your requests for assistance (however skillfully made) will always be met without conflict or difficulty. As children get older, it will make sense to explain more about your need for extra rest or assistance. Be careful not to saddle "responsible" children beyond what is appropriate for their years. Children are very sensitive to what you do and do not say. Be mindful of any potential role reversals, in which children become caretakers of the house or of you. Children adjust best when information is presented in ways that are honest and do not evoke fears (see chapter 25). As children grow into preteens and teens, you may also find it most helpful to have a closed-door policy for bedrooms (their mess, their concern).

Virtual Errands

If you have Internet access, look to the burgeoning online marketplace. It is increasingly possible to purchase whatever you need or want—food, clothing, furniture, large appliances, holiday gifts—without leaving home. Online services are designed for convenience and can include gift wrapping, card writing, and delivery. You can buy nearly anything, new or used, from local retailers, neighbors, or the other side of the world. Online auctions make it easy to find specific items, and, if you exercise restraint, at a reasonable price.

If you lack Internet access, most national chains have toll-free numbers and send catalogs free of charge. A potential downside of virtual shopping is the resulting flood of catalogs and e-mail advertisements that can follow. In many cases, you can opt out of receiving catalogs or sharing your information with other companies. Check return policies when buying through the mail, including who pays for return postage and any restocking fees for returned items.

Foraging for Food

City dwellers have limitless options; rural dwellers may face challenges in finding even a pizza delivery service. Find out what is available where you live. It is increasingly common for supermarkets to offer online shopping and delivery services. Many large chains allow you to place your orders online for later pickup and save your shopping list for future visits. Smaller grocery stores may also offer personal-shopper services for community members, which they may not advertise widely. Inquire at your local grocer about the possibility and explain your needs, as appropriate.

Another alternative, in line with the growing "locavore" spirit of eating locally grown food, is membership in a farm cooperative. Local farmers may offer memberships as a way to receive a predictable cash income. Members, then, commit to a weekly order of whatever is ripe and available, which could include a variety of fruits, vegetables, meats, cheeses, and eggs. Typically, orders are boxed up and either delivered to your door or held for pickup. The potential downside is the surprise factor, as it is the farmers and weather variables (and not you) determining the contents of your box week to week. Check with your local farmer's market about available options to support local farms and receive fresh offerings (typically at a lower price than buying them individually).

When you engage in traditional in-store shopping, come equipped with a list to eliminate time wandering around or becoming overwhelmed by the mesmerizing selection. This reduces the likelihood of finding halfway through your shopping trip that your knees or back are no longer complying with the demands. Compose your list in the comfort of your home, using a system that works with your lifestyle—perhaps a paper list on the refrigerator where everyone is expected to note desired items, perhaps a computer or phone list of usual consumables or categories to fill in as needed. Be sure to include any necessary ingredients for your week's menus and a pen to cross items from your list. Arrange your list to be intuitive and easy to interpret. For example, group items to mimic the store's layout so you can follow along the list as you shop. Use colored pens for different categories of items. Order the items on your list with the most essential items first so you can end the shopping session if your energy wanes. Or create a grocery list with tear-off sections that can be given to children, making shopping into a scavenger hunt.

Grocery stores tend to be cold and brightly lit, which may be good for ice cream and security cameras but uncomfortable for people with certain pain conditions. As needed, layer up on clothes, or keep a fleece cardigan, hat, or pair of gloves in your car. If your pain increases with fluorescent lighting, bring sunglasses. If pushing a cart hurts, guide it with your torso rather than your arms. Many large grocery stores have motorized shopping carts with seats for the shopper. Look into this option (and the times of day when they are most available) as needed. If carrying groceries can incite a flare, shop where store clerks bag the groceries and load them into your cart, and sometimes into your car. (Don't be embarrassed to stand watch while the bagging is in progress or to request lighter loads in each bag.) If your store does not offer such services, an appreciative request often brings assistance.

Consider packing the perishable items together (milk, eggs, ice cream) to unload when you first arrive home. Then you can leave the rest in your car until you recuperate or help arrives. Or, if the weather is cool (or you bring a cooler to the store), you may be able to leave the milk and eggs as well. To minimize trips to the store, stock your pantry with nonperishable items such as peanut butter, lentils, dried beans, pasta, and dried fruit. To keep fresh produce without frequent shopping, try to select fruit in various stages of ripeness—for instance, include some green bananas with the yellow ones.

When shopping with children, encourage their involvement. Very young children can assist by dropping or heaving unbreakable items into your cart or car (like toilet paper or boxes of cereal or potatoes). If their participation is enlisted from an early age, children are more likely to continue to contribute as they get older (and can carry bags and even drive to the store).

Hire Out

Deciding whether and when to hire help involves calculations of your budget, time, energy, and abilities. What aspects of life matter most to you and those you live with?

This may seem a weighty, existential question for something as mundane as housework, but consider its implications. How long does it take you to recover from engaging in housework, and what could you be missing out on? Calculate the extent to which a given task feels like a satisfactory use of your time, energy, and comfort. After scaling back and using creative measures, if you find any tasks still constitute a hardship, seek assistance. It may be well worth paying someone else to take on your most labor-intensive tasks or provide whatever services would aid you most.

Think outside the Box

The tips in this chapter are all simple. The challenge may be to approach things differently. We are creatures of habit, and sometimes we continue with behaviors even when they result in additional pain. Open yourself up to novel approaches by applying your self-knowledge from your tracking data. Treat changes as experiments. Seek simple solutions to everyday tasks and see what enhances your life.

Chapter 20

Preparing for Holidays and Travel

I t can be especially demoralizing when vacations, intended to be pleasurable breaks, are more challenging than daily life. However, for people living with pain, this is not uncommon. Leaving a more predictable environment—with its more comfortable routine, furniture, and schedule—for a less predictable one can be scary. Vacation companions will not always understand your predicament. It can be confusing to others that you can walk but not stand, or engage in something strenuous one day but not again until after a significant rest. Plus, on vacation, your well-being is often influenced by others' expectations and desires. You may be with an active bunch who greatly value your participation. The more familiar you are with your needs, the better you will be at advocating for yourself, building in needed breaks, and weighing your participation in excursions that may sound like fun but would intensify your discomfort. Traveling well relies on a combination of self-knowledge, acceptance, adaptation, positive self-talk, and assertiveness. It is particularly helpful to consider vacations and other significant forays from home as important experiments. Each trip or situation adds to your data bank on what makes a successful travel routine for you. This involves planning, as much as possible, to maximize your comfort and minimize the stress involved.

Travel Checklist

Before embarking on any trip, give yourself a quiet space to create a travel checklist that includes not only your basic necessities but also the key items for your comfort (e.g., heating pad; earplugs; special pillows; medications; travel food; information on the location and hours of the nearest pool, spa, or other facilities). Consider what will make the travel itself more comfortable, such as bringing a source of heat that you can plug into your car or use at the airport or other stops. The list can reduce anxiety associated with leaving and provide reassurance that you are prepared.

Packing, then, becomes the simple act of gathering items and placing them in a bag, which can also be carried out through collaboration—you sit comfortably, reading and checking each item off the list, while your travel mate puts each into your travel bag. Pack essential items such as medications in carry-on bags, not checked luggage, to ensure they arrive with you. Include on a pretrip list any tasks you need to do before departing, such as canceling newspaper delivery, watering plants, or arranging pet care. Once you have a helpful list, save it for future trips, adapting it as you learn or with changes—baby bottles may be replaced by sippy cups, sunscreen by gloves, and so on.

If you take multiple medications, pill caddies are helpful to make sure you bring the right number. Because travel can be disorienting, compartments with the days of the week help you make sure you've taken your pills as directed. Pack some additional days in case of unexpected travel changes. If you travel frequently, consider duplicating some of your essentials, such as toiletries, an umbrella, and sleepwear, and keeping the spares in your suitcase.

Car Travel

Significant time in the car can be uncomfortable or painful. Prepare your body for your trip by getting your best sleep the night before you leave and by engaging in exercise, meditation, or whatever measures help you feel your best before setting off. Arrange your seat for maximum comfort, such as with well-positioned pillows to support your back or buffer road vibrations and bumps; a comfortable seat cushion; or a plug-in seat cover that delivers heat, massage, and/or vibration. Schedule breaks to get out of the car to move around and stretch at whatever intervals you find most helpful. Keep in mind that deliberate breaks save time if you factor in time that would otherwise be needed to recuperate from continuous hours of travel. As a passenger, make use of the opportunity to recline or engage in creative stretches.

Traveling with others can involve negotiation skills or compromises.

Before setting off, be clear with your travel companions about adaptations that may affect them—such as the frequency of rest stops or the extent to which you can drive versus ride as a passenger. It helps to be able to explain the effect of any environmental factors that influence your comfort, such as the temperature of the car, noise levels, and the frequency and duration of breaks, without pressure, apology, or guilt. More than likely, your travel mates will want to help you reduce a pain flare-up. In the event, however, that your requests are at odds with others' comfort, come equipped with alternate ways to ensure your comfort, such as a blanket or heating pad to stay warm or earplugs or headphones to block out background noises.

Planes, Trains, and Buses

Public transportation offers the advantage of greater mobility, but with less control over the environment. Come equipped with a comfort tool kit (e.g., medication, earplugs, pillows, heat sacks, eyeshades, a soft blanket, or whatever helps you relax). If you prefer not to be disturbed, preselect a window seat and express your desires to fellow passengers, explicitly or through body language.

Avoid schlepping heavy bags; wheeled suitcases are available in all shapes and sizes. Invest in a wheeled carry-on that slides under the seat in front of you (eliminating the need to hoist it over your head) and can double, as desired, as a footrest. When possible, check larger bags, even if it may be a bit more expensive and slow you down at the end of the trip. Avoid playing the hero at the check-in counter or on board; ask for assistance with heavy bags. Leading with a compliment and a simple explanation is likely to yield positive results: "You look fit and strong. I have back trouble—any chance your back is up to lifting this bag for me?" Follow with appreciation, and use sensitivity, as others may have invisible conditions also.

Many major airports now offer massage services. If you have time, consider a back and shoulder rub before departing. Before boarding the plane and during layovers, use long periods of time to stretch, meditate, or perform other restorative activities. Seek out private spots or a quiet corner if available. Keep in mind that your priority of arriving feeling OK can help you shrug (or laugh) off any odd looks you receive from fellow passengers (seated in their hard chairs) while you engage in rejuvenating activities. Major airports now also offer private chambers; if you face a long layover and uncomfortable chairs, this investment may be well worth it.

Holidays

Holidays can be stressful for everyone. Depression and anxiety tend to spike around holidays, often due to the pressure involved and the stories we tell ourselves about what holidays "should" be like. It may help to approach holidays as exaggerated versions of everyday life; for instance, if you usually find it difficult to satisfy the handful of family and friends you see on a regular basis, expect this effect to be magnified. You are more likely to have a positive experience if you prepare by accepting what is, rather than dwelling on what you may be in your hopes or wishes. This mind-set can be physically and emotionally liberating and encourages you to take more proactive measures for your comfort. You can then relinquish pressure to uphold traditions in ways your body may not be up to, focusing instead on the spirit of the holiday, such as appreciation, gratitude, or togetherness (rather than some mythical idea of a Hallmark®-card family holiday). Even if you generally find family holidays enjoyable and pleasurable, the change in environment can increase stress. Use deliberate self-talk, mindfulness, and strategies to soothe your body to allow yourself to be present and enjoy yourself as much as possible.

Hosting Others

Weigh the pros and cons of hosting people. Some advantages include access to your usual comforts and not having to travel. Challenges of hosting tend to stem from taking on too much responsibility for other people's welfare and relinquishing needed downtime. You can reduce these potential disadvantages by fostering flexibility. If you decide to host a gathering, experiment with the following three basic rules:

Rule 1: Pace any preparations. Avoid exhausting yourself before the event even begins! Keep in mind that holiday gatherings is for visiting with others, not for impressing them with your housekeeping or culinary skills. Trying to do it all, especially while condemning your pain for intruding, will quickly exhaust you and make the entire enterprise unpleasant. Everyone benefits more from your feeling better than from a particular labor-intensive food or other tradition. However, if you are committed to offering a particular arrangement, commit also to pacing yourself. Use strategies to pace your exertions over time and in ways that will not require last-minute exertions. For example, you can prepare delicious casseroles or other homemade meals days in advance (or longer if you use a freezer). Make sure to allow yourself a long stretch of downtime before anyone arrives so you feel your best. Calculate the amount of time needed for you to feel able to welcome your guests with genuine enthusiasm, and work backward from there.

Rule 2: Share the work. Just because you are providing the meeting place does not make you a full-service inn. Consider options for reducing your workload by tapping into your community and making use of what each visitor can bring to the table, sometimes literally. Cooks tend to feel appreciated when their dishes are requested—so if a friend or relative has a specialty or crowd-pleaser, request it. Keep in mind, too, that for a price, everything can be purchased. Explore already-prepared foods from your local grocery, deli, restaurant, caterer, or ready-to-cook meal place. Consider delivery services or asking others to pick things up. Potluck-style meals offer a break to the host and foster a community feeling. Disposable plates make cleanup hassle-free, and you can select from festive to compostable varieties.

Experiment with ways to generate a "get comfortable and help yourself" attitude among your guests. Every home has a different feel. In some, the expectation is that everyone will be waited on; in others, additional people in the kitchen are a nuisance. Express the household norms that you find most beneficial. For example, let your guests know where they can find things and encourage them to explore. The more independent your guests, the more downtime you can enjoy.

Rule 3: Plan downtime. Being host does not mean you must be available at all times. Make sure to schedule time to rest and engage in beneficial practices. By helping your guests feel comfortable, you free yourself to slip away. Remember, it is your choice whether to engage in activities or outings that are challenging. When you decide these are worthwhile despite additional pain, be sure to schedule recuperative time to follow. Other times, you may decide to skip a trip and instead take a nap, meditate, go to the gym, or do whatever best manages your pain. If you feel uncomfortable doing this, examine the "should" you may be telling yourself about your role as host or family member. Talk openly with your guests. More than likely, others will be happy to excuse your presence, if it means you will be able to be fully present when you return. Keep in mind that even people who do not have pain enjoy and benefit from having time to relax and regroup. Others may appreciate the permission to take time for themselves as well. Or you may issue an invitation to join you at the gym or in other self-care activities.

Being the Guest

The main challenges in being a guest involve travel and arranging for the things you find most crucial in feeling better. Other people's places vary in the comfort they offer: some may have sleeping accommodations or lounge chairs superior to your own, while in others, you may struggle to find one place to sit that feels comfortable. For this reason, you may have to be more active than the word *guest* might imply—pack your feel-good supplies (even a comfortable chair, if it fits in your trunk), and look for ways to care for yourself in a different environment. Before you arrive, research the options for relaxation and solitude. If you benefit from swimming, walking, or massage, for example, locate the nearby pools, parks, or spas (and be sure to pack suitable gear). Toughing it out, rather than tending to your needs, not only risks additional pain but also can affect your mood and, therefore, the quality of your social interactions. If the accommodations themselves provide inadequate comfort, carefully weigh the costs and benefits of staying at a hotel or motel.

When should you say your goodbyes? Shorter trips are better trips. It is generally advisable to leave while you still feel good and can enthusiastically report to yourself and others what a great time you had.

Self-Talk and Self-Care

When people step outside their usual comfort zone, they become more vulnerable. For people in pain, this can bring up thoughts that may not manifest with as much force during the usual routine and can bring up grief. Be particularly gentle with yourself in these situations. Use your tracking data and experiments to improve your situation—but not in comparison with anyone else or some imagined ideal. It is especially important to stay mindful of self-talk during travel and holidays. Be especially aware of extreme thinking such as, "I am *never* going to leave home again," or "How pathetic that I cannot even keep up with my elderly relatives!" (See chapter 12, about generating self-talk that is realistic and positive.)

Learning Moments

Tracking your experiences can be more challenging when your routine is thrown off. But data on these unusual periods can help you improve them. Whatever your choices and experiences during travel, they offer important data for the next extended social gathering, holiday, or trip. Ask yourself:

- What were the high points for you?
- What proved especially difficult?
- What conditions took you by surprise?
- What would you have liked to change?

Then, commit to learning from your experience while it is still fresh in your mind. Rather than beat yourself up about what you "should" have done, use these lessons to help you prepare better for subsequent events. Finish the sentence, "It would have been better if . . ." and turn any regrets into learning moments. Record your insights while they are fresh—they offer valuable information you can include on your travel checklist. Otherwise, you may forget the important gems before the next holiday or vacation rolls around.

Chapter 21

Creating a Workspace That Works

When it comes to work, each of us contends with a different set of difficulties:

"My back is killing me. It's hard to concentrate."
"It hurts to sit, stand, or use my arms for very long."
"This constant pain exhausts me. My brain is overwhelmed."
"How on earth am I to 'work'? Nothing about my body feels like it is working!"

Yet there are many reasons people in chronic pain want or need to continue working (or going to school). Work is central to life. Many of us rely on the income and, sometimes, the health insurance and other benefits that may come with it. The threat of not being able to work or finish one's studies can be terrifying, and worries about financial strains compound the suffering.

Beyond material gains, work can provide nonmaterial benefits for people with chronic pain, such as:

Structure. You may find it is easier to rise from bed when you are expected somewhere. This is particularly important when pain tempts you to stay in bed rather than face the day. Work can provide a jump-start by getting you out of bed and into productive activity. (Despite the strength of the urge or need, lying in bed for prolonged periods tends to make pain and your spirits worse.)

Community. You may find work provides opportunities for social interaction, support, belonging, and friendship. This sense of community decreases the risk of isolation that people with chronic pain face.

Distraction. Work can distract you from pain and limitations. You may find that pain takes a backseat when you are successfully engaged. The more interesting you find your work, the better.

Self-efficacy. Work can provide a sense of purpose and recognition. Successes can bolster your sense of control and competence, which especially helps when symptoms seem to get the upper hand.

The potential benefits of work, however, do not mean everyone can or should be employed; sometimes a respite or retirement from work is the best strategy (as discussed in the next chapter). But if you *are* currently employed, ask yourself the following:

- How much would I like to continue in my current job?
- How am I contending with its demands?
- How does the work affect how I feel?

If you like your work (or studies), but pesky symptoms interfere with your abilities, or you leave too depleted to contemplate any life beyond work, read on. This chapter describes strategies for adapting your current work environment to make it more hospitable. (While it focuses primarily on employment, many of these are adaptable to school, and the end of the chapter offers additional tips for students.)

As I'm writing this, a litany of painful sensations begs me to be somewhere other than my office—such as curled up at home on my couch or in my hammock in the sunshine. But what keeps me going is the knowledge that the couch (and hammock) will be there, the rewards my work brings, and the various measures I've taken to increase my comfort. I appreciate, too, that I'm fortunate to have a paid position that feels good even when I don't and lets me tailor my work conditions to my needs.

The Workplace Makeover

Whenever possible, modify your work environment and responsibilities to reduce stresses and discomfort. Productive workplace changes can have significant effects. Research has shown that women with fibromyalgia who have been able to adapt their work situations to fit their needs are more likely to continue working and find their work satisfying.[1] Effective adaptation also boosts morale. When successful in making positive changes, you are also more likely to achieve a sense of accomplishment and competence.

So, how do I go about changing my work conditions? Notice the aspects of your job you find especially taxing, and brainstorm about conditions that would improve your situation. This sometimes requires thinking unconventionally. Sometimes practices become work norms by habit rather than necessity, such as tasks that are always done while standing or in a particular sequence or location. When you find yourself getting irritated, seize this feeling as an opportunity to discover a novel approach. Challenge the assumption that "what is" is what has to be. Minor changes sometimes bring significant improvements; other times, you may have to request something more substantial of your employer.

Reasonable Accommodations

As you consider workplace adaptations, know your rights. Your employer may be required by law to work with you. The United Nations Convention on the Rights of Persons with Disabilities states that disabled individuals have a right to "reasonable accommodations." This convention serves as a model for legislation throughout the world to provide equal opportunities for people with disabilities. In the United States, the federal Americans with Disabilities Act (ADA) requires businesses with at least fifteen employees to make "reasonable accommodations" to allow workers with medical disabilities to carry out their jobs. Under the ADA, individuals have the right to remain employed as long as they can perform "essential" work functions and the right to accommodations that are not "unreasonably" expensive or difficult. The ADA and similar laws in other countries improve work conditions but cannot guarantee fair treatment because of the subjective nature of what constitutes an "essential" work function or "reasonableness" for a proposed accommodation.

To be eligible for ADA protection, you have to have a disability that "substantially limits a major life activity," which includes performing manual tasks. The thorny part is that you must be able to do the job for which you were hired, even without accommodations. But once you are performing in the job, your employer is supposed to work with you to discuss available options. In the case of nonobvious disabilities, which include most chronic pain conditions, your employer can request documentation of your disability along with an explanation of why you need accommodation.

Examples of Reasonable Accommodations for Chronic Pain Conditions

Stan, a receptionist for a veterinary clinic, was missing work due to painful flare-ups. While he loved the work environment, doctors, and animals, he found that frequent phone use and continuous interactions with client families increased his pain. Because he wanted to keep his job, Stan brainstormed about what might help. He then met with the veterinarians and worked out a plan to improve his comfort and ability. His request involved less than $500 of equipment (a hands-free phone, a more ergonomic chair, a footrest, and a heating pad) and permission to take breaks for fifteen uninterrupted minutes twice a day. Stan arranged for the after-hours answering service to pick up calls during his meditative rests. These minor changes had substantial effects. Stan now looks forward to work, and his employers appreciate his presence.

Tayla had worked as a successful advertising executive for many years before developing a chronic pain condition. Her job was a huge part of her identity, and she was very upset that she could not continue the way she had been. By the end of each day spent making pitches and presentations and trying to sketch out new ideas, her body seared with pain. Determined to continue in her job, Tayla applied her creative skills to the problem. She proposed a flexible schedule, which would enable her to pace herself and work from home much of the time. She set up a comfortable workspace in her den with a computer station that allowed her to videoconference with coworkers. These changes enabled Tayla to achieve a sustainable rhythm of work and rest and once again thrive in her work.

Emmett worked on an assembly line and valued his job but found standing for long periods had become unbearable. All his coworkers were required to stand, and Emmett worried about the ramifications of asking for special treatment. To help, Emmett first talked to his doctor, who wrote a short note describing Emmett's pain condition and his need for flexible accommodations. Emmett then requested a swiveling stool with a backrest that could support his body in a standing position while reducing back strain and leg fatigue. Many of Emmett's coworkers were sympathetic to pain; however, he sometimes endured snide comments. Still, he preferred an occasional unsympathetic remark to the pain caused by unassisted standing.

Know What You Want

Before contacting your employer, think seriously about creative strategies to improve your work experience. Whenever possible, conduct experiments to test your hypotheses and track the results.

- Identify the obstacles. What bothers you most?
- Identify how these factors affect your ability to work.
- Identify desired accommodations and their anticipated cost and benefits.
  - o What simple changes can you make on your own?
  - o Are there changes requiring assistance or permission from your employer?

Improvements come from understanding the factors that would make a difference to you. This may vary substantially based on whether you spend your day standing at a cash register, driving long distances, carrying boxes or plates, sitting at a desk, or on your feet talking with others.

Fatigue and pacing. If fatigue interferes with your ability to work, experiment with strategies to rejuvenate yourself. Compare the rallying effects, for example, of a thirty-minute lunchtime nap versus five-minute meditation sessions at regular intervals. If mornings are especially difficult, you might consider working later hours. If your vitality plummets around midday, you might desire split days or part-time work. You may also find ways to modify your environment to take full advantage of rest breaks. Resting on a hard floor, for example, is likely to be counterproductive. If you have access to a private space, you might equip it with soft bedding. Or you could set up your car for midday snoozes.

Temperature and comfort. If your pain rises with cold drafts or heat, evaluate your workplace temperature. If your office is too air-conditioned, try simple strategies, such as dressing with multiple lightweight layers (or strategies to warm yourself discussed in chapter 11). If staying warm requires you to suit up like an astronaut, you might poll coworkers. If they, too, would prefer the tropics to Antarctica, you may have an easier pitch to your boss.

Ergonomics

This concept has entered the office lexicon. Employers are becoming more proactive by offering a more healthful environment. Some corporations use consultants to improve their employees' work setup. However, if you lack access to such services, assess your work conditions, including your own posture and positioning. You can also seek assistance from a physical or occupational therapist. If you spend considerable time at an office workstation, be particularly mindful of the following items. Keep in mind that products labeled "ergonomic" are not guaranteed to meet your needs.

Your chair. Evaluate your seat based on how it feels at different times in the day. Would you feel better if you got up more often? What about its features, such as back support, armrests, height, and firmness? Creative additions, such as seat or back cushions or a footstool (try phone books), may change your experience. When evaluating new chairs, make sure to try them multiple times and simulate your workday activities to find the best fit.

Keyboard, mouse, and keyboard tray. The number and variety of computer accompaniments has soared, partly in response to repetitive strain injuries from typing and clicking. Large office supply stores often offer a wide selection of displays you can try. Notice the force needed to activate different keyboards and mice and how different models feel, including split keyboards, wireless varieties, and other innovations that may increase your comfort. Consider items to increase your comfort, such as wrist rests and adjustable holders for the keyboard and mouse. Test different combinations and their effects on your hands, arms, neck, and back. Keep in mind that testing keyboards can be painful, and after a point, nothing may feel comfortable. A more realistic test may be using the equipment in your office (check the return policies).

Telephone. There is no reason to hold a telephone in your hand or between your head and shoulder (ouch!). Most desk phones include speaker options. And for private conversations, headset phones—once exclusively used by operators and rock stars—are both widely available and affordable. Most new phones of all sorts include headset jacks.

Voice-activated software. Typing pain is becoming less inevitable. Dictating may become more common than typing before too long. When comparing voice-activated products, consider their compatibility with your preferred software and the way you work. A handheld digital recorder that translates voice files into text, for example, can be used anywhere, including lying down far from your desk or computer. Even as they improve, all these products include a learning curve. You may find them frustrating at first, but they literally learn along with you. Most programs also allow seamless movement between voice and typing. Experiment to find what suits you, such as dictating new material and using the keyboard for editing

Other devices. Catalogs brim with innovative devices for people with disabilities, ranging from wide-grip pens to motorized scooters. If you're unable to find a gadget for your needs, consult an occupational therapist. A gizmo may exist for your specific situation.

Your position. Ergonomics is about not only equipment but also the way you position and move your body. Most of us feel best when we intersperse movement with rest, so experiment with your ideal ratio. Notice how you hold and move your body, your posture when you sit or stand, the way you hold or use equipment, and other ways you may position your body. Strive for smooth, unforced movements and sustainable body positioning.

- If your job is largely sedentary, explore opportunities to move and stretch: Take a lap around your building during breaks. Practice yoga postures. Take breaks to stretch your back, neck, or legs; walk to the water cooler; or engage in other frequent movement. If remembering is a problem, set a timer to ring at intervals throughout the day to remind you to move.

- If your job requires you to assume awkward positions, such as in dental work, in which you are bent over patients' heads, experiment with postures to reduce strain, and take regular breaks to stretch and recuperate.
- For jobs that involve repetitive motions such as keyboard strokes, use a gentle touch, and take frequent breaks to roll your shoulders and stretch your hands, wrists, and arms.
- If your job requires prolonged standing, consider alternative arrangements, such as a chair or footstool to rest a leg.

For assistance with these strategies, consult with a physical or occupational therapist. He or she can assess your body dynamics and your approach to aspects of your job you find difficult. The therapist may suggest specific methods to reduce strain and strengthen core muscles, such as the Alexander technique or Feldenkrais method, which teach ways to move with awareness.[1]

Transportation

If your work commute aggravates your pain, consider feasible changes.

Public transportation. If you suffer from the vibrations; bumps; or rigid seats in trains, buses, or vans, consider ways to buffer yourself. Portable seat cushions come in many varieties, including wedges with handles (which can also be clipped onto a belt or put into an around-the-waist bag for hands-free carrying).

Parking. If the walk between your car and work feels prohibitive, look into closer parking, including handicapped parking. Or, by keeping your arms free, you may be able to approach the walk instead as a therapeutic opportunity. If neither of these work, you might investigate other arrangements, such as carpooling or courtesy vans for disabled individuals.

Electric bike. The variety of motorized cycles is expanding and includes options such as sturdy three-wheeled bikes and cargo bikes that carry large loads. Among their other benefits, they allow you to park very close to your workplace.

Schlepping. Remove all unnecessary, weighty items from your bag, and stow incidentals—such as a hairbrush or stash of coins—in your car, office drawer, or wherever you are most likely to use them. In addition, evaluate how you carry your bag. Avoid the lopsided over-the-shoulder approach if it increases arm, shoulder, back, or neck pain. Roller bags may offer a good solution. Or consider personal adaptations that place the weight where you can best carry it. I tailored a hip-bag from a cheap plastic attaché case by cutting two slits in its side, then threading a belt through the slits so I can strap it around my waist like a packhorse. The funniest part is that people compliment my bag and have even asked where they could find one! Who knew that my makeshift solution would also be chic?

Telecommuting? Working from home or satellite locations is becoming more common. Consider its applicability for you.

How to Approach Your Employer

When you desire accommodation to your workplace environment, it's time to consider talking with your employer. The law is on your side, but it is still good policy to approach your employer with the intention of keeping the company on your side as well. Avoid threats of litigation as a starting point. No legislation can force employers to be reasonable, even if unreasonableness opens them to a lawsuit. The most successful strategies tend to be framed in reference to the best interests of you and your employer.

Before requesting changes, have a clear idea of what would be helpful. Employers are also more likely to respond positively to concrete ideas than to vague concerns about the difficulty of your job—plus, you may both find a discussion of the merits and costs of a specific proposal to be more helpful (and comfortable) than talking about your limits or condition. Pain, unlike disabilities that are more visible, can be confusing to employers. It is unreasonable to expect employers to offer accommodations without your input.

It is up to you how you broach the topic. The ADA does not require that you schedule a formal meeting. It is expected, however, that you inform your employer of your medical condition and the specific accommodation you are requesting. Making your initial request in writing has the benefit of serving as documentation. If you prefer to ask first in person, document the conversations with a follow-up e-mail or letter or by logging notes in a personal journal. This provides a paper trail for accountability. Once you make your wishes known, it is up to your employer to respond.

Where possible, calculate the effects of any desired adjustments on your employer and other employees (or clients). If your request poses minimal inconveniences or is neutral (or even positive) for others, then, by all means, ask. Before requesting more disruptive changes, make sure you've exhausted individualized ones (such as trying earplugs before asking for office noise reduction). When making a request, consider the following components in your request:

(a) *Warm-up.* Open with a positive statement about your experience at work to prime your employer to hear what you have to say.

(b) *Background.* Provide a brief account of your condition—just enough to support your point without unnecessary detail. Your goal is to convince your employer to take your request seriously, not to engage in a confessional, inspire pity, or raise doubt about your general abilities.

(c) *Specific request.* Ask for what you want in a clear and direct manner. Spell out what makes these accommodations reasonable (and include the phrase "reasonable accommodations" if you work in the United States, or an equivalent crucial phrase from relevant legislation in other countries).

(d) *Win-win.* Highlight the mutual benefit of accommodations. Employers are more likely to assist when they recognize their gains. Consider the positive consequences, such as an increase in your accuracy, productivity, or presence.

(e) *Listen.* Make sure to listen carefully to the response you receive. If your employer is hesitant, note the reasons. Do not feel you have to respond immediately to any concern your employer may raise. If you are caught off guard, it is far preferable to revisit the issue once you have thought it through, calmly, rather than responding with an emotional reaction, hurt, or defensiveness.

(f) *Gratitude.* Remember that you are talking to a human being. While revving up to ask for something potentially emotional, you may lose sight of the impact of the conversation on your employer. Make sure to express your appreciation. At the same time, resist apologizing or putting yourself down in any way. You have every right to make this request.

The following examples illustrate how to use the described components in a simple request. The first is a script of sorts for a face-to-face meeting. While it is unlikely that you will recite a monologue, you might write out what you would like to say as part of your preparation (or even bring notes).

> "Thank you for meeting with me, as I have something important to ask you. I have been working here for two years and really enjoy and value my job. As you may know, I suffer from a chronic pain condition called reflex sympathetic dystropy. One of the things that helps me enormously is pacing myself. Lately, I have found that by midday, my pain starts to interfere with my concentration. I would benefit enormously from a reasonable accommodation to my schedule that would enable me to take two thirty-minute breaks. I would be willing to exchange my lunch hour for a mid-morning and mid-afternoon break or work one hour later. I value this job and want to give you my best work. Taking time for rest breaks would enable me to do this. I appreciate your help."

Or, in writing:

> Dear Ms. Boss,
> I have been working for this company for one year and really value my job. As you may know, I suffer from rheumatoid arthritis. I have a couple of requests for reasonable accommodations that would greatly improve my ability to do my job:
>
> - Voice-activated software. I have researched this, and the latest version costs approximately $90.
> - A more supportive chair. I found one at Staples for $149.
>
> Thank you very much for considering ways to help me be more productive.

Note that in both cases, the requests mention the pain condition and "reasonable accommodation" and express enthusiasm for the job and the mutual benefits of the proposed changes. The way you communicate with your employer will depend on your personal style and relationship. Use what you know about your boss and yourself to put your best foot forward.

Some Other Considerations

Timing. As the saying goes, "Timing is everything." Contact your employer when you feel calm and levelheaded. While pain can be very motivating, resist any urges to burst into your boss's office during the height of pain to cry, complain, or demand a change. Negotiations can be taxing under the best circumstances; do not undertake this interaction when you feel especially vulnerable. Consider timing from your employer's point of view as well: aim to select a meeting time when your employer is most likely to be receptive. There's no harm in double-checking: "Is this a good time?" or "Would that be a good time?" If you write to your employer, let your letter germinate (and consider showing it to you someone you trust) before sending it.

Disclosure. Broaching personal issues such as your health can feel uncomfortable. While your employer needs information to understand why an accommodation is required, you need not divulge information that feels private. If your employer requires documentation from your doctor, talk with your doctor about how your situation will be described. Disclosure can involve a careful balancing act. You want your experience to be taken seriously, but without raising doubts about your ability to work. Despite ADA provisions about the illegality of retaliation for requesting accommodations, disclosure can lead to overt or covert discrimination.

It is your decision whether to disclose and how much to disclose about your pain condition to your employer, coworkers, or clients. If coworkers believe you are receiving unfairly preferential treatment, you may want to clear the air. A brief education about the realities of your experience may transform their view of you into more of a hero than a shirker. When appropriate, express your gratitude for their understanding, concern, or offers of assistance. Be aware that some naysayers may persist in the group, finding it difficult to "see" chronic pain.

Attitude. While it makes sense to feel frustrated, don't let it determine your tone. When asking for accommodation, emphasize what you have to offer, rather than any shortcomings, and the positives the changes will offer. You were hired for a reason. Focus on strategies that will enable you to continue your work—and resist second-guessing whether you are the best person for the job.

Needs versus preferences. When you propose reasonable accommodations, be clear that your requests are needs rather than personal preferences. There's a significant difference between asking for a warmer office because you "like being warm" and because cold temperatures cause burning pain in your arms, neck, and back, which affects your ability to concentrate. This also distinguishes your request from any made by coworkers with temperature preferences.

Follow-up. After your initial request, maintain documentation of any further communication. If your request does not result in your desired change, continue with written correspondence. This communicates your commitment and, if necessary, provides documentation if your employer responds unfavorably. Make sure to include explicit language such as, "I am requesting reasonable accommodations to enable me to work better with my disability," and specify a time frame within which you expect a response. If appropriate, send copies to other relevant individuals. With prompting, your employer should respond to your requests. If not, draft another letter, emphasizing the importance of these changes for you to carry out your job. If your boss dismisses or denies your request or is hostile, you can contact your nearest Equal Employment Opportunity Commission about filing a charge of discrimination.

Resources in the United States:

For questions or concerns about the ADA or reasonable accommodations, contact the Job Accommodation Network (JAN), a free consulting service of the Office of Disability Employment Policy within the Department of Labor, at http://www.jan.wvu.edu or 1-800-526-7234.

If your employer fails to grant you reasonable accommodations, contact the US Equal Employment Opportunity Commission at http://www.eeoc.gov or 1-800-669-4000.

Tips for Students

Whether you are in grade school, trade school, college, or graduate or professional school, consider the following:

Disability services. Some schools have disability service offices and require that you (or your parents or guardians) register your disability. The office may notify your instructors on your behalf about your disability and offer strategies or devices to assist with your schoolwork.

Talk with your instructors. If you need special accommodations, raise this with your instructors early, rather than when you find yourself in a pain flare-up the night before an assignment is due. Mention only what is relevant for your request—which may be simply that you have an unpredictable pain condition and may make special requests if you encounter difficulties. You might ask what their recommendation or policy would be under those circumstances.

Strategic scheduling. Keep your load light enough to graduate in a timely manner without overtaxing yourself. Consider alternatives that distribute the work over a longer period, such as summer school or part-time studies.

Brevity. Students often think longer papers are better papers. Often, it is the reverse; good writing involves succinct arguments. Conserve your energy by organizing your ideas first, and keep computer time to a minimum. Workshops in composition can help. Instructors who read and grade many papers may also appreciate brevity.

Sleep. Students sometimes choose late nights or all-nighters as a study strategy. With chronic pain, skimping on sleep tends to backfire. Experiment and see if you are more effective when you commit to a healthful sleep routine.

Self-care. Just as you schedule your classes and study sessions, schedule time for regular exercise, rest, and fun. The key to a sustainable experience is balance.

Friendships. Social life is an important part of student life. Choose your close friends carefully; you'll benefit from friends who energize rather than enervate you and who enjoy activities you find sustaining.

Chapter 22

Work Alternatives

Considering New Pathways

Working is not always a choice. Sometimes this decision is straight-forward: you simply feel too awful to work, regardless of the financial costs. Other times, unemployment occurs through a gradual process of scaling back until you find work no longer feasible. Or the decision may be made for you, due to an excessive number of missed days or other perceived shortcomings.

If you are taking a break from work due to pain, you owe it to yourself to make plans to take care of yourself and set optimistic goals. Short breaks sometimes evolve into permanent retirement; other times, they are the needed respite that enables you to regroup and consider a different career path. Whatever your situation, consider what you would like to occur in the upcoming days, weeks, or beyond. Create a plan that focuses on how you will use the time to enhance your life. Here are some examples:

(a) I plan to focus my energy on feeling better. I will experiment with different patterns of activity and rest to find the combination that is most sustaining. I will also seek out a supportive medical team and a combination of medication and therapies to bring my pain under control. When possible, I will engage in the following activities: _____ (which includes fun events to keep up my spirits). I will also explore options for affordable psychotherapy and support groups to help me contend with the stress that chronic pain has brought to my life. I hope to recover sufficiently to be able to reconsider options for work. I will give this plan three months and then reevaluate.

(b) I have decided to stop working and apply for disability compensation. My immediate goals are to file the paperwork for my disability claim and engage in behaviors to reduce my pain. I plan to focus on understanding the factors that affect my pain and finding a way to start exercising. My long-term goal is to investigate work options that would be flexible and feasible for me when my pain is under better control.

(c) I have stopped working because my job was so exhausting that I had nothing left for my family, which I also value. I plan to spend part of each day taking care of myself so that I can be more present with my children and partner. I may revisit employment issues at a later time.

Figuring out what you want—and even writing it out, as above—can be helpful for days when you feel cast adrift. Having a specific plan, with pieces to explore, can also stave off judgments, whether from yourself or others. When unemployment is involuntary, the blow may be even greater to self-esteem and finances. Losing a source of income can be incredibly stressful on family relationships.

The pressures of not working. The idea that *not* working is stressful may seem paradoxical. But a certain amount of magical thinking can arise around not working, particularly when working was a source of stress for some time. Unfortunately, terminating a job does not always bring the anticipated pain reprieve. Consider the lore of retirement. For some, it offers golden years, but not for everyone. What matters most, whether working or not, is discovering what helps the most and incorporating that into your life. This requires an active commitment. Yet, when people with chronic pain are at home without structured commitments, it can be difficult to get motivated for activities, even beneficial ones. (See chapter 13 on jump-starts.)

Unemployment from disability is not equivalent to age-related retirement, but the parallels between the two offer insight. The literature on aging points to key elements for successful retirement, which seem relevant to any form of joblessness (whether temporary or permanent):

1. *Health*. Focus your energy on managing chronic pains, and any other health conditions, as a way to fare better.

2. *Financial security*. Evaluate your resources, assets, and eligibility for disability compensation. Consider ideas for part-time or modified income-generating activities.

3. *Social support.* Unemployment can reduce social connection. Staying home and feeling awful can be a recipe for isolation. Regardless of how you feel, stay connected and tend valued relationships.
4. *Positive attitude and coping.* With chronic pain, your attitude and coping strategies are continually challenged, and these challenges are important to take on, over and over again, to improve your experience.
5. *Meaningful activities.* Without a job to structure your life, you are condemned, as French philosopher Jean-Paul Sartre described, to the freedom of having to create your own meaning. Figure out what matters most to you, and each day, focus on at least one meaningful thing you *can* do.

Additional pressures of staying at home. If you are home on account of pain, a significant part of your job is engaging in behaviors to improve how you feel. This involves building a solid medical team, if you don't already have one, and actively experimenting with approaches to increase comfort and satisfaction. But if you are part of a household, you can become vulnerable to others' ideas about what "getting to stay at home" may mean. As described in chapter 19, you can become something of a de facto housekeeper. At times, this may work, but when it does not, talk with family members. Keep your goals realistic, without guilt. Remember, you left your job because of a painful disability. Relinquishing the breadwinner role can be especially stressful; then, not feeling up to the fix-it chores or the heavy lifting at home can be doubly demoralizing, particularly for men. Keep in mind that your capabilities are likely to fluctuate from day to day, and do not judge yourself on what you can or cannot accomplish. Adapting to your new circumstances is a process. You may need considerable downtime to feel better. At the same time, seek ways to stay engaged, whatever this may mean on a given day.

Exploring New Career Avenues

My Story

When an old friend learned that my career as an academic sociologist was waylaid by chronic pain, he responded enthusiastically, "What a great chance to do something really interesting!" You may be thinking, "What a lousy friend." My initial thought was, "He's *got* to be kidding!" I had spent years preparing for a career that I could no longer contemplate because I hurt all the time. What "interesting" thing would I be able to do? But he was not being facetious, nor was he a lousy friend. I often reflect on his words and smile as I contemplate the career path I have since taken. Sometimes, in the ending of one dream lies the makings for another.

As I accepted that I was no longer built for the rigors of a full-time academic position and its "publish or perish" culture, I began contemplating alternatives. Let me emphasize that this was not easy. Not in the least. My identity at that point was very much bound up in becoming a sociology professor, and I had invested many years of schooling toward this objective. It was painful to surrender this ambition. I revisited the reasons that had interested me in this career:

- The work felt interesting and meaningful.
- I enjoyed writing.
- I enjoyed teaching.
- I appreciated interactions with others.
- I appreciated the flexibility in the schedule and projects.

These reasons still rang true. Next, I reflected on how I might continue in this career in a less intense way. I searched for part-time appointments with less pressure, and I found several options for teaching as an adjunct or visiting professor that I previously would not have considered. I also found opportunities to teach water aerobics classes for rehab patients and older adults with arthritis; the compensation included a pool membership, something I would have found difficult to afford at that time.

Slowly, I began opening myself up to other types of work. During this time, I happened to tap into an online discussion board on chronic pain that mirrored my suffering. I wanted to participate, and, rather than describing my struggles, I found myself crafting a message with the strategies I had found most helpful. This felt good, even therapeutic, and I enjoyed the response I received from others. Soon after this, I came across an advertisement for a flexible position at Emory University in Atlanta, Georgia, as an advocate and liaison with academic, patient, and medical communities around emergent illnesses. My application about invisible disabilities was accepted, and the position at Emory launched this book. I want to emphasize that up until that time, I would not have imagined choosing work that involved pain as a focus. However, I discovered that self-help writing and advocacy work felt even more satisfying to me than academic pursuits.

This steered me toward social work. I figured, too, that a job that largely involved listening to others would be a good match for my physical state. In my midthirties, pain and all, I returned to school to pursue a master's degree in social work. I had the tremendous benefit of family support for this change, and I reasoned that the investment of time, money, and pain would be well worth it. Since then, I've cobbled together a career in clinical social work as a part-time instructor, part-time writer and advocate, and part-time psychotherapist. I feel truly blessed.

Your Story

Each of us is distinct. We have different desires, interests, strengths, needs, and resources. Your options and experiences will also differ by your age, prior experiences, training, career history, family circumstances, culture, and health. Yet many people with pain share the pivotal experience of contemplating a life transition. If what you have been doing or hoping to do no longer seems feasible, look inward and all around you. Keep in mind Plato's observation that "necessity is the mother of invention." Your story, too, is about re-creating employment options that can be sustaining and rewarding.

Realistic assessment. Begin with a sense of what you *can* do and your best prediction of what it would take to fare well in a job. You may have to adjust your definition of what a full workday or workweek looks like for you. Be realistic in assessing your needs, but realize at the same time that they can continue to change. No matter what you do—and whether or not you receive a paycheck—you, like everyone else, will experience twenty-four hours in a day. What do you want your day to look like? Ask yourself:

- What type of schedule best suits me?
- What set of conditions allows me maximum comfort?
- What does my ideal use of time look like?
- What percentage of my day do I prefer to be sitting, standing, lying down, and sleeping?

- How much of my day would I like to spend in solitary pursuits? How much engaged with others?
- What would my ideal workday or workweek look like?

The key is to identify things you enjoy and explore related work possibilities. Set realistic goals for yourself, and know your own limits while keeping your focus on what you are able to do. Sometimes, when you feel particularly bad, it is hard to imagine engaging in much. You may feel overwhelmed by pain and exhaustion and may wonder, despite your best efforts and motivation, how you can succeed in any work. Or you may feel hard-pressed to find an existing job with sufficient flexibility to meet your needs, both creative ones and financial ones. Take it one step at a time. Your worst moments are not the times to contemplate a new career.

At the same time, recall the power of the jump-start described in chapter 13. As a peer with fibromyalgia shared with me, "I tend to keep going and going because as soon as I stopped, I would crawl back under the covers." Turn to your experiments to remind yourself how you do while engaging in different activities. Often, your best days are the ones in which you did something satisfying, pain or not. Use your tracking tool to experiment with the conditions that enable you to function best. The better you come to know yourself, the easier it will be to find something suitable. If you decide you would like to find employment, the central task becomes matching your current abilities with a desired job.

Gratefulness. Nobody wants chronic pain. Yet the intrusion of illness can deliver unlikely gifts. Becoming unable to continue in your current job can open otherwise unexplored career paths or new avenues for growth, as it did for me. Without such a catalyst, many people might continue in their current jobs, year after year, without questioning their choices, even if they are not particularly happy. Try to be grateful for this break in routine and for the chance to look deeply into what matters most to you.

Creativity. Use your imagination. You may be thinking, "No kidding—I'll need imagination to think of anything I can do with this pain." But there are endless possibilities. Ask yourself, "Given my set of circumstances, what would represent meaningful work for me?" Who knows? You may discover a hidden talent or return to a childhood occupational dream. There are famous authors who first set pen to paper in their fifties or sixties. Use your condition to reflect on your choices, view the larger picture, and examine your priorities. You may remember a career ambition you relinquished years ago or a wholly new direction you find intriguing. Dancers who are no longer able to dance may find meaning as teachers, choreographers, costume designers, or consultants. Professionals may turn a hobby into a vocation and become artists, writers, or entrepreneurs. Use your creativity to envision the possibilities. Clients of mine have, after years in various corporate jobs, found satisfying experiences in opening their own businesses caring for animals, tutoring high school students, making jewelry, and maintaining pools.

Pacing. Approach your goal in manageable steps, and avoid being weighed down by the size of the challenges you face. Find small tasks that feel appropriate to your energy level. Don't let bad days dissuade you from your goals. Accept that you will have times that feel too painful or exhausting to work. At such moments, engage in restorative activities and maintain your perspective.

Priorities. Reflect on what would give you the greatest job fulfillment. Try to identify exactly what you have found satisfying in previous jobs or other activities. Are you seeking creativity? Productivity? Do you value the identity or status linked to your position, or the sense of connection to an organization, or having a place outside the house where others value you and your contribution? As you answer these questions, refocus your energy on the priorities that emerge.

Research and resources. Talk with friends, family, and colleagues; they can be valuable resources. Visit the library. Search online. There is an entire industry dedicated to the pursuit of the right job, including self-help books, occupational therapists, career counselors, and life coaches. Occupational therapists offer adaptive solutions, including gadgets to complete tasks you find difficult, and often their work is covered by medical insurance. Career counselors and life coaches help with career issues, such as feelings of discouragement, long-term goals, and interpersonal matters that may arise when you think about the kind of work you want to do. These professionals are not linked to any particular jobs, and you are not hiring them to find you a job. Instead, they help evaluate your capabilities and the impact of various activities on your ability to function, and they help you determine the work that may best suit you. Their services are generally not covered by medical insurance.

Among the most popular self-help books is *What Color Is Your Parachute?* by Richard Nelson Bolles. This book encourages people to figure out the type of work they most want and use strategies to pursue it. Bolles's later volume, *Job*

Hunting for the So-Called Handicapped (or People Who Have Disabilities), explores life questions while addressing constraints and fears. If you feel stuck, consider talking to a professional. It is a hefty enterprise to search for a new career path while contending with pain.

Some Career Possibilities

Consider the ideas below to help you get started in thinking about jobs that can allow for flexibility and incorporate your personal creativity.

Flextime positions. Flexible work arrangements are becoming more common, particularly in smaller organizations. Many opportunities exist for part-time and as-needed positions as well as job-sharing positions, in which you divide work responsibilities and salary with another employee, either by task or by day. Having a less demanding schedule opens possibilities, whether you desire to remain in the same organization or field or embark on something entirely new.

Freelance. Another option is hiring yourself out as a freelancer for work that appeals to you. (Local Internet lists, such as Craigslist®, can provide free advertising.) This work allows you to explore the market for your ideas and to choose which jobs to accept and when. These flexible arrangements, however, do not include benefits, such as health insurance or retirement pay.

Retraining. If there is something that feels right for you, it may be worthwhile to invest in further education or training. Take a long road's view. Even if your next career requires a significant time investment, you'll have your remaining years to reap the benefits.

Consulting. The market for consultants of all types is wide and expanding. Consider what you may have to share with others, whether your know-how is in computers, gardening, farming, childcare, genealogy, construction, investment, or cooking. The odds are that you can market your expertise or experience, either directly to the public or through an organization.

Working from home. With the help of the Internet, it has become increasingly possible to work from the comfort of your own home. The examples below apply to jobs in which you hire yourself to a large organization or set out as an entrepreneur. There are many professional associations and networks that can assist you. Consider the following work-from-home options:

- *Market research* predates the Internet and is often conducted over the telephone. If you are comfortable on the phone and appreciate work that does not carry over into other parts of your day, this may be for you. Market research jobs can be full- or part-time. The work typically involves asking questions over the telephone from a script and recording people's responses. Look for established firms, and beware of scams.

- *Copyediting.* If you have editorial skills, you can market your services for a wide range of services, including résumés, advertising copy, and organizational newsletters. You can advertise your proofreading skills locally or internationally and work as part of an established organization or as an entrepreneur.

- *Virtual assistants* are part of a growing international field. This new profession provides Internet-based administrative, clerical, creative, and technical services on a contractual basis. The work can be done from home and on your own schedule.

- *Direct sales* allows individuals, with the help of the Internet, to operate home-based businesses. Consider your passions—perhaps an art, craft, talent, or particular interest in collectibles. Start small and, over time, explore ways to grow your company. This is the strategy used by "mama's cookies" type operations that have moved from kitchens and garages to national markets.

- *Graphic design.* If you are artistic and creative, there is a never-ending need for brochures, flyers, business cards, logos, and website design. The Internet contains associations of freelance designers, photographers, writers, architects, fashion and video designers, and more.

- *Personal shopping.* It may surprise you to know that you can make a career out of shopping online for busy professionals. Networks of personal shoppers are paid to assume the shopping tasks of selecting everything from special or personal gifts to business items. If you enjoy shopping and are Internet savvy, this may be for you.

- *Retail sales.* If you are interested in sales, consider opening an Internet storefront. You can turn a shopping obsession into a moneymaking business that you can run from home on your own schedule. The online company eBay offers training services on getting started; maximizing your sales; and improving, streamlining, and sustaining a profitable business.

- *Other entrepreneurial jobs.* Being your own boss has certain advantages, including control over the volume and pace of your work. On the flip side, the availability of jobs—and, thus, pay—can be unpredictable. Whatever your strengths, you are likely to discover multiple niches. Scores of online articles and magazines report success stories and suggestions for starting small and eventually turning a passion into a profitable enterprise. Some examples include:

o Event planning (professional conferences, family reunions, weddings, toddler birthday parties)
o Artistic enterprises (scrapbooking, online photo albums, Power-Point® presentations, specialty bookmarks, custom candy wrappers, woodworking)
o Caregiving (house-sitting, pet-sitting, childcare)
o Tutoring (assisting grade-school students, teaching English as a second language to adults, helping student athletes)
o Food preparation (homemade dinners, specialty cookies)
o Resale (buying in bulk and selling individually for profit)

And the lists go on. You may discover an untapped niche and build a substantial company from the comfort of home. Unleash your creative juices, and take it one small step at a time. A client of mine who used to own franchises but was unable to maintain a full-time schedule is creating a niche by marketing his expertise in managing schedules for other establishments (which he can do from the comfort of home).

Employment, however, is not for everyone. If you have already invested years in a career, early retirement may be more appealing. Sometimes workplaces offer financial incentives for early retirement. This can free you to explore your next stage, whether fly-fishing, writing a memoir, minting commemorative coins, or refocusing on family or volunteer activities. Or you may realize you need a hiatus from work due to pain and related limitations and, thus, seek disability compensation to help you during this period.

Disability Compensation

The topic of disability compensation is vast. This section provides basic information on the types available in the United States, discusses the problems inherent in having to "prove" one's disability, and offers tips to endure the process. If you live in a country with a more developed social welfare system, some of this may be unnecessary.

Individual private insurance. In the United States, private disability insurance plans may be part of individual disability income policies, group policies, group association policies, and riders attached to life insurance policies. Some employees, including civil service workers, veterans, and other government employees, receive private disability income insurance as part of their benefits package. Some employers provide disability insurance to all employees; others offer it for an additional fee, or not at all. Individual policies tend to be expensive and insure people with the means and foresight to purchase a private plan for unexpected illness or disability.

Check whether you carry private disability insurance, and, if so, its specifics, including what you need to do to apply. Policies can include short-term disability benefits, long-term disability benefits, or both. Generally, eligibility for short-term disability begins when you become disabled and lasts approximately three to six months. If your disability continues, you may then qualify for long-term insurance, which usually starts at the conclusion of the short-term disability period. Most policies have deadlines and strict timing requirements, so start filing as soon as you can. If the policy is offered through your work, your employer should be able to assist you and sometimes file the paperwork on your behalf. Either way, stay on top of the process because it is time sensitive. If you have more than one disability insurance plan, initiate the paperwork for all.

Check, also, whether you happen to live in a state with a state disability insurance program. These programs tend to be run by the same agency that administers unemployment insurance. Contact your state's unemployment office to see what is available. If your state has a program, check whether you are eligible to apply through automatic payroll deductions while employed.

The definition of disability varies from policy to policy. Review your insurance company's plan carefully. If you are denied coverage, you may appeal. At that point, you may want to seek legal advice to help navigate the process.

Social Security Disability Insurance (SSDI). The federal disability insurance in the United States is offered through the Social Security Administration and referred to as Social Security Disability Insurance. Contributions to SSDI are made through the Federal Insurance Contributions Act (FICA), the same fund that supports retirement benefits. You may have noticed FICA deductions on your paycheck. Individuals become eligible to apply for benefits if they have paid FICA taxes for a certain period of time and are unable to perform substantial work for at least one year due to a "medically determined physical or mental impairment."

SSDI offers long-term benefits only (no short-term coverage). The application process for SSDI is lengthy. As soon as you anticipate that you will be unable to work for one year or more, start building your case. Research the application process, organize your materials, and talk with your healthcare professionals. You can then file for disability benefits online or by visiting your local Social Security office. Before filling out any paperwork, assemble your materials. Your disability case will be judged largely on the medical records in your file that describe your inability to work. Thus, it is important that the appropriate documents are included in your file and that the medical records accurately report, in detail, your abilities and disabilities as they pertain to activities of daily living and employment. Talk openly with your healthcare professionals about documenting your limitations in your medical records and in any correspondence they direct to the Social Security Administration (SSA).

Then, be prepared both to wait and for possible rejection. The SSA generally takes several months to issue a decision, and most applications are rejected. If your case is denied at this stage, you can appeal. Unfortunately, it is also common to receive a second rejection, at which point you can request a hearing with an administrative law judge. This process can be long, and during this time, people may have little in the way of financial support. However, the odds of a positive ruling increase when you go before an administrative law judge—so stick it out if you can. And even if your appeal is denied, your case may be presented to higher courts.

Legal representation can be helpful at any step of the process. Your local Social Security office can supply a list of lawyers who specialize in disability law. Most disability lawyers accept cases on contingency—that is, you pay only if you win, and their fee is typically a percentage of your award. Be resourceful in finding an attorney or law firm with a good track record and reputation. Before hiring an attorney, schedule an introductory meeting to get acquainted. Ask questions to determine the extent to which the lawyer sees your case as legitimate (there is no point to working with a biased representative) and can explain his or her strategy and the basis of your collaboration. Lawyers view "disability" in this context as a legal construct, not simply a medical one, and should understand what is essential in presenting your case. Lawyers can reassure you, assist with paperwork, and represent you if your case goes before an administrative law judge.

If you are granted SSDI, you are entitled to a monthly paycheck and Medicare health insurance. You should also receive retroactive payments for the period during which you were awaiting an outcome and possibly from the date you became disabled. In some cases, you may have access to vocational rehabilitation or other programs intended to help you return to work. The amount of your monthly check is determined by the amount you contributed to FICA over the years—so the higher your income and the more years you worked, the higher your check.

While receiving SSDI, you can also work under two conditions: (1) if your monthly income does not exceed a specific amount, and (2) if you are engaging in a trial work period, which, under SSDI regulations, means you can work for a specific number of months without jeopardizing your benefits. Any month in which you earn more than a specific amount counts as part of your trial work period. If you complete your trial work period, you are no longer entitled to SSDI payments, as this is interpreted to mean you are capable of gainful employment. As you are experimenting with your ability to work while on disability, keep track of your income each month. Report the months in which you make over the threshold amount, and make sure to refund SSA for checks you receive during these months. You will be accountable for SSDI overpayments unless you can demonstrate that (a) the mistake was not your fault, and (b) repayment would create a hardship. After you complete your trial work period, if you later become unable to work due to disability, you can reapply for SSDI.

While you wait for the SSA determination of your case, the financial strain and uncertainty can create great stress. Conserve finances and be frugal as much as possible, and try to avoid unnecessary debt. You may be eligible for services such as food stamps or a food bank. Check with state and federal government offices.

Supplemental Security Income (SSI). The SSA offers another program for people who are unable to work and lack financial resources. SSI is funded by general federal tax revenues and is based on financial need, unrelated to your work history. SSI pays monthly benefits to individuals with disabilities who have little or no income and minimal savings (or household assets, if married). In contrast,

SSDI does not consider assets; people with substantial savings or a gainfully employed spouse can be granted SSDI, as long as they are judged to be disabled.

SSI does not have the requirement that applicants must be disabled for a year. People who are temporarily disabled or successfully manage their pain and resume working after a few months can still apply for SSI to cover their limited period of disability. As with SSDI, decisions may take several months, you can appeal if denied, you may seek legal representation, and payment can be awarded retroactively for the period in question. Medicaid, a federal health insurance program, may be an option for those who are disabled or whose income falls below federal poverty levels.

More than one disability payment at a time? Generally, insurance systems are not set up for you to receive full disability payments from more than one source. If you have been receiving benefits from your private disability insurance and are then awarded state disability insurance, your private insurance payments will likely decrease based on your supplemental benefits. For this reason, private insurance companies often pay for legal representation to help you obtain state disability insurance. If you are eligible for both SSDI and SSI, Social Security will determine which program will support you (and, in some cases, one may be used to supplement the other).

Having to "Prove Disability"

Applying for disability in the United States can be a demoralizing process. By design, the burden falls on you to prove that you are unable to work and deserve compensation. It can feel as if the outcome bestows a judgment about the magnitude of your suffering or the legitimacy of your experience. Refrain from believing this. Disability decisions are based on legal formulas and a series of negotiations that include some random elements—not on a purely objective assessment of your pain and struggles. From my personal experience, work with clients, and correspondence with many people with "invisible disabilities," I have observed that the process can be quite confusing and discouraging and sometimes seems to defy common sense.

By understanding the obstacles and biases inherent in the process, you can be better prepared to cope with rejections and attribute them to the system, rather than accepting them as your just deserts.

1. *Doctor bias.* Disability cases rely on the expertise of medical professionals who speak on behalf of their patients. Unfortunately, doctors, who are trained to value lab tests, may be less inclined to give legitimacy to chronic pain conditions that have few observable signs. Such doubts can surface in your medical files, undermining your credibility. If your doctor has noted disbelief of your condition or the severity of your pain in your file, this is passed along. Even physicians appointed by Social Security to conduct examinations or evaluate your case may show similar preconceptions.

2. *Subjectivity of (dis)ability.* Disability is a subjective concept. The SSA has a list of recognized illness categories eligible for disability. Being included, however, does not guarantee that your disability claim will receive a positive ruling. According to federal requirements, people are disabled based not on a diagnosis but on how it affects their ability to work. For example, an individual who is legally blind but can earn a substantial income as a massage therapist or musician is ineligible for disability compensation. With something as amorphous as chronic pain, the burden of proof becomes twofold: (1) proving the existence of a potentially disabling condition, and (2) proving that the condition prevents you from working.

3. *Difficulty of documentation.* The invisibility of chronic pain makes it difficult for others to perceive. There are no agreed-upon, objective indicators of pain. Assessments are based, instead, on self-reports of patients to their healthcare professionals and on the professionals' interpretation of these reports. Tools and tests intended to measure pain or strength may not assess a person's ability to perform work, especially over a long period of time. The best evidence comes from doctors' notes over time consistently describing your limitations, such as, "Reports pain at an eight and is unable to sit or stand for more than five minutes."

4. *Variability in our presentation.* Chronic pain conditions often present confusing pictures. Sufferers can look perfectly "normal," despite sizable struggles, and symptoms vary considerably over time. Someone who can walk a mile one day may be unable to rise from bed the next, and people may be able to engage in many activities, but not for a sustained period. These inconsistencies present a confusing case to judges.

This subjectivity also means that proof of a disability depends on the perceived credibility of the claimant, the specificity of notes documenting disability by the treating physicians, and the discretion of the judge. This leaves ample room for judicial and medical biases to surface at any step of the evaluation.

5. *Mismatch between process and symptoms.* The process of applying for disability benefits is ill suited to people suffering from chronic pains. Pain that is severe enough to keep people from working also interferes with the arduous application process, which requires substantial concentration and stamina. Moreover, the long wait for a verdict and the frequent rejections are stressful. People with chronic pain may face skepticism about their suffering and lack social or financial support to persevere in their fight for a just and positive verdict.

Keys to Survival

Bear in mind that while obtaining disability compensation can be an uphill battle, it is also very possible. The following survival tips can help you tolerate this process and increase your odds of success.

Check your emotions. If possible, separate your emotions from the application process. Resist the temptation to attribute any symbolic value to the correspondence you receive from the disability administration. Remind yourself that you are dealing with a bureaucracy with a confusing set of procedures. More than likely, you will receive at least one rejection letter that misrepresents your situation. Expect this, and be prepared to keep going and file the next set of papers. *Do not let rejection letters represent anything about your value or difficulties.* You would not be applying for disability compensation if you were not struggling. Also, ignore the harshness of any rejection letters. Remind yourself that they are computer generated and not really about you.

Start early. It is common for people to hesitate before contacting Social Security, as it may feel like an act of last resort. Some people even wait until their resources are completely depleted. It may be that they hope to improve and not need assistance or that they fear the application process will cause further suffering. But, whatever your reasons, do not put it off. Begin the application process for SSDI or SSI (or both) as early as possible. If the application seems too difficult, seek assistance. Whatever your qualms, forge ahead. Time will pass, and your health and finances may change. If it turns out that you no longer need the help, you will not be in any worse a position for having applied or started the process.

Be persistent. Expect to have your first application denied. Then, if you are in the minority of individuals who receive compensation with the initial application, you can be delightfully surprised. In most cases, persistence pays. Do not let a rejection letter slow your response or resolve. Continue to respond in a timely fashion, submitting whatever additional information you see fit. Be like the Little Engine That Could.

Documentation. A major part of your application comes from your physicians' records. You will be asked to sign medical releases to authorize your healthcare providers to share documents with SSA. Make sure to include any and all doctors you have seen who can attest to your medical condition. Beyond this, you can contribute to the documentation representing your experience through your personal PAINTRACKING records and by providing your doctors with documentation, such as letters detailing your experience, that they can incorporate in your medical file. Chapter 16 describes the value of submitting written notes to your doctor that succinctly summarize your current experience; such notes not only help in your treatment but can serve as evidence in your disability case. Also consider how you can represent your tracked data in a comprehensive, readable document that highlights your symptom severity, limitations, and attempts to work.

For an evaluator or judge reviewing your case, the most relevant medical records contain a detailed description of the limitations you experience on account of your diagnosis. It can be helpful, therefore, to come to appointments equipped with a list of your main symptoms and a description of how they may interfere with activities of daily living, including dressing, eating, bathing, housework, employment, and relationships. Make this a routine part of your visit with any healthcare professional, such as psychotherapists, physical therapists, occupational therapists, gynecologists, or any other specialists you see. Records can get lost or misplaced. Keep copies for your own records just in case they are needed.

Because doctors' records hold the most weight, it is crucial they clearly document the severity of your symptoms and impairments. Unfortunately, having a supportive physician does not guarantee the relevant information will be included in your file. If you have not been providing a note at each visit, consider composing a summary for your doctor of what a typical day is like for you. It is important that Social Security have a clear idea of your symptoms and difficulties, such as how pain affects your concentration and stamina. Typically, any document you provide your doctor becomes part of your medical file. It does not hurt to ask your doctor if, and in what way, the information you have provided has been incorporated into your medical chart.

Talk with your doctor and other healthcare professionals. Talking with your doctor about disability may feel uncomfortable, but having these conversations is essential for your case. If you are starting fresh with a new doctor, it may help to establish rapport before asking for assistance with a disability claim. Doctors may experience bias against new patients seeking to collect disability, especially if that is the first thing you talk about, but as your relationship develops, this bias will likely diminish. You contribute to your disability case with a new doctor by being a responsible patient. Be honest and up front about your limitations and difficulties as you work together on improvement. Refer to chapter 16 for how to compose a background letter for a first appointment with a new doctor. Make sure to include information on pertinent experience, as described above.

It is your right to view the contents of your medical charts or records. While at the doctor's office, ask to see your medical file, and look for clear documentation of your complaints, abilities, and limitations. It is helpful to have the doctor look over the chart with you so you do not misinterpret medical words, abbreviations, or jargon. If you believe important details are missing, talk with your physician about submitting a letter to Social Security on your behalf. Physicians are busy professionals; be mindful of the time involved in any request you have. You might offer to help by drafting a letter or listing bullet points on your daily experiences. Most important is that your doctor include a description of your symptoms and abilities—the more detailed, the better. The declaration that you are "disabled" carries little weight without details that would satisfy the legal definition. Doctors may not know it is not up to them to judge your disability status. Their role is to provide sufficient data to assist a medical evaluator and a judge in reaching a fitting conclusion.

Assistance and support. Even on your best days, applying for disability can be challenging. It consists of deciphering rules and procedures, filling out forms that can be time consuming and emotionally as well as physically draining. Given that you feel too awful to work, why go it alone? If you are lucky enough to have a close acquaintance or family member who is organized and available to shepherd you through the process, solicit that person's help. If you are concerned that you are taking advantage of a friendship, compensate them with a kind act when you are able. Support groups may offer helpful tips and opportunities to vent your frustrations. They may also put you in touch with individuals who have successfully navigated the process. Some national organizations, such as the Fibromyalgia Network, provide tool kits that include helpful advice about applying for disability insurance, including information for your physician. Working with a disability attorney from the beginning, or from any point in the process, can provide support, reassurance, and valuable feedback and guidance.

The Big Picture

Receiving disability compensation does not mean you will not be able to return to work at some point or in some other capacity. You may collect disability compensation while retraining or figuring out how to work on a part-time or trial basis. Because you can earn up to a certain monthly income without reversing your disability status, you may end up finding part-time work that is satisfying and can supplement your disability check. Taking a hiatus from work can free you to focus on improvement and discovering more creative and flexible work arrangements. Take one small step at a time and see how it feels.

Chapter 23

Approaching Social Relationships

I magine a group of porcupines huddling together for warmth on a cold winter day; as their quills poke one another, the porcupines disperse, only to find themselves cold once again. After alternating between too much proximity and too much distance, the animals eventually discover they fare best by remaining at a little distance from each other.[1] As the German philosopher Arthur Schopenhauer represented with this parable about porcupines, all relationships require back-and-forth movement as we seek our comfort zones. *Everybody* has preferences, sensitivities, flaws, and quirks; throwing chronic pain into this mix makes relationships even more complex. At times, you may find yourself trying to negotiate interactions while feeling pained, exhausted, or misunderstood.

Sometimes, you may prefer to be alone at home, where you can prioritize your comfort, tend to your symptoms, set your pace, and control your environment. Isolation can seem appealing because it frees people from having to explain, compromise, or make special requests. But, as with the porcupines out in the cold, it has major drawbacks. The challenge, instead, is to devise effective strategies so you can engage in interactions with minimal pain.

Chronic pain may affect your current and potential relationships in any number of ways. You may struggle with how to engage socially despite pain. You may suffer from insecurities or fears about your ability to be a good partner or friend. You may engage in unhelpful comparisons, which can upend relationships. In romantic relationships, developing pain early presents different challenges than after many years together, and these challenges differ from the ones you face if you are single and searching for intimacy. With people you knew before developing pain, you face the task of maintaining the relationships despite changes. With new relationships, you face questions of disclosure. Your focus will also continually change as your relationships grow and develop. The more you understand about your own needs, the better able you will be to engage in an effective relationship.

"Understanding": Separate Myth from Reality

It is a common lament that "nobody understands what I'm going through." For people with chronic pain, understanding can mean a lot. To be understood is to be validated.

During a casual conversation, a friend of mine mentioned how she had explained my health condition to an acquaintance: "You know when you work yourself really hard so that you feel totally exhausted and ache from top to bottom so bad that you cannot even get up? Well, that's how Debbie feels. Only it does not go away." I was floored. Tears filled my eyes as I realized that my friend *really* understood my daily reality. If she were an anthropologist, she would have successfully achieved a deep understanding of the "native's experience."

Yet it is unfair to expect others, even those closest to you, to comprehend the whole of your experience. This goes against the popular myth "If you loved me, you'd understand." Even with love, understanding is not automatic. Instead, it requires deliberate and clear communication and, to some extent, a common experience upon which to draw.

The invisible and fluctuating nature of chronic pain makes this even more difficult. Understanding often comes from what can be observed, but how you look and how you feel may have little in common. Moreover, people with chronic pain often engage in activities despite their pain, making their experience harder to decipher. Consider your own difficulty gauging your own well-being from one minute to the next. Imagine the difficulty facing outsiders. The fact that everyone experiences pains also invites people to make comparisons that may or may not be relevant.

Understanding is a loaded term. Consider the meaning you may attach to "being understood." It may have emotional components, such as receiving acceptance or recognition for your struggles or permission for your responses. You may expect understanding to free you from being second-guessed or misjudged. With understanding, you could decline invitations or requests, for example, without being challenged or criticized. Or you may think understanding would provide practical help, such as freeing you from having to explain or ask for help because others would be more apt to offer a hand or give you a break.

But before you ponder how well others understand you, contemplate *the extent to which anyone really understands another person's experience.* Start with the people in your life. Would you say you fully comprehend what it is like for your neighbor in the middle of a messy divorce, college roommate suffering from an eating disorder, colleague battling substance abuse, friends who have been trying for years to conceive, acquaintances grieving the death of a child, or coworker caring for a spouse with Alzheimer's? To what extent do you understand what they are going through or need?

It may be generally unrealistic to believe we can walk in another's shoes. Social scientists debate whether an "outsider" or "observer" can comprehend the experience of a "native," despite the depth of their observations. Experiencing similar circumstances or losses can heighten your ability to comprehend others' experiences. But even then, your experiences and reactions may differ. We each bring with us a unique history and vantage point.

The good news is you do not need an intimate understanding to provide sympathy, validation, or assistance. Thank goodness people can learn to be supportive of those in pain without enduring the same painful experiences. In fact, the goal of "understanding" may be off base. Instead, it may be more useful to think about the importance of a road map or set of scripts to guide responses. Consider those times you may have felt unsure of what to say or do in the face of another's grief. Wouldn't it have been helpful to have had a set of guidelines or desired responses? This is precisely the kind of information you can provide to those who care about you.

Ask for what you want and need! This significantly reframes the issue. Rather than seeking or hoping for "understanding," focus on ways to express to others what you seek from them. Most people respond well to clear requests, particularly when made with warmth and gratitude. Consider these examples:

> "I'm having trouble with _____ today. It would be helpful to me if you could _____."

> "My back is killing me and I would benefit from some downtime. Would you be able to _____ for me?"

"I'm having a 'poor me' moment. I know I'd feel better if you'd
_____."

This framework places the burden on your shoulders. To receive your desired response, you need to understand your own needs and be able and willing to make a clear request. It would be unfair to expect others to anticipate wants or needs that are unclear to you. The more you learn from your tracking experiments, the better equipped you will be to ask for what you need. Positive reinforcement from your successes also makes it less difficult to ask the next time.

In addition to self-knowledge, making requests requires the acceptance of your current situation and the willingness to advocate for yourself. Let's say, for example, that you were invited by friends to a restaurant or a party and that you realize having a comfortable place would greatly improve your experience. You could choose to interact as "everyone else." Or you could request a particular restaurant that you know has comfortable chairs, or you could ask whether there will be a quiet room at the party should you desire a meditation break. It's your call what to ask for and how much to divulge. When you make requests, others do not need to "understand" everything about your experience. You can choose what you convey to others. In this way, making requests holds certain advantages over seeking understanding.

Understanding, in contrast, can be double edged. It is common for people with chronic pain to fantasize at some point about what it would be like if others felt their pain, even for an hour, so they would really "get it." But be careful what you wish for. Understanding can result in positive or nonjudgmental responses, but it is unrealistic to expect this to be the rule. People could react in any number of ways if they *really* knew your situation, such as with pity, discomfort, or anxiety. Understanding can also elicit biases. Social invitations might dwindle as "understanding" friends try to protect you from exertion. Sympathetic friends may also prefer to limit time with you because they would feel sad knowing that you are struggling while in their company. Understanding coworkers and employers may feel uncomfortable working with you. Consider your own personal history—at any time, have you responded awkwardly to knowledge about someone else's difficulties?

Keep in mind, too, that requests for understanding or for having your needs met both focus on *your* situation. The people in your life also have their own needs, desires, and reactions. As you focus on your important needs, don't lose sight of theirs. It helps to check if the other person is in a position to offer what you seek. When appropriate, ask about the effects of your request on others. And be mindful to reserve sufficient energy to be attentive and supportive of those in your life.

Limit Illness Talk

Nobody wants to listen to grievances all the time, yet limiting illness talk can be difficult, especially when pain is intense. Consider other avenues to vent, distract yourself, or otherwise let go of suffering. As you gain control over your experience, your need for pain-related talk will decrease. As needed, try the following strategies to limit illness talk without bottling it up or becoming resentful or withdrawn.

Focus elsewhere. Some pain sufferers will lament, "But when I feel horrible, what am I supposed to do—ignore it?" To some extent, yes! Just because pain sometimes screams for attention does not mean you have to give in to it. First, make use of your best strategies to increase your comfort. Then, practice focusing your attention elsewhere and observe the result. Successfully engaging your mind decreases your perception of pain. Plus, talking about pain is tiresome. You risk not only turning away others but boring yourself.

Seek connection. Experiment with deliberate focus on others—engage your senses and observe, listen, and experience what they are sharing. Interactions can take on a more satisfying quality, further increasing intimacy. By their nature, relationships are based on reciprocity and mutual caring. Make a point of asking people close to you how *they* are doing, and *listen*. Remember, your behavior establishes norms. When you ask about others, you let them know that your pain has not robbed you of your compassion or your ability to be good company. Deeper connections will likely improve how you feel. Test it and see.

Identify safe outlets for venting. It is a legitimate need to express your struggles. Consider talking with a psychotherapist, counselor, or other professional or joining a support group. Or consider channeling your frustration into a creative pursuit, such as expressing yourself through art, music, journaling, or prose.

Make a venting list. Compile a list of people with "friendly ears," those you can talk to frankly and vent with when necessary. Leave off anyone who would not appreciate being on this list, would be too affected by your travails, or may be invalidating or offer unsolicited advice. Always check whether someone is up for venting. If not, move down your list. Inform others when you would like to have a hearty unloading session so they can prepare themselves. Be mindful that venting shifts some of your burden to the recipient. While your need to unload may be great, respect others' boundaries. Even those who may welcome an occasional vent session will burn out if you forget your manners. Be mindful that the worse you feel, the greater the risk of becoming self-absorbed. Always check in to see how the other person is doing and assess their cues.

Set guidelines for venting. Some illness-related talk may be necessary. Consider strategies that allow you to broach topics with the assurance that they will not spill over into all your time together. With a partner, for example, you might create rules about off-limits contexts, such as mealtimes, in the bedroom, or before heading out for the evening. You can also designate specific times of day that are best for pain-related discussion. It also helps to be clear about the type of response you seek: do you desire assistance solving a particular problem or just a sympathetic ear? People are less likely to feel overwhelmed with problems when they feel prepared. Clarity increases the odds that both parties will receive the response they crave.

Allow others to vent too! Be willing to reciprocate. Your valued friends may also need a caring person to unload on when they are frustrated. Be willing to listen and commiserate. Those closest to you are likely to experience grief over what your pain condition means for them. Strive to be present to hear about any difficulties they may be having and provide ample reassurance that their problems matter. When feasible, create a way to grieve *together*, without comparison. Explore judgmental thoughts that may impair your ability to listen, such as seeing others as insufficiently grateful for their health or judging others' problems as relatively trivial. Judgmental thoughts become problematic when they hinder your ability to support other people. Seek ways to boost your empathy, such as reminding yourself that everything is relative, including your own pain. Be mindful of the potential ramifications of judgments. When others feel judged or invalidated, they will share less. When you are unable to listen, request a rain check until you are more comfortable.

Balance venting with positive. Research shows that people tend to flourish when they express a greater ratio of positive to negative emotions (see chapter 12). Be sure to get your good venting in. Then, strive for a balance of positive reports. When people inquire how you are doing, include signs of improvement, however small, or other accomplishments. For each complaint, share as many or more positive observations of any kind.

Seek out fun alternatives. You may gain more from an evening of indulging in silly games with friends or watching a movie than from a venting session. Whenever you engage in enjoyable distractions, you improve how you feel. Test this by deliberately engaging in activities that buoy your spirits.

Seek topics of interest to share. Don't let the pain cut you off from the outside world. Make a project of jotting down tidbits you come across from the radio, Internet, newspapers, TV, books, friends, or work. By searching for and sharing items you find interesting, you become more interesting as well. Being ready with a provocative or amusing story equips you for conversations outside of your pain experience, regardless of how you feel. This practice also reminds you that you continue to be a multifaceted person who lives in a larger world. Pain is only one dimension of your experience—even if, at times, you lose sight of this.

Problem Solve Together

Engaging in problem solving with people who care about you offers a chance to connect in a positive pursuit, which can be satisfying for everyone involved. Consider the strengths of the people in your life. Those with fix-it approaches may be grateful for an opportunity to brainstorm about innovations for annoying problems. For me, assistance over the years with creative engineering from family and friends has resulted in many innovations, from a simple contraption for hands-free hair drying to an enormous project involving tons of gravel, sand, and bricks, which eliminated my need to climb steps to leave my house. I have also benefited from others' insights into ways to increase my comfort while socializing, traveling, and parenting. This sort of creativity is mutually beneficial because it allows loved ones to be engaged and effective in finding ways to improve your life.

Instead of lamenting how difficult certain things can be, devote thought to exactly what makes them difficult. Complete the following sentence: "It would be a lot easier if _____." Then, consider what can be done. Focusing on specific factors, rather than potentially overwhelming emotions, allows for achievable remedies. Solutions can be simple, such as equipping your car with seat warmers or creating private signals to use in social situations to communicate when you are ready to leave.

You may also welcome assistance in devising your tracking system or interpreting its data. While such involvement can be a gift, be aware of potential pitfalls. The more involved others are with your data, the more watchful they may be—noting, for example, when you deviate from your most salubrious schedule. While it can be helpful to have someone in the role of watchdog, it can also become intrusive or create relationship strain. Be sure to discuss the terms of your collaboration and how to keep goals realistic. Keep a healthy supply of fun on hand to prevent your relationship from becoming illness oriented.

It may also be helpful to visualize your pain condition as something separate from you and the relationship. This can free you and your partner to brainstorm in a collaborative enterprise, without blame, shame, or guilt, about ways to tackle problems created by "the illness."

Socializing with Others

Social engagements are supposed to be fun. But with chronic pain, they can feel exhausting and not worth the effort. Yet this is not inevitable. You can increase your enjoyment by prioritizing and planning. It may sound counterintuitive to approach fun in a calculated way; however, knowledgeable planning can actually enhance spontaneity. Consider the well-planned vacation. It often takes research, reservations, and even assistance from professionals to create an ideal vacation. Then, once there, you can kick back, enjoy, and be spontaneous, rather than waste time and energy searching for creature comforts. Apply the principle of the well-planned vacation to a well-planned social life. For people with chronic pain, planning for routine socializing may allow for relaxation and greater pleasure.

Step 1: Prioritize. Chronic pain can operate as a relationship test. Assess which relationships are worth a "pain investment" and which are not. Let your pain help you weed out draining relationships and focus on satisfying ones. Whenever possible, reserve your time and energy for activities and people you adore. Decide which engagements you want to attend, and, when possible, politely decline the rest. People cancel for all sorts of reasons. A polite,

"Thanks for the invitation. I am not up for it," typically suffices. For social engagements that you feel obliged to attend, weigh the consequences of your decision. Keep in mind that just because you *can* participate despite discomfort does not mean that you always must. For the obligations you must honor, limit the visit. As my grandfather, Jacob, always said, "Never stay too long. It keeps people wanting more." With him, they always did.

Step 2: Plan. Be a good scout and come prepared. For activities you choose, consider what would increase your comfort, and arrange for those conditions. It can help to keep a handy checklist of comfort tools or a packed bag ready to grab on your way out. If you plan to meet at an unfamiliar venue, phone ahead to inquire about any conditions that would help you prepare. Consider other relevant information. If you are sharing a ride, check whether or not the driver would mind leaving early. Or ask a party host if there's a place where you would be able to lie down for a while. Asking in advance reduces the vulnerability you may feel when making requests in your moment of need. Backup plans can also assuage fears about participating. Remember, friends will prefer that you are comfortable, particularly if your request poses little inconvenience and you ask in an appreciative manner. So, speak up. If you will benefit from meeting inside rather than outside, let your friends know.

Difficulties can arise when you desire more substantial modifications, particularly when others have competing preferences. Avoid requests that appear too aggressive or demanding. Requesting a sturdier chair may not be difficult, but asking a party of twenty to change plans is likely to be unreasonable. In these situations, come prepared and use creativity. Excuse yourself as often as needed to meditate, stretch, run hot water over your hands—whatever helps.

Common Roadblocks to Asking for Help

Unfortunately, requesting assistance is not always simple. It depends not only on your relationship and situation but also on the meaning you might associate with making requests. I used to find that the worse I felt (and, thus, the more I needed help), the less able I was to ask. Examine your comfort level with accepting help. Then, check the following list for what may account for your hesitation:

You fear that accepting help means you are "weak." People are typically much harder on themselves than they would be on others. If you are judging yourself as "weak" or "vulnerable" for needing help, try to imagine the shoe on the other foot. More than likely, you would provide assistance for someone in the same situation, willingly and without judgment. Asking for help can be a sign of strength—particularly when the request feels more difficult than enduring additional pain. Experiment by making small requests. See how it feels. You can also ask people about their experience of your request. This helps you decide whether it feels worth it. (Keep in mind that some people want to help you but don't know how, so your request will be met with relief and help them feel useful.)

You have difficulty identifying your needs. It is nearly impossible to request help when you don't know what you want. Feeling needy but unable to identify what you need can foster a feeling of helplessness. You owe it to yourself and others to figure out what would increase your comfort and well-being. Specific requests are easier to make—and to hear—than vague cries. Specific, doable things—like carrying your chair or massaging your neck—give people specific ways to contribute to your comfort. Figuring out what you need creates a more satisfying experience for everyone.

You prefer to bite the bullet. There may be times when you prefer to do something for yourself rather than ask for assistance, even when it is challenging for you. This is your choice. You may be enjoying the sense of pride or accomplishment that can come from toughing it out or from masking your difficulties in certain situations. There's no problem deciding in a clearheaded fashion to engage in a pain-escalating behavior. Keep in mind, however, that you may not be the only one affected by your decisions (as you may be out of commission as a result later).

You feel shameful for asking. Self-judgments can inhibit requesting help. You may feel uncomfortable when you seek help for things you think you should be able to do. Recognize this for the emotional reasoning it is, not a realistic assessment of the situation. Explore the extent to which your worries come from feelings about yourself rather than anticipated responses from others. It may help to think through a specific example, including how you might word the request and what you expect might happen. Remember, you can reveal just enough information to allow others to understand your request. For example, you might tell a grocery store clerk that you have back trouble and would appreciate a hand with your bags.

You don't know how to ask. When asking for help feels difficult, plan the request. Landing on the right wording can be liberating. Strive to generate a request in language that is polite, direct, and specific; shows your appreciation; and includes a brief account of your reasons for asking.

You fear rejection. You may worry that once you rally the courage to ask, you may be turned down. This is a risk. We cannot expect others to comply with every request. It helps to keep requests reasonable, have a sense of the person you are asking, and have an alternate plan should you be turned down. If you find the possibility of being turned down prohibitive, examine your beliefs.

You believe you shouldn't have to ask. Occasionally, people may succeed in figuring out what you need or want before you ask. As nice as it may be to have someone anticipate your needs, expecting such mind-reading capabilities is unreasonable. Do your part and communicate directly.

Assistance threatens your independence. Asking for help relinquishes some of your control. Weigh the costs of sacrificing some control against the benefits of sparing yourself physical pain. When assistance is provided, accept it *just as it is provided.* The next time you request help, you may decide to specify with greater detail what you want. However, criticizing the way others assist you is a surefire way to prevent further assistance. As you become more competent in delegating to others, your feelings of independence may increase. Keep in mind, too, that nobody is wholly independent. We *all* depend on others.

You feel embarrassment for being different. In some circumstances, you may decide passing for "normal" feels worth a certain amount of suffering. This depends on many factors, such as your plans for the day and your estimation of the repercussions of passing. You may prefer the pain that follows standing in line to the embarrassment of requesting permission to move an available chair to the line.

You worry you ask for help too often. It makes sense to fear that too-frequent requests will wear out your welcome or overburden others. But, rather than worrying about it, ask! It's a good practice to check in routinely with others to see whether your requests extend beyond their comfort zone.

You worry your request will put others out. It can be difficult to request special accommodations that involve sacrifice from others. Imagine, for example, that you arrive at a meeting and all the good chairs are taken. Do you sit in a chair that ensures a painful flare-up or ask someone to trade chairs? Like the bad chair, this decision can be hard! It may well be that people in the better chairs prefer to remain in them. However, unless they, too, have pain, they may not feel strongly about the chair, particularly if they know how much the trade would benefit you. Try a simple and direct approach without being demanding or encouraging guilt: "I have chronic pain, and these chairs are lousy for me. Any chance you'd swap chairs?" If someone relinquishes a chair, accept it with gratitude.

When contemplating a request of any kind, figure out the specifics of what you want and then express it in a way that is simple, direct, and appreciative. It helps to ask with a pleasant voice and expression. If your request is turned down, be a good sport. This is easier done when you have an alternate plan to safeguard your comfort. The more often you ask for help—and receive an affirmative response—the easier it becomes over time. Remember, even if others say no (and they have this right), you are no worse off for asking.

Dating and Disclosure

Dating can be a tricky business. During the "getting to know each other" phase, people try to present themselves in the best light possible. Admittedly, it is not very sexy to advertise that you suffer from pain or physical limits. It helps that chronic pain is not a communicable disease! No matter how intimate you become, nobody will catch your symptoms. Therefore, you will not harm anyone or put them at risk if you decide to withhold information until you are comfortable sharing. This situation is not unique to pain—that someone suffers from diabetes, depression, constipation, or a thyroid condition is not typically the material of scintillating conversations. The aim is to wait long enough so as not to overwhelm the other person before you each have a sense of the other, but not so long that it feels dishonest.

Be proactive in planning social opportunities you would find comfortable. To some, dating may conjure up raucous parties or a club scene. However, many people, even young ones, would love an excuse to exit loud, smoky bars or nightclubs and spend a quiet, more intimate evening. Be resourceful in offering alternatives you would find more comfortable. Know the local theaters and restaurants. Survey the weekly papers for activities you can participate in, such as a short show at the planetarium. You can also engage in activities you find painful, but otherwise fun, by limiting the time you spend, using your medications proactively, or planning a follow-up activity to restore your comfort, such as visiting your favorite coffeehouse with oversized chairs.

When your health becomes relevant as the relationship develops, provide context-specific information. This does not mean dropping a medical textbook into your date's lap. But you might reassure your date if your reluctance to hold hands is due to hand pain rather than your sentiments. Then, offer an alternative, such as linked arms or a hug or kiss, if appropriate. Or, if you are invited for a hike, you might share that you prefer to walk briskly, may require rest breaks, or whatever the case may be.

For someone who is getting to know you, trading noisy bars for a comfortable space to relax and talk may sound more romantic than off-putting. However, in the sometimes-brutal dating world, it can be "one strike, you're out." Whatever reaction you receive provides data about that person and some feedback on your approach. Some people will find it admirable that you live with pain—a testament to your strength—while others may feel intimidated or overwhelmed. The response you receive will depend on the other person's age, experience, and maturity level, as well as how you portray your situation. As painful as rejection can be, it is important to know if someone is mature enough to contend with your reality.

The more at peace and accepting you are of yourself, the more attractive you become to others. If you are conflicted about your identity or what you have to offer, this will come through. How you present your condition is significant. Keep in mind that everyone has quirks. It may not be immediately relevant whether you prefer something because of pain or some other reason. Strive to convey your self-care measures in a positive light. You can explain, for example, that you feel best when you are well rested. The issue of living with pain becomes more relevant if and when the relationship becomes more serious. But then, if you find you are compatible and interested in each other, your pain condition becomes one of your many attributes.

Do not shortchange yourself! Nobody's perfect. We all come with unique attributes that make us who we are. Through no fault of your own, you hurt. This may mean you may not be able to be as spontaneous as you would like at all times—or, at least, not without paying for it later. When you meet someone you would like to know better, enhance your interactions by limiting complaints and seeking out amusement and distraction. We all take a risk when we reach out to others. You, like the rest of the dating world, will suffer a certain amount of rejection, which may or may not have to do with your health condition.

How to Respond to Questions about Your Health

People often ask questions without expecting a response, such as in the pro forma, "How are you?" In that case, a detailed medical account would violate social norms. Other times, people may inquire with interest, often hoping for reassuring news. When I encounter old friends who ask about my pain (with that hopeful glint in their eye), I might respond with a smile, "I'm happy." Unless you have a specific reason for sharing details, long explanations are seldom warranted. Provide a quick response that feels comfortable to you, and then move on. It is remarkably easy to deflect attention from yourself. You might say, "I still hurt, but I'm managing," or "I'm doing well enough, but that's boring," and then introduce a new subject: "I read the funniest thing yesterday . . ." or "How is that adorable son (or boyfriend) of yours?" or whatever topic is likely of mutual interest.

Most often, people ask about unexpected reactions or behaviors out of mild curiosity and are not looking for elaborate reasons. For example, when you are confronted with a hand to shake, a quick account such as, "I hurt my hand," is unlikely to set interactions off-kilter. Or you may skip the explanation altogether with a simple, "Oh, I'm sorry, I can't shake hands today. . . . It's *very* nice to meet you." Use nonverbal gestures to your advantage—such as an apologetic shrug toward your hand, paired with a welcoming smile. Devise your own ways to keep social interactions smooth.

When you divulge information, other questions may follow. People may ask:

- How did your condition develop? Is it genetic?
- Is it going to go away?
- Do you hurt right now? Do you hurt all the time?
- What does it feel like?
- Is it degenerative?
- Are you going to die from it?

It is human nature to be curious. It helps to be equipped with brief, honest, and reassuring answers. Your reaction helps others to gauge theirs. They want to know how sorry to feel for you, whether they can feel relieved that you may recover or improve, and what sort of assistance you may need. Your answers provide them with a way to categorize your experience, such as, "OK, you are not dying, but it sounds pretty unpleasant." It may suffice to say something vague like, "I have good and bad days." You can elaborate further depending on your relationship, your desire to assume the role of educator, and your assessment of the other person's genuine interest. Turn to humor to keep it light.

Chapter 24

Improving Committed Relationships

Contending with chronic health problems while in a committed relationship raises difficult concerns and questions. You may worry about:

- the effect of your problems and needs on your partner;
- letting your partner down;
- whether your partner loves you as you now are;
- whether you still have enough in common;
- your ability to be a valuable, contributing partner;
- your partner's ability to handle the difficulties; or
- changes in your sexual relationship.

These are legitimate worries. It is noteworthy that traditional wedding vows include phrases such as "for better, for worse" and "in sickness and in health." We enter committed, intimate relationships for many reasons. People may be able to list the qualities in their partner that attracted them. But what happens when things change?

Part of the task couples face when one member develops a chronic difficulty is to create a new couple narrative. Love does not depend on how well someone sleeps or whether they can carry heavy objects. Consider Christopher Reeve, who embodied his screen character Superman in the way he adapted to paralysis after a tragic horse-riding accident. In one moment, his circumstances changed from substantial privilege to disability. His memoir, *Still Me*, captured his two selves with its double entendre—the continuation of his former self along with his changed self, the "still" one. Mr. Reeve deserves much credit for the adaptation that enabled him to continue in his roles as an active father and husband, actor, and director, as well as new roles as author, advocate, and spokesperson for people with spinal cord injuries. His family members likewise deserve credit for finding ways to continue to incorporate the "still Reeve" into their lives, exemplifying the dynamic nature of relationships. It's important not to downplay their struggles, which must have been considerable. However, the Reeves found ways to shift in their roles. No doubt, their financial resources aided with logistics, but the fortitude and commitment came from within.

Effective partnerships are based on trust. It helps tremendously when you feel confident that you have each other's best interests at heart. If not, conflict will be inevitable (and counseling may be crucial). However, if you trust your partner's intentions, the question becomes how best to move forward together. During crises, relationships require extra sensitivity and reassurance. Find ways to reassure yourself and your partner that your symptoms will not divide you. Knowing that nobody plans to jump ship helps you both muddle through uncharted waters. Pain is an inevitable part of life. With adjustments, life can and will go on with all its joys and messiness.

Create Space for Your Partner's Response

It is often difficult for well partners to express difficulties they may be experiencing. There are many reasons for this. Well partners may struggle with the following:

- Feeling guilt or shame about their own thoughts: "I don't have pain— what do I have to gripe about?"
- Feeling apprehensive about further burdening an ill partner: "It doesn't feel fair to complain about how this affects me."
- Struggling with issues of blame: "If I complain about how this affects me, it sounds like I'm blaming you. Even though I know your illness is not your fault, I still get angry about it. And then I would also feel selfish."
- Feeling their ill partner is unable or unwilling to provide support: "You are just going through too much to be there for me."

Be deliberate about opening communication lines for your partner to talk about difficulties he or she may be experiencing. Let your partner know you care and are (still) available. Reassure him or her that you are not too fragile to offer assistance and comfort. When you notice your own inner turmoil interfering with your ability to listen, let your partner know, rather than being inattentive or responding unsupportively. When you increase your own comfort and satisfaction, it is easier to be present for others. But, however you feel, do your best to provide space and support for your partner as you reshape your lives together. Let your partner know you understand this is difficult for him or her also. As appropriate, encourage your partner to talk with compassionate friends or family members or a therapist, counselor, or support group.

Renegotiate Roles

Chronic illness often throws a wrench into how people see themselves, and this extends to relationships. Before your pain began, you may have been "Self-Sufficient Man," who supported his family financially and never required help with physical tasks, no matter how arduous, or "Multitasking Supermom," who held two jobs, cultivated the family's social life, and shunned prepared foods. When chronic pain upends your sense of self in a relationship, adaptation is more challenging. Change, however, is an inevitable part of relationships. Healthy relationships adapt with expected as well as unpredicted life changes.

Chronic pain presents a life transition, which will take place alongside other common transitions, such as changes in employment or residence, parenthood (with its many phases), or the decline or death of a parent. Adaptation involves an intricate dance. It helps to acknowledge the challenges you experience in trying to maintain prior roles or grieving over losses you experience as a couple or family. Implicit gender roles may become explicit or be called into question. For men in pain, becoming more reliant on women in their lives for physical tasks or financial support may be challenging. Similarly, women whose identity involves nurturing may struggle in relinquishing tasks they had found affirming. Yet people's roles are not synonymous with the tasks they perform. You can continue to be the dependable or strong or nurturing member of the family by adapting the way you enact your role. Flexible-mindedness helps bridge prior roles with emergent ones.

When illness enters committed relationships, couples are challenged to discover and use coping strategies that allow them to adapt. Locate your sources of strength and resilience as a couple (or family) to carry you through, such as your sense of humor, your ability to persevere, your passion, the depth of your history and bond, your mutual respect, and the support you receive from others in your life. Reflect on what has helped you as a couple in the past. In the event that illness has made some of these resources less available, use your creativity to locate new ones. Experiment together.

Role Snafus: How to Navigate Roadblocks to a Balanced Partnership

What you or your partner may feel—fear, despair, worry, hope, apprehension, or helplessness—will seep into the relationship whether or not you directly express these sentiments. As each of you confronts difficulties, old coping patterns may become more deeply entrenched, and new roles can emerge. Be on the lookout for signs your relationship is in need of attention:

Denial. A certain amount of denial is to be expected and can work as a protective mechanism. People sometimes cope by not accepting the reality of the situation. This reaction typically comes from fear or discomfort; it is hard to bear the fact that someone you love is in pain. It can also be difficult to believe things you cannot see or understand. Denial is often considered an early phase in the grieving process (see chapter 26). When it persists, however, denial can undermine trust. If your partner seems to be discounting your reality, decide what it is most important that he or she accept, and then choose your approach. Would your partner respond best to written material, an explanation delivered with humor and reassurance, or a meeting with a trusted professional? When you share information, be mindful of your own reaction. Do not exaggerate the severity of your struggles in order to get your partner's attention or let another's disbelief create self-doubt. By keeping a balanced perspective and presentation, you increase the likelihood that your partner will come around.

Caregiving. Well-intentioned partners sometimes embrace the role of caregiver, particularly when your suffering is great. While assisting each other is part of the give-and-take of any relationship, assuming a continual caregiving role can threaten the balance of the relationship, foster unhealthful dependency, and lead to resentment. Be on the lookout for signs your partner is overly cautious or protective or treats you as if you are incapable of doing anything for yourself. This can result from a failure to clarify what you *can* do for yourself. When your pain feels overwhelming, you might reinforce caregiver behaviors. But no matter how severe the disability, everyone has things they can do for themselves. Talk openly about trends that may be interfering with you maintaining an equal partnership, one in which you both provide and receive support in whatever forms are feasible.

Embitterment. Over time, partners can feel bitter, put-upon, or neglected. They may resent having to do more than their fair share of work or feel their experiences are treated as relatively unimportant. Resentment can destroy relationships. If you suspect your partner feels aggrieved, take action. Inquire about your partner's experience, and validate concerns that he or she may raise. Help problem solve as appropriate, and encourage honest discussion by staying present. Seek ways to help your partner reduce his or her workload burdens and feel valued. It is often less important that tasks are divided fifty-fifty than that partners feel adequately recognized and appreciated.

Detachment. Some partners may feel so troubled or overwhelmed that they retreat or try to avoid you altogether. People who retreat are likely to have a history of using that reaction as a coping mechanism. If your partner seems detached, reflect on what may have helped in the past to draw your partner back and reengage with you. Most people respond well to tenderness, joyfulness, and reassurance in words and behaviors. (You will also benefit from exhibiting these.) Consider sharing with your partner the very things you would like to hear, and know on some level to be true, about your ability to improve, adapt, and grow as a couple.

Identify Your Worst Problems and Work Together to Improve Them

Acknowledging problems can feel threatening. People living with pain may feel too overwhelmed to face additional difficulty, and partners may be averse to raising troubling topics. However, unspoken problems can become the elephant in the room. In other words, the problems we try hardest to avoid have a way of growing in size. Both members of the couple may be masking their worries or grief out of compassion for the other. However, acknowledging the difficulties that chronic pain brings to the relationship enables couples to support each other and work as a team to confront challenges. The following are common "elephants." Look for any that are relevant to you or your relationship.

Inward focus. At times, pain commands attention and consumes all other thoughts. When people are wrapped up in their own misery, there's room for little else. Be aware of the extent to which your thinking or interactions focus on pain. No matter how rotten you may feel, a continual preoccupation with yourself or your suffering is destructive. Intentionally cultivate a more outward focus. This improves not only your relationship but also how you feel, which then decreases your desire to focus inward. There will be times when pain interferes with your ability to engage. When this happens, say so, and reconnect after a hiatus to improve how you feel.

Alienation. Pain feels lonely, and ironically, when people are in most need of support and companionship, they may push others away. Do not let yourself fall into a lonely existence. Maintaining social connections is also important as a couple. Seek out relationships and social situations that keep you connected with people you enjoy. It is important for partners to support each other, but relying too much on one person can create an unfair burden. Cultivate and look to your wider social network to connect with others.

Distress. Chronic pain creates physical, emotional, and, often, financial distress. The paradox is that the greater the distress, the fewer resources we have to contend with it. Start by acknowledging to each other the stress of chronic pain, and then experiment with ways to reduce it, such as by increasing calm, tender moments and by sharing activities you enjoy together. Approaches that help you reduce pain—such as exercise, meditation, or massage—can provide restoration as a couple. You may also decide to take part in individual, couples, family, or group therapy.

Limitations. Physical limitations facing one individual also affect the couple. Prioritize activities as a couple. Decide which are most meaningful, and then consider ways to take part in them. Try to brainstorm situation-specific solutions. This may involve role renegotiation, shifting expectations, and compromises when straightforward solutions are elusive. It can be especially frustrating when a couple's identity or lifestyle involved certain activities. If you were a "skiing couple," for example, winter vacation may mean that while one partner skis, the other will be relaxing in the lodge or nearby spa. Be open, at the same time, to new pursuits you can share.

Guilt feelings. Chronic pain elicits many emotions, such as sadness, frustration, and anger. Experiences of guilt and shame, however, tend to come more from what people may be saying to themselves about their reactions or from judgmental self-talk about what they should be able to do. For example, people with chronic pain may experience shame over not being a "good partner" or a "good parent." Partners may feel guilty over their bouts of anger, grief, or compassion fatigue. Guilt and shame are unjustified and destructive when they arise about circumstances beyond one's control. When you experience feelings of unjustified guilt or shame, investigate these. Check your assumptions, and help liberate each other from unwarranted emotional suffering.

Lack of curiosity. Do not force a library of information on a partner who may already feel overwhelmed. If you feel dejected that your partner is not more inquisitive about your health difficulties or experience, investigate your reasons. While some people cope best by delving into literature and becoming medical experts, others may prefer you share only what is absolutely necessary. Supply information only on a need-to-know basis. If you desire a more empathetic response, address this directly. Others' interest in your medical condition does not necessarily correlate with their interest in you as a person or their "belief" in your experience. Respond gently. You may learn their personal reasons for shielding themselves from the facts of your condition.

Communication problems. Addressing difficulties you face as a couple requires communication. However, talking about problems does not necessarily improve them. It depends on how the topics are raised, as well as both partners' receptivity and responses. Timing is also crucial—pain can interfere with concentration and increase emotional vulnerability. Take note of difficulties either of you might have regarding the raising or discussing of critical topics. Effective communication can ease the challenges of chronic illness.

What Makes Communication Effective?

According to internationally renowned relationship expert John Gottman, there's no one "best way" of communicating. Dr. Gottman, a psychologist who has studied the interactional patterns of more than eight thousand couples over three decades, has devised a method to predict whether or not couples will stay together.[1] The method is so reliable that Gottman and his colleagues (who include his wife of many years, Dr. Julie Gottman) can predict with a high level of accuracy whether a couple's marriage will endure or end by observing their interactional style as newlyweds. While a "therapeutic" style of talking, in which each member listens quietly and then validates the other, can foster closeness, they found that other styles can be just as effective.

The crucial features for couples are to remain actively engaged (not detached), enjoy each other, make use of humor (not sarcasm), and prevent negative talk from escalating into hostility and put-downs. Couples with volatile styles, who raise their voices and interrupt each other, can sustain satisfying relationships *if* they are able to "kiss and make up." All couples fare better when they can accept or resolve their differences, even when this follows from a raucous or dramatic episode. The most destructive patterns involve detachment or the harboring of hostility.[2]

Chronic distress adds challenges to good communication, such as increased negative feelings, uncertainty, and stress. To counteract these forces, experiment with the following strategies derived from Gottman's findings:

- *Use humor.* Strive to approach difficulties with humor, rather than a morose tone. If you think there's nothing funny about chronic pain, expand your thinking. Laugh as a couple whenever possible.
- *Stay open.* Feeling lousy makes you more vulnerable to closing off. Strive as a couple to respond to feelings of detachment as reminders to reach out rather than retreat.
- *Foster closeness.* Make it a priority to engage in things you enjoy as often as possible. Keep it simple: Make dates to watch a favorite TV show. Invite friends over for "game night." Turn up the music and dance, even for a few moments. Make love.
- *Air grievances before they build.* Humor can be a great tension diffuser. But when you are not quick with a healing joke, don't wait long before trying to resolve a problem. Timely sharing reduces the chance of harboring negativity.
- *Share constructively.* Do your best to raise issues in a constructive manner, and listen when your partner does the same. Strive to stay positive, limit criticism, and locate opportunities to offer praise. Expressions of contempt are highly destructive.
- *Keep away the negatives.* Avoid hurtful talk such as name-calling and portraying problems as character flaws. This is easiest when you nurture trust and see yourselves on the same side. When needed, take a time-out from a difficult discussion, rather than risk blurting out something

blaming or damning. After a meditative break, revisit the issue more constructively. Examine any feelings of hostility, which may be better directed at the illness and not your partner, who is weathering the storm with you, even if ungracefully at times.

- *Take responsibility.* No problem is one-sided. Find and acknowledge the role you are playing when problems arise. Avoid self-righteousness, speaking from a position of superiority, or blaming the other person.
- *Be present.* Try to stay attentive, even when it is difficult to do so. Retreating or shutting down exacerbates problems by creating emotional distance. Take a break when needed; then, return with your full attention.

Deliberate Listening Exercises

A common mistake in intimate relationships is to expect others to know what you are thinking. This mind-reading myth causes much suffering. As discussed earlier, expressing your needs clearly is much more effective than hoping for "understanding." Yet effective communication can be difficult, particularly with emotionally charged topics. You may worry about hurting others' feelings, putting them on the defensive or into retreat, or otherwise not receiving the response you seek.

Effective communication is not simple, and misunderstandings are common. Communication has three parts: (1) what you intend to convey, (2) how you actually express it, and (3) how others interpret what you say. At any one of these points, the message may be obscured. People often make assumptions about what was meant, rather than investigating the original intent. Misunderstandings not cleared up in a timely manner can be damaging.

Think about how you talk to the people closest to you. Conversations sometimes happen as people enter and exit rooms, rather than face to face. Requests sometimes come through verbal and nonverbal hints rather than directly. And with the omnipresence of technology, much communication takes place virtually, with "emoticons"—small typed face icons, such as ;) to represent a wink—standing in for nonverbal cues.

When understanding really matters, you may benefit from active listening, a therapeutic style of communication intended to ensure mutual understanding. If this approach is new for you, experiment with the exercise below, in which one person assumes the role of "talker" and the other of "listener." Stick to the ground rules.

Ground rules for the *talker*:

1. Look directly at the listener and state what is on your mind.
2. Avoid the words "always" and "never," as these exaggerations place blame and often elicit defensiveness.
3. When bringing up the other's behavior, start with "I" and include your feelings. For example, instead of saying, "*You* don't listen to me," try something like, "*I feel sad* when you . . . don't appear to listen." Using I-statements removes blame and accusation and focuses, instead, on your feelings and experience.

Ground rules for the *listener*:

1. Look at the talker.
2. Use nonverbal cues to show you are listening, such as maintaining eye contact; nodding your head; and making soft, affirming sounds.
3. Do not respond otherwise to what is being said. Your job is to listen carefully. Do not interrupt, ask questions, or argue. Do your best to stay calm and supportive. Focus on the talker's words, and avoid composing responses in your head. (You will have a turn to be the talker.)
4. When the talker is finished, give a brief summary of what you heard. This allows both people to find out what was communicated. You can begin with a phrase like, "What I heard you say is . . ."
5. The talker then has a chance to clarify as needed, until the listener has clearly understood the talker's precise intent. Then, feel free to switch roles.

This exercise deliberately slows down conversation to ensure understanding. Its artificial manner can feel strange, frustrating, or silly at first. You might observe how hard it can be to listen without jumping in. One or both of you may feel resistant to the exercise or require a reminder of the ground rules. But be patient. The benefit of clear communication may be worth initial discomfort. As you experiment with this strategy, note its effects.

Active listening is particularly helpful with sensitive topics. If you notice that you feel angry or sad about what you heard, you can make sure your interpretation was the intended one. As you become more comfortable with the exercise, you can transfer the skills into a more natural conversational style.

Sex and Intimacy

Self-help articles on sexuality and chronic illness are often akin to Victorian views of women's sexuality, as if sex is a duty to be tolerated. Even the most positive writings focus on ways to minimize the difficulties of sexual activity. While this approach makes sense—sex may seem beside the point when you're in pain—it downplays the *benefits* of intimacy and sexual activity for your well-being.

Benefits! Sexual connections not only strengthen relationships, they can reduce painful symptoms. Consider this from a physiological view: People experience a multitude of sensations as nerve synapses transmit information to the brain. At any moment, your brain will attend to some messages over others. Substantial research demonstrates the calming effect of touch, which also intensifies with emotional connection. Both touch and orgasms increase opioids (the body's natural painkillers) like endorphins and enkephalins,[3] decrease levels of cortisol (a hormone secreted with stress), and stimulate oxytocin (which evokes feelings of attachment, contentment, and calm).[4] It has also been suggested that the chemicals associated with orgasms reduce pain for a wide range of problems, including lower back pain, migraines, arthritis, and premenstrual pain.[5] Therefore, if you are lucky enough to have someone to share an enjoyable sex life with, by all means, indulge! Rather than letting pain keep your partner at arm's length, seek comfort in your partner's arms. Let your experimentation include the impact of intimacy. Explore the effects of sensual touch and intimacy on your well-being and the relationship.

Obstacles. Sometimes, however, you may need to take steps to prepare yourself to indulge in the salubrious effects of sensuality. Let's face it—pain can be a turn-off. When you're preoccupied with bodily pains, you may struggle to see your body as a source of pleasure. Or you may, before developing pain, have viewed sex as something carefree (rather than careful) and resent this change. Or you may worry that your illness detracts from your attractiveness—a feeling that may be compounded by the weight gain or loss or blows to your self-esteem that can accompany chronic pain. Or your relationship may have changed, and it may feel challenging to reintroduce sexuality. Obstacles can also come from your partner's experiences. Caretaking roles can feel incongruous with sexuality. Your partner may worry about your fragility or feel selfish "bothering" you or angry or frustrated over changes he or she does not understand. Moreover, medications can reduce libido and sexual function.

Tend to the relationship. Relationship problems can inhibit physical intimacy. Sometimes what we say to ourselves can interfere with intimacy. Notice any negative self-talk. If you are preoccupied with relationship problems, address them. Sometimes individual or couples counseling can be helpful. Increasing feelings of closeness reduces barriers to sexual intimacy.

Intimacy issues. Raising issues around sex and intimacy can feel uncomfortable. Consider ways to decrease the potential awkwardness. For example, choosing a neutral place and a time when you are relaxed, comfortable, and fully clothed may reduce the pressure. Consider active listening to ensure you understand each other's feelings. Focus on the positive, and avoid accusatory language. For example, you might express that it "feels wonderful when you hold me close," rather than lamenting that your partner no longer touches you. Give your partner space to reflect and respond, with assurance of your affection.

Comfort. Create an environment that feels conducive to intimacy. Use your tracking data to enhance your comfort by ensuring that you have sufficient rest, medication, exercise, restorative downtime, or other helpful measures. The better you feel, and feel about yourself, the easier it is to enjoy intimacy. Feeling comfortable and safe also increases your ability to be spontaneous and present. Enhance your comfort by using supportive pillows and the sexual positions that are most comfortable for you and by pacing yourselves. Talk with your partner about whatever will liberate you from worries about discomfort or otherwise prohibit your sexual expression and closeness. Unite in the quest to create a satisfying sex life.

Getting started. When you hurt or feel spent from the day, intercourse may sound like painful calisthenics. But, just as with exercise, getting started may be the most difficult part, but you will likely feel (much) better once engaged. It may help to concentrate on your positive feelings for your partner or visualize what would feel good. Focus your attention on this feeling or image (rather than your pain) to move closer to your partner. It may help to reinvent foreplay rituals. Consider ways to help you relax and feel more comfortable, such as music or massage. Be careful, however, not to let foreplay resemble a physical therapy session. Intimacy is about making and sharing pleasure and closeness. Consider what helps put you in the mood, and incorporate this into your routine.

Start slow. If you have not engaged in sexual activity for some time or are feeling apprehensive, address this with your partner. It may be useful to start slow, perhaps with an agreement to touch without immediately moving toward intercourse. The partner who desires a slower pace can provide signals to change the pace or direction as desired. It can also be helpful to agree what will or will not happen and when. This does not mean keeping to a rigid schedule: "Five minutes of kissing, one minute rubbing shoulder, thirty seconds earlobe nibbling…" As you each clear your mind of worries about disappointing or pressuring the other, you can focus specifically on how good it feels to be together. Take advantage of the release of serotonin and endorphins. Take turns exploring each other's bodies in a sensual, nonsexual way. By slowing things down, you can rediscover the sensuality of gentle touch and kissing. As the positive sensations increase and feel-good chemicals flood your system, your desire may intensify.

Focus on the journey, not the destination. You play a significant part in your pleasure by focusing on your immediate experience and being mindful of distracting thoughts or sensations (see chapter 10). Deliberately focus your attention on positive sensations—the smoothness of your partner's skin, the softness of your partner's hair, the pleasant smells and tastes, and the feeling of your emotional bond—the more you engage all your senses, the better. If you notice distracting thoughts, let them drift away. Observe the effect of staying in the moment and focusing on your pleasure.

Be creative. Couples who have been together for some time may develop something of a sexual routine. Chronic pain might be an invitation to try something new. Take the opportunity to mix it up. It may make sense to change your approach to intimacy, such as who tends to initiate, how, and the sequence and pacing. Explore positions that take the stress off your arms, neck, or other sensitive areas. Consider sexual accoutrements that may enhance your experience. Don't let the pain beat you—use this as an opportunity to explore your sexuality more deeply. Consider how people who live with chronic pain could benefit from some "chronic pleasure."

Experiment. You may find that pain can create new sources of pleasure. Rubbing a sore back or neck may incite ecstasy, particularly if you know your body well and can communicate your preferences to your partner; attention to painful feet can be blissful. Another strategy is to take the focus off your own body and attend fully to your partner's. Touching your partner and concentrating on his or her response frees you from thinking about your own physicality. Indulge in the pleasure your partner experiences. Your involvement may spur you to become more active as well.

Additional considerations. If you suspect that medication is negatively affecting your libido or sexual function, talk with your doctor. You may benefit from a change in medication, dose, or timing. Keep in mind, too, that people's sexual desire typically varies with the phases of a relationship. Being parents of young children, for example, is a common reason for decreased sexual activity. People may emphasize sexual activity less as they age. But whatever your situation, your sexual expression is your choice as an individual couple.

It may sound unsexy to apply science to your sex life. However, data on the physical and emotional benefits of sensuality support the value of investing in an intimate life filled with sensual pleasure. Add your own data to this by experimenting with intimacy and its effects. When you're laid out by pain or exhaustion, you may have to remind yourself of these benefits and act opposite to your immediate instinct. However, the more often you indulge in intimate relations with your partner, the easier it becomes to get started, no matter how bad you may feel. More than likely, too, the pleasure you generate will spill into other areas of your life together.

A Final Note

What does it mean to you to have a rich life? When people reflect on their lives, among other things, they reflect on their relationships. You deserve credit for the positive relationships in your life, as do those who have stuck by you and struggled and celebrated alongside you. Even the best relationships take work, and this work is compounded by chronic pain. Consider ways to attend to your relationships in a sustainable manner so that you can reap the greatest benefits without depleting anyone.

Chapter 25

Navigating Parenthood and Other Caregiving Roles

Becoming a parent is a significant, life-changing event. In the best of cases, along with much joy, new parenthood brings significant responsibility, worry, exertion, and fatigue. Contemplating whether and when to have children can raise significant questions and doubts. Living with chronic pain introduces additional concerns, worries, and fears:

> "How might chronic pain affect pregnancy and delivery?"
> "How will chronic pain affect my ability to parent?"
> "What if I were to pass this horrid condition to my child? I wouldn't forgive myself if my child hurt like I do."

Although it is understandable that you might experience guilt if your child were to develop your pain condition—particularly if you pondered that outcome before conceiving a child—no one has a crystal ball. Everyone carries the risk of inheritable conditions, such as diabetes, heart disease, allergies, asthma, autoimmune disorders, obesity, and psychiatric disorders, among a long list of others. While certain chronic pains may cluster in some families, nobody can predict whether a child will inherit pain any more than your many other attributes, such as your looks, talents, or disposition. What makes you *you* is much more than your pain condition. In addition, the reason some people develop pain conditions is complicated; genetics are only one piece of the puzzle.

The decision of whether and how to have children is highly personal. Becoming a parent is much more than reproducing one's genes. If you have significant reasons to worry about your family history or about the effect of pregnancy, medication, or childbirth on your (or your partner's) body or health, you can consider alternatives. Adoption and foster care also provide the option of rearing an older child, skipping the most physically labor-intensive first months or years. Most important is to figure out what feels right *for you*.

What If My Child Develops Chronic Pain?

Keep in mind the pace that research is advancing. We are likely to face a very different landscape for pain treatments ten or twenty years from now. The things you can *deliberately* pass on to your children are ways to care for and respect their bodies—such as good sleep habits, regular exercise, and stress-management techniques—which reduce the likelihood of developing medical problems of all kinds. Should your child develop "invisible pains," you will be ready with empathy, moral support, information, and guidance. Much suffering comes from the difficulty of obtaining a prompt diagnosis and from unsympathetic responses. Early detection and treatment can make conditions more manageable. Without this period of uncertainty and corresponding deterioration, the prognosis may be much better. You can help him or her to learn the adaptive techniques that may have taken you years to acquire.

From a young age, children can reap benefits from understanding their body and its patterns and having feedback mechanisms to guide their attitude and behaviors. You can work with your child to craft a simple tracking form that is relevant and commensurate with his or her maturity and interest. Children can be amazingly resilient, particularly when we model a matter-of-fact attitude in which difficulties are seen as challenges and we help them view themselves as capable individuals. Children living with pain can learn skills early on to understand the ways their behavior affects how they feel. This can carry over into positive coping skills and an increased feeling of empowerment.

In addition to nurturing and sustaining his or her children, a parent's job is to promote independence. No doubt it would be painful for you if your child hurt, and you might want to coddle or shield him or her as much as you can. At the same time, consider the benefits of helping him or her to be emotionally and physically sturdy. Parents continually struggle between protecting their children and letting them contend with difficulties. Consider what happens when toddlers fall. Before deciding to brush themselves off or to commit to a wail, they search out others' responses. Whether the parent gasps, laughs, or gently says, "You're OK," will shape the toddler's behavior and inner story. Children also learn through observing adults as role models.

When it comes to pain, a parent's central task would be to validate the child's difficulties while encouraging him or her to rise beyond them. It is important to express your love, support, and compassion and to model empathy. At the same time, children benefit from being able to interpret bodily cues in a constructive way, develop skills to cope, and redirect their attention elsewhere, as needed. This can come from gentle and consistent reminders from data that the child supplies through implicit or explicit data tracking. Your child does not have to fill out tracking sheets for you to observe patterns that you can share. Notice, for example, when your child is engaged and content, and reflect this: "You look like you are having a great time!" Encourage him or her to acknowledge it as well. This helps your child capture positive experiences. You can then reference that experience to encourage your child as needed: "I know you don't feel great right now, but remember that once you get together with your friends (or whatever had worked before), you'll have a great time."

Children also benefit when adults appropriately name their experience. This helps them to understand their experience and feel validated. Consider giving nicknames to patterns that become apparent. For example, "the before and after thing" could refer to a common occurrence in which your child dreads doing something beforehand (due to pain) but ends up enjoying it. If the nickname makes sense to your child, use it. "Oh, this is the before and after thing. You know things will turn around." This provides an understandable framework for your child's experience, which can foster lifelong adaptation.

Young children often benefit from concrete exercises. Consider working with your children to create appropriate tools, such as a sticker chart, that can reward them for adaptive responses. Certain stickers could represent accomplishments in your child's struggles. For example, reinforce instances in which they:

- succeed in tricking their minds to focus on something other than difficulties,
- engage in self-care behaviors to feel better,
- use "happy thoughts" to improve their mood and experience,
- engage in a realistic pep talk to move past an impasse, or
- achieve a second wind by pacing themselves and resting as needed.

Help your children feel proud. You can reinforce their skills by "catching" them using coping strategies, such as self-care and positive self-talk. Dole out deserved compliments. As a parent, it is your responsibility to celebrate your children's accomplishments. Another way to assist children, once they have developed some self-knowledge and skills, is by asking them, "What will help you feel better?" This sort of question empowers children to recognize their own ability to influence the way they feel.

Tactics such as helping children name their experience, develop coping strategies and insight, and consider their strengths and abilities are generally helpful. If you have more than one child, consider ways to use these approaches with them, as well. This also helps you to treat your children in a similar manner, regardless of their health. All children struggle with their emotions, and no doubt children would be affected by having a sibling with pain, as well as your reaction to it.

Chronic Pain and Pregnancy

Some women may experience pain relief from the influx of hormones. Others, however, may find that pregnancy stresses, exacerbates, and compounds their symptoms. This may not be surprising. Pregnancy has dramatic effects on women's bodies, including weight gain, fatigue, and sleep difficulties, along with other assorted discomforts. But however miserable your pregnancy may be (and keep in mind that you may be among the lucky ones who feel terrific), it is time limited and for a specific purpose. In addition, living with chronic pain may offer something of a pregnancy boot camp. For healthy women, pregnancy may the first time they have to contemplate daytime naps or figure changes related to their physical well-being into their daily lives. Women with chronic pain, however, are familiar with discomfort and fatigue as well as self-care.

Medications and pregnancy. Talk with your doctor about medications you are taking, and create a strategy to try to reduce or discontinue them, as appropriate. While it may be ideal to discontinue medications before conceiving, it is not always feasible. Some people are uncomfortable taking *any* medication while pregnant, but for many of us, this option would leave us in intolerable pain. What is best for you depends on the particular medications you are taking and your well-being without them.

Each drug is rated with a letter indicating the degree of risk posed to a fetus, with A being the lowest. Some are known to be safe; others are known to be unsafe, with the remainder falling in the gray area in between. Most research on in utero effects of medications are carried out by administering very high doses to laboratory animals; thus, for many prescription drugs, the effect of small doses on human development remains unclear. Discuss with your doctor the medications you should try to reduce or wean from completely; then, proceed gradually and under careful doctor supervision. Given that there are no simple answers, you may want to explore any questions with more than one doctor or specialist, or even the pharmaceutical companies themselves.

Ideally, the best time to experiment with reducing or discontinuing medications is *before* you become pregnant. If you became pregnant while on medication, talk with your doctor right away. The general aim is to take the lowest doses that will provide adequate relief. Keep in mind that you need to feel well enough during pregnancy to take good care of yourself. After much struggle, I felt reassured by the words of my obstetrician: "There is no such thing as a risk-free pregnancy. It is more important for fetal development that you sleep and feel reasonably well than that you avoid all medication."

Talk with your own doctor about what he or she would advise for you. Although sacrifice may be an element of both pregnancy and parenthood, martyrdom need not be. Work with your doctor to establish your optimal medications and dosages and then to accept your decision and avoid second-guessing it. The odds are in your favor that any child carried to term will be born healthy. You can reduce the likelihood of problems by following prenatal guidelines for diet and supplements (e.g., with folic acid) to ensure your own nutrition and that of your forming and growing baby. Of all birth defects, a minimal number (about 1 percent or less) are likely to be related to exposures to chemicals during pregnancy. Most birth defects result from random factors over which we have no control.[1]

Yet be prepared to encounter judgments from others who have strong opinions (regardless of their knowledge on the subject). In the United States, opinions about risks to the fetus can be fairly stringent. Unlike in Europe, the American public generally shuns *any* alcohol consumption during pregnancy, despite evidence that fetal development is negatively affected by significant amounts and not the occasional drink.

Surviving pregnancy. Your fetus reaps the benefits of whatever kindnesses you give yourself. Get enough sleep, eat a healthful diet, and continue to pace yourself with moderate exercise and naps, as needed. Because your body is likely to undergo dramatic changes, attend to your tracking data to see what helps during different phases. You may want to alter some of the categories you track to fit specific questions you have. As your sleep patterns change, you might conduct experiments to improve your sleep, as well as measure the effect of sleep quality and daytime naps on your well-being. You might also experiment with the effects of diet and exercise as your body changes.

It is generally recommended that once pregnant, women continue existing exercise routines but do not begin new or more vigorous programs. Consider exercises you will be able to continue throughout your pregnancy. Whenever possible, establish a reasonable exercise program for yourself *before* becoming pregnant. Walking offers cardiovascular fitness and strengthens key muscle groups that support your changing physique. Water exercises are kind to the body, particularly during the later months, when you may gratefully welcome a respite from gravity. Experiment and see what feels best for you.

Pregnancy can be very hard on a woman's body—a good reason to consider redoubling your usual efforts toward self-care. You may benefit, for example, from increased massage or other treatment throughout your pregnancy. Enjoy other people's reactions! Unlike suffering under the invisible strain of chronic pain, pregnancy is public. It is not uncommon for people to attend generously to the comfort of a (visibly) pregnant woman.

Chronic pain and delivery. Our society places great significance on the dramatic but fleeting event that marks the transition from pregnancy to parenthood. Professionals teach classes for expectant mothers and partners to prepare for labor, including strategies for pain relief such as purposeful breathing, guided imagery, and meditation or hypnosis. Women who live with chronic pain are no strangers to pain, which may make labor less frightening. You may already be familiar with the pain-control techniques taught in childbirth classes; if not, such classes may also prove useful for your daily life. Whatever labor entails, it lasts at most a day or two, involves breaks between contractions, and, if all goes well, ends with something of a miracle. In addition, strong medications are often available. I remember fondly the feeling when my epidural took effect; I felt better during that moment than I had in years.

Beware of an existing subculture that distinguishes "natural" labor from childbirth that is assisted by any pain medications. Debates on this topic often take a moral stance. If you feel yourself caught up in the debate about what is best, remind yourself that living with chronic pain is plenty ennobling—there's no need to prove anything to anyone during labor. On delivery day, the goal is to deliver a child. Recovering from childbirth takes time, and with a baby counting on you for sustenance and care, it is no time for *additional* heroics.

Bottle or breast? Breast-feeding is one of the most charged issues facing new mothers. The scientific pendulum supports the benefits of breast milk; however, an entire generation grew up just fine on formula. Allow yourself to make the decision that feels right for you. For women with chronic pain, breast-feeding raises additional issues. For one, any medications you are taking will continue to be transmitted to the baby. If you would like to breast-feed, talk with your doctor about how to minimize any harmful effects of medications—such as monitoring the dosage and timing of feedings—and what to look out for in your infant. Your doctor may recommend that you aim for a short-term goal, such as one or two months—long enough to provide the immunizing benefits of breast-feeding, while limiting the exposure to medication. Discuss strategies with your doctor to wean your baby gradually from your breast in the event that drug withdrawal may occur.

Another consideration is your comfort. Make use of specialized pillows and supportive furniture so nursing your baby does not bring about significant added pain. Experiment with positions that allow for hands-free feeding. Keep in mind that there is no one way to breast-feed. It is a personal decision if and how you decide to supplement feedings to allow yourself some downtime without the baby. By pumping or using formula, you also allow others to share in the feeding, while you get needed rest. Discuss with your doctor or a trusted consultant how to take advantage of a more varied approach. One benefit of breast-feeding is that it compels downtime by forcing new mothers to sit down and relax. The release of hormones can lull you to sleep along with your baby.

Recovering from childbirth. It is reasonable to expect that childbirth will cause a pain flare-up. Do your best to prepare for this. Minutes after greeting my first son, I scheduled a recuperative massage for later that week, which I recall being one of the best massages I've ever experienced. While in the hospital, make use of the assistance. Let yourself sleep while your baby is in the nursery. If you decide to breast-feed, consider allowing the nurses to bottle-feed, whether by pumping or with formula, so you can sleep. The La Leche League might have a cow over this advice; however, once mothers become skilled with the "latch on," babies are adept at extracting what they need. Lactating women produce milk on demand. The key ingredients are sufficient rest and hydration. Sleep may be more important than avoiding bottle-feeding. Just as with other aspects of parenthood, figure out what feels most comfortable to you.

Parenting with Chronic Pain

Parents with chronic pain offer their children many gifts:

- We can model the importance of living a healthful, balanced lifestyle with plenty of self-care.
- We understand the role of stress. We strive to reduce stress in our home and in our children's lives as much as possible.
- We value quiet time. We can focus on ways to reduce chaos and carve out quiet time for calm interchanges. Infants and young children have no limit on cuddling, a practice we can value for the comfort it provides all of us.
- We can help children accept differences and show them the ways we experience difficulties and have adapted.
- We benefit from fostering self-reliance, which contributes to children's self-esteem and confidence.

The first year. The greatest physical challenge of parenthood arrives with newborns. During their first weeks, sleep deprivation is inevitable as you recover from pregnancy and childbirth (even if you are the father). Before your child is born, create a plan for backup and assistance with childcare and household tasks. Discuss with your partner a schedule that will be kindest to you both, in which you have the opportunity to care for yourselves as well as the baby. Infants need to eat, sleep, be held, and be cleaned, and it doesn't matter to them which caring adult assists. In many cultures, extended family and community members rally around new mothers and take over many of the responsibilities that often become the solitary duties of mothers (and fathers) in the United States. There is no reason to feel bad about needing or accepting help.

Members of your network of family and friends may be happy to help in many ways, both large and small. Remember, what may seem like a tremendous effort to you, such as preparing dinner, is likely to be a simple task for friends who are well and rested. Don't feel shy about making requests when people ask to visit: "I'd love for you to stop by to meet the baby. How about coming at noon and bringing lunch?" Anyone who has had a baby knows how disorienting the first weeks are (even in the absence of chronic pain). The prospect of seeing the new baby may also make friends more generous. If you are able, it is worth the expense to hire help to run errands, and do other chores or childcare.

Becoming a parent is an emotionally charged time. Surround yourself with people you find peaceful and who contribute to your well-being. Before accepting assistance, consider how the person affects you. If you find your parents comforting, and they want to help, take them up on their offers. However, if you suspect that particular people would introduce additional stress, then you may need to create some rules. Be clear when you are in need of time by yourself. If your partner is available, you may decide to impose a moratorium on overnight guests (unless they are extremely helpful) so you can focus on recovery and becoming acquainted with your baby. Friends and family should not expect you to entertain or otherwise care for them, particularly if they are there to assist you. It is additionally important to carve out space for your own downtime. Sleeping when the baby sleeps is good advice. If you are unable to sleep during these hours, at least try to relax. Cultivate a relaxation method such as meditation or a hot bath to help you reach a deep state of tranquility.

Because virtually all new parents experience the tremendous fatigue that comes with an infant, forgetfulness is treated as expected, even socially acceptable, by healthy peers: "Oh, that's because you just had a baby." Enjoy this reprieve. At least waking up for a baby is a wonderful reason to feel lousy. Babies are adorable for a reason, and, if all goes as planned, they grow big enough to sleep through the night.

Ignore anyone who insists you *must* be able to carry your baby around. Babies are content to lie down and cuddle with a loving caregiver. Configure an environment and style to take advantage of your strengths. Diaper changing can be done at any height that works for you. A stroller or bassinet on wheels provides an easy way to transport your baby from room to room. Keep in mind that there is *never* a reason to carry a car seat, particularly with a baby in it. They are terribly heavy, awkward, and cumbersome. You can gently lift the baby out of the seat and into a lightweight stroller. If you are determined and able to remove the car seat, consider investing in a stroller frame that holds the seat. Once you insert the seat into the frame, you can push it as a stroller. If vibrations bother your arms, look for a stroller with good shock absorbers. Motorized strollers exist if pushing is difficult. Think about what tasks may prove troublesome, and then experiment to find out what works for you.

Young children. You do not have to carry your children around or rough-house with them to be a "good parent." Children are adaptable and will accept whatever you present as perfectly normal. As long as it involves love, you're doing fine. Children learn about their parents' styles quite easily, such as knowing that Mom only sits on soft surfaces, or Dad plays while lying on the floor or bed. Emphasize the positive: "I would love to read your new book. Bring it over to me, and I'll read it to you in bed."

Communicate regularly to your child that everyone requires downtime. Set aside short breaks for yourself as you need them. Inform your children gently and consistently that you are taking time to relax from the day, and encourage them to do the same. Help them engage in activities that require minimal supervision. Children rise to the occasion. Create an environment in which children can explore and cultivate their independence. You can make snack foods and drinks accessible and instruct them on the rules for helping themselves. Teach them to pick out clothes and pick up after themselves (see chapter 19). Interact with your children in ways that allow you to relax, such as lying down on a mat and sharing about your day or doing yoga together. As children get older, they become increasingly independent, and the physical demands of parenthood lessen.

Disclosing to Your Children

Children may be afraid to confront their parents' vulnerability. At each age, consider what you want your children to know about your condition. For young children, the most important thing to convey is the rules, such as, "No jumping on Mama." Most often, there's no need to explain the rules. As they get older, children will have questions. Seeing you take medications, they may become curious, worried, or even frightened that you will die. Use appropriate language to quell their fears and to reassure them, as realistically as possible, that you will continue to be available for them. As appropriate, explain what helps you feel your best and how they can contribute in small ways to help you be more available for them. Emphasize the positive: "You really helped me out by putting away your coat and shoes." Be careful to avoid guilt: "I felt lousy all day because *you* woke me up!" Strive to display a positive example of coping with illness, and your children will reflect your attitude.

Caregiving for Others

Unfortunately, living with a chronic illness does not provide a magical "free pass" that guarantees that you or others in your life will escape other health problems. When you find yourself in the role of caregiver, it is especially important that you care for yourself as well. Some tips for your arsenal:

Avoid heroics. Nobody benefits if you wear yourself out trying to help. As hard as it may seem, the more needed you are, the more important it is to care for yourself. Reserve time for exercise, restorative downtime, and fun activities to keep yourself feeling whole. Think of the safety instructions that airlines make before takeoff: In the event of an emergency, secure your own breathing mask before assisting others. Without sufficient oxygen, we are no good to each other. This is equally good advice when you are in a long-term caregiver role, as may be the case with an aging parent or a spouse or child with a chronic condition.

Be clear, be kind. It is unfair to overextend yourself and then blame others. Be aware of your limits, and let people know what you are able to do. In the case of a partner with a pulled muscle: "I will rub your back for five minutes, then do it again later." You may add, "I wish I could do it longer now, but I need to do it in small bits."

Be sympathetic and caring. People appreciate special treatment when they feel lousy. A cold or other temporary setback can feel totally debilitating to someone who is generally healthy. Keep in mind that everyone has a different physical status quo. Refrain from unhelpful comparisons or criticism when others feel needy. Manage negative feelings that may arise. For example, you may feel resentful or jealous that your otherwise healthy partner can opt out of activities until he or she feels better. While it may be true you do not share that luxury, that's not the other person's fault. Avoid the urge to respond, "*Now* you know how I feel all the time." Strive to help those in your life to feel better, not burden them with guilt.

Nobody would choose pain or illness, and most respond appreciatively to kind treatment. As a partner, it is part of your job to support and sustain the other. You know what it is like to feel lousy. No doubt, there are many times your partner engages in extra care for you. Try to view their temporary setbacks as opportunities to nurture.

Aging with your partner. There is a tremendous range of experience as people age. Some remain active and healthy, and their functional age remains well under their physical age. As people become older, it is more expected to suffer aches and pains. People with chronic pain have practice for this aspect of old age. As your partner ages, it is more likely that he or she will need assistance or come to rely on you in new ways. It is important to be a careful caregiver and to look, whenever feasible, for outside assistance and additional support.

Chapter 26

Grief and Acceptance

The adaptive strategies in this book are based on the assumption that you are psychologically able to make such adjustments. However, chronic pain can be devastating. People often need time to adjust to the news that they have a chronic problem before they feel ready to think about adaptive strategies. Chronic illness triggers grief. People may mourn for their former self—a person, for example, who could engage in activities spontaneously with energy and stamina, even a naïve sense of invincibility.

Grieving is a necessary process in which you face painful emotions and eventually move past them. Before you feel ready to adapt to your changed circumstances, you may need to express how difficult this transition is for you. It is important to be able to vocalize your sadness and receive validation and comfort. Suppressing feelings of sorrow can increase depression and isolation. Through grief comes acceptance, which is essential if you are to move forward and rebuild your life.

Accept the Reality of the Loss

Accepting that you have a chronic condition can feel heavy and depressing, especially if you interpret this to mean there's no hope of improvement. You may have been told, "You have to learn to live with it," a message also implicit in the term "chronic." Accepting chronic pain, however, is not the same as resignation or being stuck. Beware of any practitioner who harps on the permanence of your condition without encouraging a realistic hope for change. Acceptance of your current experience is essential to the process that enables you to move forward and contemplate positive measures to improve.

Paradoxically, the more you come to accept the reality of your situation, the less suffering it involves. Acceptance is a realistic acknowledgment of the current situation. It does not mean that you are happy about it or that it will not improve. Through acceptance, you can stop fighting; spend less time wishing things were otherwise; and focus on what you can do to improve the moment, rather than on the injustice of the situation. In contrast, denying reality and suffering the consequences is exhausting. Acceptance involves patience and a willingness to let go. Whatever your religious beliefs, the message in the Serenity Prayer by Reinhold Niebuhr encapsulates this: "God, grant me the serenity to accept the things I cannot change, courage to change the things I can, and wisdom to know the difference."

Many theorists write about the grieving process through which people reach acceptance. Among the first, and most famous, was Elisabeth Kübler-Ross, who interviewed patients with terminal conditions about their experience. From her research, she described five stages of grief: (1) denial, (2) anger, (3) bargaining, (4) depression, and (5) acceptance.[1] Note that acceptance comes after emotional vicissitudes and struggle. Dr. Kübler-Ross and subsequent researchers report that grief takes many forms. You may skip some of the stages, experience them in a different sequence, or return to certain ones repeatedly. Still, the Kübler-Ross model can provide a road map for considering your own reactions and how they change over time.

> Denial: "This can't be happening."
>
> Anger: "Why me? It's not fair."
>
> Bargaining: "I'll do anything to make the pain stop—like quit smoking, promise to be a nicer person, or cut off my left foot."
>
> Depression: "This is too hard. I feel desperate and want to give up."
>
> Acceptance: "It's going to be OK. I can do this."

How do you know when you have "accepted" your situation? This is a good question, especially because acceptance can look different for different people and does not mean you are forever finished with the other stages of grief. If you think of grief as an open wound, acceptance is the scar that forms once you have healed; the scar remains but no longer demands the attention of a fresh laceration. Evidence of acceptance can be seen, for example, in your ability to talk about your situation without distress.

Early on in my pain, I remember that watching a dance performance left me wallowing in self-pity because I was comparing the dancers' agility and strength to my pain and restriction. At some point later, I realized I no longer made these comparisons when watching such shows and was instead able to enjoy the beauty of the performance. Acceptance may also mean that certain self-preserving behaviors become instinctual. You might develop the habit of standing up at the table to pass a heavy serving plate rather than lifting it from a sitting position, which would strain your arms. Or by accepting that standing aggravates your back pain, you give yourself permission to sit down. Acceptance is a thousand small things that indicate your acknowledgment of yourself as you are.

Grief can well up, however, even when you have long since accepted your situation. As with all losses, some days will be harder than others, and particular events or thoughts can trigger an emotional response. In general, however, as you gradually achieve acceptance, stories of your past can become joyous memories rather than morbid testaments to what you have lost. Sadness may come in waves but no longer interfere with your ability to engage in life.

Work through the Pain

Therapeutic approaches to grief emphasize the importance of being in a safe place to delve into the pain that surrounds loss. Grief can operate like a pressure cooker: without the release of steam, you risk explosion. By mourning your losses, you can gradually release steam and lessen the emotional pressure. Allowing yourself to grieve is part of the healing process.

A strategy described by psychologist Marsha Linehan to reduce the intensity of negative emotions is to experience them as waves without minimizing or exaggerating your experience.[2] When you observe yourself feeling down, try to identify the main emotion and then imagine it washing over you. Refrain from trying to push it away or deny it. Remind yourself that you are not the emotion and it does not define your experience. Confronting your feelings will help reduce them and free you to consider strategies to improve how you feel.

Early in my relationship with pain, I joked with friends about my exhaustion with stories about the triumphs of people living with limitations—the armless artist who painted award-winning landscapes with her feet, the one-legged cross-country skier, the paraplegic scientist who pens groundbreaking books. Instead, I craved a club that complained about difficulties. Perhaps I was onto something. At that time, I needed to be able to express my frustration, grief, and exhaustion. I wasn't yet ready for a pep talk. I craved compassion.

Yet grief can be stigmatized as unhealthy, a sign of weakness, or wallowing in self-pity. Well-wishers may be uncomfortable with the emotional suffering that can accompany chronic pain. Furthermore, even when complaints are justified, no one wants to be known as a whiner. How, then, are people to find outlets for their grief?

Consider the venting strategies described in chapter 23 to process your grief with family and friends without overburdening them. Journaling, for example, offers a way to express your deepest despair, anger, or fears without affecting anyone else. Or select another medium in which you feel comfortable expressing yourself. Releasing painful feelings is cathartic, whether in the form of "sketches of the dark side," "poems of fire," "pain comics," "confessions of suffering," or "letters to my pain" or to "my lost self." In addition, being able to observe what you have recorded allows you to externalize your experience. You can later return to your words, images, or recordings and, over time, shape a narrative that emphasizes positive themes, such as your hope, strength, humor, empathy, and resilience.

Because grief involves a community, contemplate ways to make yours a *collective* experience. When someone dies, people band together. Memorial services tend to celebrate the life lived. Consider gathering with people closest to you for whatever feels appropriate. This could be a meal in which people express empathy and grief, share stories about your strength, or ask questions that allow you to clarify and unload your experience. People may value the opportunity to engage in a collective ritual. For example, friends of a cancer patient undergoing chemotherapy may shave their heads in a symbolic gesture of support and grief. Talk with people in your life about creative ways to join together.

I came upon a healing ritual unwittingly when pain drove me to relocate from San Francisco to my parents' house in Pennsylvania with two suitcases and several boxes of books. After my abrupt departure, my dear friends and brother held a garage sale, which they filmed, replete with ad-libbed comments for my benefit. The film turned out to be a hilarious, poignant, and very meaningful tribute to the end of a chapter in my life. I watched the recording repeatedly and now realize it represented a sort of memorial service that helped me move forward.

You can also work through the grief brought about by your pain with the help of trained professionals. Many mental health professionals have specific training to help navigate the grief process. Feel free to ask prospective counselors about their professional (and personal) experiences with grief. It is essential that you feel safe to process deep feelings. A support group can provide another avenue for grief work. Seek one in which you can commiserate over losses and give and receive empathy and validation. (Review chapter 18 for more information on individual and group therapy.)

Rituals around death not only support the mourners but also drive home the reality of the loss. When it comes to accepting chronic illness or pain, receipt of an official diagnosis or disability compensation can have the same effect. Being denied legitimate recognition of your suffering by the medical establishment, legal system, government, employers, or family members can interfere with healthy grief. Others' failure to acknowledge your experience of loss may complicate your own acceptance and adjustment. Research has found that the stigma experienced by chronic pain sufferers is highest when they have not been diagnosed and that experiencing this level of stigma negatively affects their outcomes.[3] Public acknowledgment can make losses easier to bear.

People who have suffered for years without recognition may accept a diagnosis readily and with relief. In contrast, individuals who recently developed symptoms may be more likely to fight against a chronic label and prognosis. When I first developed pain, I remember feeling too upset and frightened to consider the reality before me. Whatever your losses signify, acceptance comes more willingly when you also receive acknowledgment, social support, and the belief that you will be able to craft a life that feels meaningful and whole.

Forge ahead! When no longer bogged down by grief, you will be in a position to apply the principles of this book and create a life that is meaningful, despite your pain. There was a time I could not have imagined what that meant. But living well with pain is exactly what I am doing. By accepting your current situation, you can examine it for what it is and find realistic ways to improve. PAINTRACKING puts you squarely in the driver's seat. You become intimately aware of the potential consequences of any choices you make. From that position, pain is no longer frightening, even at its worst, because it becomes predictable. Pain no longer controls your life. When you know what's coming, you can plan. This includes pulling out your best coping strategies when pain promises to be strong. This also includes making use of effective therapeutic approaches to increase your comfort and abilities. How you feel, within realistic parameters, is within your control.

Living well with chronic pain, especially in its early stages, requires vigilance and dedication. Your initial tasks involve collecting and analyzing data so that you understand the particulars of your experience. This includes experimenting to determine what medication, physical therapy, exercise, pacing of activities, and cognitive mechanisms work best for you. Next, you must make changes—some small, some profound—to the way you live in order to reduce the role pain plays in your life. You must learn to listen to the data instead of your instincts or body until you succeed in retraining yourself to respond to what will actually help (and not what you may feel like or wish for). As you internalize these responses, the road becomes much, much easier to navigate.

At a support group meeting during my first year with pain, I remember a woman dabbing her eyes as she shared with us that it was ten years that month since she developed chronic pain and fatigue. She was clearly expressing grief, and it was valuable to her that we acknowledged the significance of her milestone. As I anticipate my upcoming twenty-year anniversary with pain, I imagine the party I will throw myself.

Facing pain with acceptance and understanding requires strength. Give yourself "pain credit" for your daily perseverance, struggles, and achievements. Living with chronic pain can feel like a continual test, even when you know the answers. Make sure you acknowledge your hard work in living with pain and strive to create the life you want. You really can do it!

Acknowledgments

*P*aintracking has taken many years to write. In the life I have created during these years with family, work, friends, school, pain, and self-care, I safeguarded small blocks of time to write. This book has been part of my own healing journey. How ironic that my painful condition has both inspired and interfered with my writing.

Many people helped shepherd *Paintracking* from idea to bound volume. Because this project spanned nearly fifteen years, listing *everyone* who has sustained me isn't practical. I'll begin with a thank-you to Emory and the community of Atlanta, Georgia, where, in 1997, as a Rockefeller Foundation fellow, I joined together medical, patient, and academic groups to grapple with invisible illness—which inspired this book. I'm also indebted to patient advocates who asked me to write material for their local support groups and later, national organizations—articles that evolved into book chapters.

At times, I felt like quitting; then, inevitably, I'd receive an appreciative note about my writings. I owe tremendous gratitude to those who have reached out to me over the years, shared their stories, encouraged my work, and waited patiently. I would also like to thank:

- The handful of vocal skeptics who "don't believe" in diffuse chronic pain and the doctors who personally mistreated me, disparaging my complaints and refusing to prescribe needed pain medication so I could "get used to it." They helped fuel my commitment to produce a comprehensive guide that would empower chronic pain sufferers.
- The compassionate physicians who helped me gain control over my symptoms. They include my longtime family doctor and other healthcare professionals who treat me with respect and without judgment.

- The massage therapists who have given me tremendous relief and hope while I lay on my stomach, peering through that little round face hole.
- My friends, for treating me "just like everyone else," arguing and laughing with me and, when needed, offering a hand or a hug. Special thanks to my dearest old friends for acting as a lifeline during my most challenging period, helping me grieve and reminding me of the ways I was still myself, and gratitude to my "post-pain" friends who accept my quirks and provide treasured laughs and intimacy.
- The many groups that people my life—the ladies of the Y water aerobics class; members of my playwright and academic writing groups; my students and colleagues at UNC; my therapy consult team and community; and my clients, who have taught me courage and resilience.
- The people who read and offered thoughtful feedback on many chapter drafts: medical doctors Barbara Bergdolt, Louise Greenspan, Chrissy Kistler, Alan Spanos, and Denniz Zolnoun; clinical social workers Martha Diehl and Marne Meredith; editor Diane Wyant; and the experts who wrote "book blurbs," many of whom also shared valuable feedback. The book profited greatly from each reader, and, as is often said, any remaining errors are mine alone.
- The team at Prometheus Books, including Steven L. Mitchell, who saw promise in this book (I will cherish the existential chats that followed from my "quick question" phone calls); copyeditor Jacqueline May Parkison, who engaged in enjoyable late-night exchanges with me; and Jennifer Tordy, Jade Zora Ballard, and Meghan Quinn for their professional finishing-line work.
- And finally, my family for caring for and supporting me. It was my older brother, Dan, and sister-in-law, Lisa Feldman Barrett, who set PAINTRACK-ING in motion by gently prodding me to figure out what was going on with my body. My younger brother, Ben, nurtured me through my most desperate times, and my parents took me back into their home, years after they thought they had launched me; fought for my improvement; and subsequently edited drafts of this book. My aunt and uncle for their constant support. My deepest thanks go to Charlie, my partner in all senses. Thanks also to his kin for embracing me warmly and nonjudgmentally and to our sons, who remind me every day that it is all worth it.

I hope you all like the book.

Notes

Chapter 2: Pain Positive?

1. See Dan Ariely's books *The Upside of Irrationality: The Unexpected Benefits of Defying Logic at Work and at Home* (New York: Harper, 2010) and *Predictably Irrational: The Hidden Forces That Shape Our Decisions*, rev. and expanded ed. (New York: Harper, 2009), and his website, http://danariely.com.

Chapter 4: Committing to the Process:
Addressing the "yes, but . . ."

1. See Inflexxion (http:/www.inflexxion.com) and its websites that offer information and tools for people with pain conditions: painACTION (http://www.painaction.com), and, for professionals, painEDU (http://www.painedu.org).

2. Synne W. Venuti et al., "The Role of a Pain Tracking Tool: A Survey of Healthcare Providers and Patients" (paper presented at 2011 Annual Meeting of the American Academy of Pain Medicine, National Harbor, MD, March 24–27, 2011).

Chapter 6: Tracking Your Well-Being

1. Department of Veteran Affairs, *Pain as the 5th Vital Sign Tool Kit* (Washington, DC: Veterans Health Administration, 2000), http://www.va.gov/PAIN MANAGEMENT/docs/TOOLKIT.pdf (accessed August 13, 2011).

2. Eula Biss, "The Pain Scale," *Seneca Review* 35 (Spring 2005): 5–25.

3. See the work by psychiatrist Yukio Ishizuka on the power of tracking positive outcomes, particularly couple closeness to bring more general life improvements, regardless of the source of pain, at http://positivementalhealthfoundation .com.

Chapter 10: Strategies to Focus and Calm Your Mind

1. Jarred Younger et al., "Viewing Pictures of a Romantic Partner Reduces Experimental Pain: Involvement of Neural Reward Systems," *PLoS ONE* 5, no. 10 (October 13, 2010): e13309.

2. Susan Schaffer and Carolyn Yucha, "Relaxation and Pain Management: The Relaxation Response Can Play a Role in Managing Chronic and Acute Pain," *American Journal of Nursing* 104 (2004): 75–82.

3. Samuel Yeung Shan Wong et al., "Comparing the Effectiveness of Mindfulness-Based Stress Reduction and Multidisciplinary Intervention Programs for Chronic Pain: A Randomized Comparative Trial," *Clinical Journal of Pain* 27, no. 8 (July 12, 2011): epub ahead of print.

4. Jon Kabat-Zinn, *Full Catastrophe Living: Using the Wisdom of Your Body and Mind to Face Stress, Pain, and Illness* (New York: Delta Trade Paperbacks, 2005).

5. Thich Nhat Hanh has written extensively on embracing pain as a way to relieve it. You might start with his *Being Peace* (Berkeley, CA: Parallax Press, 1987) for wisdom on self-acceptance or *The Miracle of Mindfulness: A Manual on Meditation* (Boston: Beacon, 1999) on approaching the present moment mindfully.

Chapter 11: Strategies to Soothe Your Body

1. Bryany G. Cusens et al., "Evaluation of the Breathworks Mindfulness-Based Pain Management Programme: Effects on Well-Being and Multiple Measures of Mindfulness," *Clinical Psychology and Psychotherapy* 17 (2010): 63–78.

2. Marsha Linehan, *Skills Training Manual for Treating Borderline Personality Disorder* (New York: Guilford, 1993).

3. William F. Fry, "Humor and the Brain: A Selective Review," *International Journal of Humor Research* 15 (2002): 305–33.

4. Andrea D. Furlan et al., "Massage for Low-Back Pain," *Cochrane Database of Systematic Reviews* 2008, no. 4 (October 8, 2008): CD001929; Daniel C. Cherkin et al., "Comparison of the Effects of 2 Types of Massage and Usual Care on Chronic Low Back Pain: A Randomized, Controlled Trial," *Annals of Internal Medicine* 155 (2011): 1–9; JoEllen M. Sefton et al., "Physiological and Clinical Changes after Therapeutic Massage of the Neck and Shoulders," *Manual Therapy* 16, no. 5 (May 13, 2011): epub ahead of print.

5. Tiffany Field et al., "Cortisol Decreases and Serotonin and Dopamine Increase following Massage Therapy," *International Journal of Neuroscience* 115 (2005): 1397–1413.

6. David G. Simons, Janet G. Travell, and Lois S. Simons, *Travell and Simons'*

Myofascial Pain and Dysfunction: The Trigger Point Manual, 2 vols. (Media, PA: Williams and Wilkins, 1992–99). See also *Travell and Simons' Trigger Point Flip Charts* (Baltimore, MD: Lippincott, Williams, and Wilkins, 1996), a book of illustrated flip charts geared in part for patient education.

Chapter 12: Strategies to Shape Your Self-Talk

1. Barbara Fredrickson's *Positivity: Groundbreaking Research Reveals How to Embrace the Hidden Strength of Positive Emotions, Overcome Negativity, and Thrive* (New York: Crown, 2009) presents research on significant effects of maintaining a 3:1 ratio of positive to negative emotions.

2. Matthias J. Koepp et al., "Evidence for Endogenous Opioid Release in the Amygdala during Positive Emotion," *NeuroImage* 44 (2009): 252–56.

3. Arthur W. Frank, *The Wounded Storyteller: Body, Illness, and Ethics* (Chicago: University of Chicago Press, 1995.)

Chapter 13: Strategies to Pace Yourself

1. Karl-Gösta Henriksson et al., "Women with Fibromyalgia: Work and Rehabilitation," *Disability and Rehabilitation* 27 (2005): 685–95.

Chapter 15: Strategies to Exercise More Effectively

1. See meta-analysis of research in U. M. Kujala, "Evidence on the Effects of Exercise Therapy in the Treatment of Chronic Disease," *British Journal of Sports Medicine* 43 (2009): 550–55.

2. See, for example, Angela J. Busch et al., "Exercise for Treating Fibromyalgia Syndrome," *Cochrane Database of Systematic Reviews* 2007, no. 4 (October 17, 2007): CD003786; Hanne Dagfinrud, Kåre Birger Hagen, and Tore K. Kvien, "Physiotherapy Interventions for Ankylosing Spondylitis," *Cochrane Database of Systematic Reviews* 2008, no. 1 (January 23, 2008): CD002822; A. Murtezani et al., "A Comparison of High Intensity Aerobic Exercise and Passive Modalities for the Treatment of Workers with Chronic Low Back Pain: A Randomized, Controlled Trial," *European Journal of Physical and Rehabilitative Medicine* 47, no. 3 (May 23, 2011): epub ahead of print.

3. Lars L. Andersen et al., "Effect of Two Contrasting Types of Physical Exercise on Chronic Neck Muscle Pain," *Arthritis Care and Research* 59 (2008): 84–91.

4. Mary E. Sanders, "Bridging Land and Water Exercise," *Journal on Active Aging* (July/August 2003): 52–54.

Chapter 16: Collaborating Effectively with Your Doctor

1. American College of Rheumatology, "What Is a Rheumatologist?" http://www.rheumatology.org/practice/clinical/patients/rheumatologist.asp (accessed March 30, 2011).

2. Association of American Physiatrists, "An Introduction to PM&R," http://www.physiatry.org/Field_Introduction.cfm#specialty (accessed March 30, 2011).

3. American Academy of Neurology, "Working with Your Doctor," http://patients.aan.com/go/workingwithyourdoctor (accessed March 30, 2011).

Chapter 17: Strategies to Make Sense of Prescription Medications

1. Jeremy A. Greene, "What's in a Name? Generics and the Persistence of the Pharmaceutical Brand in American Medicine," *Journal of the History of Medicine and Allied Sciences* (September 21, 2010): epub ahead of print, http://jhmas.oxfordjournals.org/content/early/2010/09/21/jhmas.jrq049.short (accessed May 11, 2011).

2. US Food and Drug Administration, *Approved Drug Products with Therapeutic Equivalence Evaluations*, 31st ed. (Washington, DC: Food and Drug Administration, 2011), http://www.fda.gov/Drugs/DevelopmentApproval Process/ucm079068.htm (accessed May 11, 2011).

3. Daniel Carpenter and Dominique A. Tobbell, "Bioequivalence: The Regulatory Career of a Pharmaceutical Concept," *Bulletin of the History of Medicine* 85 (2011): 93–131.

4. Russell K. Portenoy, "Therapy for Chronic Nonmalignant Pain: A Review of the Critical Issues," *Journal of Pain and Symptom Management* 11 (1996): 203–17.

5. Ibid., p. 203.

6. Peggy Compton, "The OIH Paradox: Can Opioids Make Pain Worse?" *Pain Treatment Topics*, August 20, 2008, http://pain-topics.org/pdf/Compton -OIH-Paradox.pdf (accessed May 5, 2011).

7. For a readable review of medication used in the treatment of chronic pain, see Hue Jung Park and Dong Eon Moon, "Pharmacological Management of Chronic Pain," *Korean Journal of Pain* 23 (2010): 99–108.

8. "Adverse Effects of Benzodiazepines," Web4Health, http://web4health .info/it/bio-benzo-sideeffects.htm (accessed November 10, 2011).

9. Compton, "OIH Paradox."

10. Barbara Martinez et al., "Merck Pulls Vioxx from Market after Link to

Heart Problems," *Wall Street Journal*, October 1, 2004, http://finance.wharton.upenn.edu/~acmack/merck0.pdf (accessed July 26, 2011).

11. Allan I. Basbaum and David Julius, "Toward Better Pain Control," *Scientific American* 294 (May 22, 2006): 60–67.

12. Hansen Wang et al., "Identification of an Adenylyl Cyclase Inhibitor for Treating Neuropathic and Inflammatory Pain," *Science Translational Medicine* 3 (January 12, 2011): 65ra3.

13. Reza Sharif-Naeini and Allan I. Basbaum, "Targeting Pain Where It Resides . . . In the Brain," *Science Translational Medicine* 3 (January 12, 2011): 65ps1.

14. Mark J. Zylka, "Pain-Relieving Prospects for Adenosine Receptors and Ectonucleotidases," *Trends in Molecular Medicine* 17 (2011): 188–96. Section also augmented by conversations with Dr. Zylka in May 2011.

15. "Former GSK Exec to Lead UNC Drug Discovery Center," Eshelman School of Pharmacy, University of North Carolina at Chapel Hill, October 12, 2007, http://www.pharmacy.unc.edu/news/schoolnews/former-gsk-exec-to-lead-unc-drug-discovery-center (accessed May 11, 2011). Section also augmented by conversations with Dr. Stephen Frye in May 2011.

16. Nanna Goldman et al., "Adenosine A1 Receptors Mediate Local Anti-Nociceptive Effects of Acupuncture," *Nature Neuroscience* 13 (2010): 883–88.

17. Mark J. Zylka, "Needling Adenosine Receptors for Pain Relief," *Nature and Neuroscience* 13 (2010): 783–84.

18. Andreas S. Beutler and M. Reinhardt, "AAV for Pain: Steps towards Clinical Translation," *Gene Therapy* 16 (2009): 461–69. Section also augmented by conversations with Dr. Beutler in May 2011.

19. D. Roberson et al., "Targeting of Sodium Channel Blockers into Nociceptors to Produce Long-Duration Analgesia: A Systematic Study and Review," *British Journal of Pharmacology* 164, no. 1 (September 2011): 48–58.

20. Arthur Gomtsyan and Connie R. Faltynek, *Vanilloid Receptor TRPV1 in Drug Discovery: Targeting Pain and Other Pathological Disorders* (Hoboken, NJ: Wiley, 2010).

Chapter 18: Strategies for Working with Mental Health Professionals

1. American Psychiatric Association, *Diagnostic and Statistical Manual of Mental Disorders*, 4th ed. (Washington, DC: American Psychiatric Association, 2000).

2. The following books, written for students and professionals, are accessible:

Joan Berzoff et al., *Inside Out and Outside In: Psychodynamic Clinical Theory and Psychopathology in Contemporary Multicultural Contexts,* 3rd ed. (Lanham, MD: Rowman and Littlefield, 2011); and Nancy McWilliams, *Psychoanalytic Psychotherapy: A Practitioner's Guide* (New York: Guilford Press, 2004). For information on the tradition that underlies this approach, visit the website of the American Psychoanalytic Association (http://www.apsa.org) and select "About Psychoanalysis."

3. For accessible information on this approach, see Aldo Pucci, *The Client's Guide to Cognitive-Behavioral Therapy: How to Live a Healthy, Happy Life . . . No Matter What!* (Bloomington, IN: iUniverse, 2006); or Rhena Branck and Rob Wilson, *Cognitive Behavioural Therapy Workbook for Dummies* (Hoboken, NJ: For Dummies, 2006); or visit the website of the American Institute of Cognitive Therapy (http://www.cognitivetherapynyc.com).

4. Johan W. S. Vlaeyen et al. found that people with fibromyalgia struggled to complete homework in "Cognitive-Educational Treatment of Fibromyalgia: A Randomized Clinical Trial," *Journal of Rheumatology* 23 (1996): 1237–45.

5. For practical materials on dialectical behavioral therapy, see Matthew McKay, Jeffrey C. Wood, and Jeffrey Brantley, *The Dialectical Behavior Therapy Skills Workbook: Practical DBT Exercises for Learning Mindfulness, Interpersonal Effectiveness, Emotion Regulation, and Distress Tolerance* (Oakland, CA: New Harbinger, 2007); or the website put together by individuals who have gone through DBT at http://www.dbtselfhelp.com/.

6. Described in the first text on DBT by its founder, Marsha Linehan, *Cognitive-Behavioral Treatment of Borderline Personality Disorder* (New York: Guilford, 1993).

7. For more information, read Jackie Gardner-Nix, *The Mindfulness Solution to Pain: Step by Step Techniques for Chronic Pain Management* (Oakland, CA: New Harbinger, 2009); listen to Jon Kabat-Zinn's audiobook *Mindfulness Meditation for Pain Relief: Guided Practices for Reclaiming Your Body and Your Life*, read by the author (Louisville, CO: Sounds True, 2009); or visit the website of the Center for Mindfulness in Medicine, Health Care, and Society at the University of Massachusetts for information, resources, and programs at http://www.umassmed.edu/cfm/home.

Chapter 19: Taking Care of Your Home

1. Karen Pryor, *Don't Shoot the Dog! The New Art of Teaching and Training*, rev. ed. (New York: Bantam Books, 1999).

Chapter 21: Creating a Workspace That Works

1. Several researchers have studied the relationship between chronic pain and work, particularly for women with fibromyalgia; see: Carol S. Burckhardt et al., "The Impact of Fibromyalgia on Employment Status of Newly Diagnosed Young Women," *Journal of Musculoskeletal Pain* 13 (2005): 31–41; Gunilla Liedberg and Chris Henriksson, "Factors of Importance for Work Disability in Women with Fibromyalgia: An Interview Study," *Arthritis Care and Research* 47 (2002): 266–74.

Chapter 22: Work Alternatives: Considering New Pathways

1. For information on these movement methods, visit http://alexander technique.com and http://www.feldenkrais.com.

Chapter 23: Approaching Social Relationships

1. Arthur Schopenhauer, *Studies in Pessimism: A Series of Essays* (London: Swan Sonnenschein, 1908), p. 142.

Chapter 24: Improving Committed Relationships

1. For information on the Gottman Institute, visit http://www.gottman .com.

2. Books by John M. Gottman include: *The Science of Trust: Emotional Attunement for Couples* (New York: W. W. Norton, 2011); *The Relationship Cure: A Five-Step Guide to Strengthening Your Marriage, Family, and Friendships* (New York: Three Rivers, 2002); *The Seven Principles for Making Marriage Work*, with Nan Silver (New York: Crown, 1999); and *Why Marriages Succeed or Fail, and How You Can Make Yours Last* (New York: Simon and Schuster, 1995).

3. For evidence of naturally occurring opioids upon orgasm in animal experiments, see Gabriela Rodríguez-Manzo et al., "Evidence for Changes in Brain Enkephalin Contents Associated to Male Rat Sexual Activity," *Behavioral Brain Research* 1–2, (2002): 47–55; and S. P. Yang et al., "Involvement of Endogenous Opioidergic Neurons in Modulation of Prolactin Secretion in Response to Mating in the Female Rat," *Neuroendocrinology* 72 (2000): 20–28.

4. Dixie Meyer, "Selective Serotonin Reuptake Inhibitors and Their Effects on Relationship Satisfaction," *Family Journal* 15 (2007): 392–97; Donatella Marazziti et al., "A Relationship between Oxytocin and Anxiety of Romantic Attachment," *Clinical Practice and Epidemiology in Mental Health* 2 (2006): 28.

5. Kathleen Doheny, "10 Surprising Health Benefits of Sex," WebMD, http://www.webmd.com/sex-relationships/features/10-surprising-health-benefits-of-sex (accessed May 15, 2011).

Chapter 25: *Navigating Parenthood and Other Caregiving Roles*

1. US Department of Health and Human Services, *Reviewer Guidance Evaluating the Risks of Drug Exposure in Human Pregnancies* (Rockville, MD: Center for Drug Evaluation and Research, 2005).

Chapter 26: *Grief and Acceptance*

1. Elisabeth Kübler-Ross, *On Death and Dying* (New York: Macmillan, 1969).

2. Marsha Linehan, *Skills Training Manual for Treating Borderline Personality Disorder* (New York: Guilford Press, 1993).

3. Pia Asbring and Anna-Liisa Närvänen, "Women's Experiences of Stigma in Relation to Chronic Fatigue Syndrome and Fibromyalgia," *Qualitative Health Research* 12 (2002): 148–60.

Index